# The Herbalist's Way

# The Herbalist's Way

*The Art and Practice of Healing with Plant Medicines*

NANCY AND MICHAEL PHILLIPS

Foreword by Rosemary Gladstar

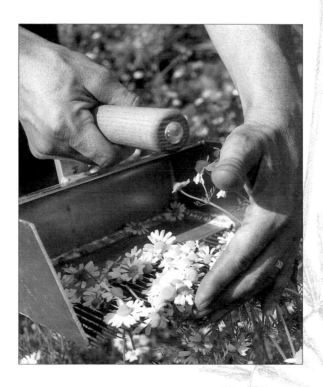

CHELSEA GREEN PUBLISHING
WHITE RIVER JUNCTION, VERMONT

Library of Congress Cataloging-in-Publication Data
Phillips, Nancy, 1957-
The herbalist's way : the art and practice of healing with plant medicines /
Nancy and Michael Phillips ; foreword by Rosemary Gladstar.
     p. ; cm.
Rev. ed. of: The village herbalist. c2001.
Includes bibliographical references and index.
ISBN 1-931498-76-8 (pbk. : alk. paper)
1. Materia medica, Vegetable. 2. Medicinal plants. 3. Herbs--Therapeutic use.
[DNLM: 1. Medicine, Herbal--methods. 2. Phytotherapy--methods. 3. Plant Preparations. 4. Plants, Medicinal. WB 925 P562h 2004] I. Phillips, Michael, 1957- II. Phillips, Nancy, 1957- The village herbalist. III. Title.
RS164.P5335 2004
615'.321--dc22
                         2004028996
Chelsea Green Publishing
85 North Main Street, Suite 120
White River Junction, VT 05001
(800) 639-4099
www.chelseagreen.com

*For* GRACE ELENA
and all those in the next generation.

*Honor the Earth.*
*Give glory to the Creator.*
*Cherish that sweet connection with the plants.*
*And your medicine power will be*
*deep and strong.*

# Contents

# Foreword

I consider it an honor to be writing this foreword for one of my favorite herb books, written by two of my favorite herbalists. Michael and Nancy Phillips personify the image of the traditional, yet thoroughly modern "village herbalist," and their homestead in the north woods of New Hampshire has become a place of pilgrimage for many other herbalists and herbal students. Here one finds a plant lover's dream, an herbalist's oasis—an old farmstead that has been lovingly restored and is surrounded by forested hills, lush gardens, and a year-round mountain brook running down through the field. Michael and Nancy and Gracie, their budding young herbalist daughter, "walk their talk" easily and with joy, and what they write about they actually live. Their experience lends substance and insight to the words they spin on paper in the late nights after the gardens are tended, meals cooked, animals bedded, and the chores of the day are put to rest.

I have been excited about this project almost from the moment of its conception, when Nancy and Michael first mentioned that they were thinking of writing a book about herbal healing for would-be practitioners. I knew without doubt that this would be more than simply another herbal "how-to" book. That it would reach down to the heart and spirit of herbalism and capture the essence of this great tradition of healing. That it would address the issues of being a family or community herbalist and of "practicing" herbal medicine in the modern world. Knowing the quality of everything that Michael and Nancy do and the honesty and soulfulness they put into their endeavors, I fully expected they would create a great book. As it happened, though, they have exceeded even my greatest expectations.

This is an immensely practical book. In the context of being a community herbalist, *The Herbalist's Way* instructs the reader how to harvest, prepare, and use a variety of useful healing plants. Wonderful recipes are provided—some of Nancy's favorite preparations, as well as step-by-step instructions on how to prepare home medicine from the plants. But that's only the beginning, a fine appetizer to the feast that awaits the reader.

The book is also wonderfully clear-eyed and straightforwardly honest—even brazen—and it jumps right into the core issues surrounding herbalism: what it means to be an herbalist; what "practicing" herbalism is all about; and the various paths before us, whether we are grower, wild crafter, practitioner, medicine maker, manufacturer, or store keeper. And it doesn't stop there. The realities of the FDA. Standardization. Certification. Scientific validation. These are critically important topics that most herb books gingerly step around. Nancy and Michael wisely refrain from providing all the answers, but rather pose intelligent and necessary questions. They provide important facts to ponder and allow us, the readers, to think for ourselves. Ah, such a refreshing and respectful approach.

And finally, *The Herbalist's Way* is beautifully written, poetic in its substance. Michael and Nancy interviewed herbalists across the country and used their words to paint pictures of the community herbalists of today. We are allowed glimpses into the lives of leading herb growers, medicine makers, and practitioners. We hear and learn from their tales, their experiences, and their often very spicy versions of what they feel the issues facing modern medicine and herbalists are today. It's a wonderful read, and it leaves one inspired, renewed, and invigorated.

In the last decade there have been a plethora of herb books flooding the marketplace. Some are good and find a spot on my heavily laden bookshelves, to be gleaned in future for bits of herbal information. Others are destined to gather dust, not worth the trees it took to produce them. And then there are those—only a few, a rare book here and there—that are destined to become herbal classics, treasured like old friends, thumbed through again and again for their depth of herbal wisdom, for their teachings, and for their inner brilliance that illuminates this ancient field of plant study. Michael and Nancy Phillips have created such a special and inspirational work.

ROSEMARY GLADSTAR

# Acknowledgments

*We are like a couple of strong draft horses and sometimes one of us decides to go a different way than the other one, but ultimately we can't, because we are yoked. After a little tugging and pulling we get rolling together and make a good team.*

SO BEGAN a letter Nancy wrote to a friend halfway into the writing of *The Herbalist's Way*. She describes the tumult of a husband and wife collaboration quite well. Lord knows, she had a particularly ornery stallion to deal with at times. Yet now we have arrived at our journey's end, as evidenced by this book. We have quite a few people we'd like to thank for helping us in this horseplay.

Our parents, for their enduring love and encouragement. Mom, Mom, and Dad, you're the best. Alan, you saved us from numerous computer glitches that continually defied our down-to-earth wisdom. Gracie, for surviving with such aplomb our daily tussle about having quiet time to write. Now you can play the piano all you want.

Rosemary, for being a model herbalist, teacher, friend, activist, and an inspiring human being. Your wisdom and generosity are extraordinary. Having you as our mentor has been a precious blessing in our lives.

The teachers and students at Sage Mountain who have stretched our minds, fed our souls, and enriched our lives. All you "homework team sisters" especially bring such joy to our hearts. Amy, your honesty and coaching are a special blessing. Karl, your weavings of ceremony throughout warms the heart. Robert, thanks for taking such good care of the mountain and "the boss."

All the herbalists that responded to our survey way back when. We especially acknowledge and cherish those of you who went that extra mile and shared your life story and herbal insights for the profiles provided throughout this book. This collaborative effort hinged on the openness and trust so many herbalists showed us along the way. Earth is a richer place shared with all of you.

Editorial guidance is a must for any book. Thank you, Ben, for doing right by our healing vision. We're honored to be part of the Chelsea Green home team bespeaking a friendlier world and a sustainable way of life. And Frank, no back-to-the-land couple ever had a more committed photographer!

The support we received along the way from our good friends and neighbors truly speaks for the connection of community. Many of you who kept checking in about "the book" would ask perceptively in the next breath about "the marriage." A certain carpentry partner particularly deserves applause for understanding that tight phrasing equates to tight joinery. Daniel, may our herbal humor always make up for having a building buddy equally dedicated to growing plants greener than green.

Last, but furthest from least, we are grateful to the plants and all the creatures in our Earth family. The precious bond between all beings makes life complete.

We hope you find this guide everything we intend. Don't hesitate to give us suggestions for improving future editions. *The Herbalist's Way* truly belongs to all in the herbal community.

GREEN BLESSINGS!
NANCY AND MICHAEL

# Introduction

None of us becomes an herbalist overnight. Learning the spiritual teachings and healing qualities of the plants takes more than a lifetime to experience. We need to discover for ourselves how to grow and harvest the herbs we use and how to make effective preparations from them. We need to probe a seemingly endless pool of knowledge about the body, mind, and spirit. Learning a huge range of healing techniques and therapies enhances our work with the herbs. Of course, a truckload each of wisdom and common sense is needed to complete the package. Wow! Try to balance all of that and find time to raise a family and then make yourself available to people. I constantly fall short of my ideal. ℘ At times I am so enthralled with being an herbalist that I want to catch up, to be as experienced and knowledgeable as my wisest teachers. As a child, I wasn't handed down this knowledge, yet the ancestral roots are a deep part of my being. ℘ I have the vision of what I want to become, but I must learn to be patient with myself and enjoy the journey. We serve and blossom when we can. We grow and nurture our roots through all our days. A sapling doesn't become a big solid oak in a few years or even a decade. Yet I can begin to create some shade and protection for others. I can drop my leaves and begin to nourish the soil for the community around me. I can lend my branches for others to find shelter and respite from the high winds and storms of life. I can make the world a bit more beautiful by sharing a bright healing spark, like green leaves do in springtime. Each experience makes me stronger, more solid, more deeply rooted in Mother Earth. My heart continually opens to the guidance of the Creator.

*Increasingly I am more able to be of service to others from this strong foundation.* ❧ *If your passion runs deep, and you have that strong desire to learn as much as you can about herbs, health, and healing, and to share that wisdom with your community, then you are on the right track. This book is intended to help you move more quickly along the engrossing and rewarding path to becoming an herbalist.* —N.P. ❧

D ISCOVERING THAT our medicine can be found in the fields and woods that surround us is empowering. So many of the good things in this life are simply intended as everyday blessings. Our culture has promoted our food, our health, at times even our spirituality, as centralized economic commodities. Professions deliver the goods, relieving us of the responsibility for knowing more about ourselves and our delightful place on Earth. Carried to the extreme, this vision of health care has devolved to one where health management organizations (HMOs) approve extremely profitable pharmaceuticals to support isolated and failing body systems. Aren't we missing something here? The healing process is misunderstood by those who believe it is the doctor or drug, or both, that makes us better. Not so. Our bodies have a natural ability to work their own cure. A healer uses compassion, intuitive experience, restorative therapies, and medicines to bolster another person (being the sum total of body, mind, and spirit) in his or her recovery. We are all healers as much as we are all in need of healing. Here to assist us on that journey is an incredibly complex, beautifully simple, always inspiring world of healing plants.

Herbal medicine is more about a deep relationship with the plants—and ourselves—than it is about a dusty jar of distant leaf that happens to retain enough vitality to serve as a specified remedy. The current infatuation with herbal capsules and food supplements available at the nearest superstore` misses this mark on several counts. An herbalist begins with the healing plants growing outside the door, whether they are grown in the garden, approaching bloom in a wildflower meadow, or growing in a shaded woodland glen. Local medicine provides both a livelihood for the healers within our communities and a direct experience of the plants that help heal those in need. Such neighborly circles are also our best bet for healing the impact of *Homo sapiens* on our planet home. We left the Garden of Eden with its promise of all we need. Isn't it time we return?

We begin our journey by linking back to what was good for our communities in the past. People who grew up intimately involved with Nature had a generational handle on the good foods and medicines available to them. Reverence for these great gifts filled the human heart. The village herbalist often served as a midwife, family pharmacist, and spiritual guide all rolled into one. Communities honored their healers throughout most of history. The call to serve, to be an instrument of healing, did not lead to glory or riches. Barter and sliding scales of payment made it possible for everyone in need both to benefit from and support those local people who dedicated their lives to this good work. Such mutual caring worked in days when community circles balanced individual desires with a deep understanding of the generations to come and the sacredness of Creation.

Human ingenuity is a combination of traditional wisdom and ever expanding consciousness and discovery. Speaking appreciatively of past medical practice is not a call to use leeches to absorb the "ill humours" of the body.* Nor do we imply that modern heroic medicine should be shunned. Antibiotics, surgery, and technology all have a place in today's health care systems. Our goal is to join with others in shaping a sustainable future by drawing on what is usable and honored from the past and mixing it with the enlightened choices of today. We are blessed to live in a time when so many healing modalities are available. More and more people are beginning to realize that modern allopathic medicine is not always the best choice for every situation. Yet many are in the lemminglike habit of following the usual routine when presented with a health concern.

Taking responsibility for family health begins with a conversant herbalist in each home, someone who has learned the basics about eating right and tonic herbs and healing baths and poultices. The appeal of herbs for most people lies in this simple approach, one that embraces everyday health. We can fend off the flu, relieve a stress headache, and nurture vitality with herbs all on our own. Home herbalism is a basic life skill.

Today's community herbalist fills a bigger role than the home herbalist: teaching mothers and fathers the first principles of the herbal healing art, suggesting healing approaches for a wide array of illnesses, having plant remedies available, and recognizing personal limits when the advice of a more experienced practitioner is advised. Later in this book, we will take an encompassing look at the question of licensing or certifying herbalists. For now, suffice it to say that people who assume responsibility for their own health, and who exercise their own free will, will be drawn to healers who resonate with love and community approval.

Integrating an herbal livelihood within the context of a sustainable community is of critical importance. Learning the plants and their healing properties comes most of all through direct experience. Weekend courses, in-depth seminars, and apprenticing with an herbal mentor can round out one's knowledge base. Practitioners can learn to network with local growers, who in turn realize the quality considerations we've listed to keep medicinal herb customers returning to the farm. The potential joys and concerns of setting up shop—be it tips on label design for a line of tinctures or handling government regulations in heartening fashion—are detailed for budding herbal entrepreneurs. Such neighborhood apothecaries often serve as educational centers where the proper use of healing herbs can be taught by local herbalists.

The drift of any book ultimately rests on the viewpoint of its authors. Ours, we suspect, is obvious. Unhindered by a string of letters behind our names to indicate intellectual worth, we embrace local plant medicine and an Earth-centered lifestyle with unwavering verve. Gut feelings and heartfelt

---

*In truth, even the oft-despised leech has found a place in modern medicine. Reconstructive surgeons have found blood-sucking *Hirudo medicinalis* most effective at cleaning up venous congestion when replaced skin tissue needs capillary circulation reestablished. More than 10,000 leeches were sold for medicinal purposes in the United States in 1988. For a fascinating look at how traditional healing knowledge continues to show merit, see Robert and Michèle Root-Bernstein, *Honey, Mud, Maggots, and Other Medical Marvels* (New York: Houghton Mifflin, 1997).

passion matter. We don't speak with unquestionable authority about options you have with your own body. Personal responsibility to discern what's right for each of us remains paramount throughout our time on this planet. *The Herbalist's Way* bespeaks both a personal path and a cultural journey. We wrote this book to add medical care to the ongoing discussion of sustainability in these mad and impetuous times. The wisdom to move forward in a direction that honors the past, holds the present moment in awe, and leaves room for the seventh generation to come shall guide us all to lives worth living.

# The Herbalist's Way

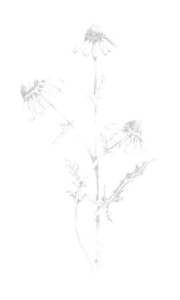

# CHAPTER ONE

# The Medicine of the People

COMFREY
*Symphytum officinale*

*C*ommunity herbalists are the mainstay of herbalism, the nurturers and protectors of good health. We may look a bit weedy compared to the flashy cultivated garden flower or a properly trained and pruned hybrid rose. We appear gentle and very commonplace. But we can make a powerful difference if our ways are heeded. Our role complements the work of other holistic care providers. A community herbalist can be invaluable in educating people about good health practices and in helping them recover from common family ailments. We're first in line to give people answers about how the plants can assist in their basic care. ❧ One of the concepts taught in an introductory course on the use of medicinal herbs is that herbs are not all used or categorized the same way. I learned to visualize this concept much like a clothesline: The tonic, or nourishing, herbs are all hung at one end, the specific medicinal herbs are in the middle, and the low-dose herbs are at the opposite end of the line. The sequence—oats, raspberry, nettles, chamomile, echinacea, black cohosh, goldenseal, lobelia, poke, digitalis—reflects an increasing specificity in plant medicines. We call on the nourishing herbs at the left the most often, using these as food and health-giving teas. These mainstays of herbal tradition are gentle and yet highly effective. Occasionally, when things get out of balance, we need to go to the more specific medicinal herbs. And in rare situations, we need to use low doses of very strong, potentially dangerous plants and expertise is critical. ❧ Surely there is a continuum of health care practitioners in the same way that there is a continuum of herbs. All of us promote well-being and treat *specific illnesses. Yet, just as with the plants, it isn't always possible to draw firm and strict lines where each one fits. Each of us serves some good purpose and is chosen for particular situations. One of the foundations of herbalism is to use nourishing herbs regularly over time to build overall health. The community herbalist will always be the tonic provider for a people's medicine. I'm certain the clothesline has room for plenty more.* —N.P. 

ENJOYING GOOD HEALTH is everyone's birthright. Plants offer a healing relationship in which we can find good foods and medicines to keep ourselves on track. Comprehending these gifts—both for everyday use and for specific therapeutic purpose—has long been the province of the community herbalist. However, many people today have lost this healing link with Nature. An incredible transformation awaits those who bring open-minded intention to the "Green Nations" of the plant realm. To be alive is to be able to heal. Immersing ourselves in the wonderful offerings of the plants brings far more than a cure for what ails us. True healing restores the life circle of body, mind, and spirit. An herbalist works with the life circle of the plant world to help people experience their own innate wholeness in an infinite universe.

The desire for a simpler and more natural lifestyle grows as human experience becomes more complex and further removed from Earth-based reality. Western culture pushes incessantly for more riches, more comfort, more individuality, more science. Yet *more* will always be balanced by *less* somewhere else. Any of us can ponder the other side of the ledger for these materialistic times: less peace, less community, less health, less holistic understanding. This curve ball we've collectively pitched to ourselves needs examination from every angle if we are to bring wholeness into all areas of our lives. Thankfully, contemporary patterns and group thinking do not need to carry the day for any individual. Human consciousness continues to evolve despite generations of cultural blunders and affairs of the ego. Honest. Hope begins in understanding the broader currents, where spiritual insight can lead to heartfelt thankfulness for the present moment. Context matters. Looking at our medicine—how we care for ourselves—reveals the need for gentler ways that recognize all aspects of mind, body, and spirit.

A medicine of the people will, first and foremost, take place nearby. Caring begins with the people who know us. A cellular harmony exists between the plant and animal species who share the same environment. Certainly, conventional medical care serves a good purpose in apt situations. We want our seven to nine minutes with the doctor should the need arise.[1] Yet somewhere between our body's innate ability to heal itself and conventional medicine's high-dollar attempt at a cure lie many situations that can be bridged by common sense and a compassionate connection to the world into which we are born. This is a bridge that knowledgeable herbalists can provide—a world that the plants are ready and willing to share.

More than 83 million Americans reported tuning in to so-called alternative medicine in 1998, according to a nationwide survey published in the *Journal of the*

*American Medical Association.* The therapies most commonly used were chiropractic, herbs, massage, and relaxation techniques. Yet the numbers are not the telling consideration here. People are turning to healing modalities that work effectively, cost less, and do the desired good with fewer side effects than mainstream medicine. The term *alternative medicine* is revealing, for now we broach the political and economic forces that shape choices deemed "conventional" and "on the up and up." History shapes all cultural destiny, and medicine is no exception. We shall examine the thousands of years of herbal knowledge garnered from plant-based experience that preceded the allopathic doctoring to which many now turn in times of illness or injury. Today's swell of so-called conventional medicine rides on a healing ocean of innumerable depths, both explored and unexplored. Ultimately, to get well, we swim in waters that no one wave can claim exclusively as its own. The point is that we get well.

Doctor friends have told us that a good three-quarters of the people coming to see them have come to the wrong place. Patients often come at the first signs of discomfort or irregularity, expecting a quick fix for obvious symptoms. Over-the-counter medications possess all the glitter that advertising can muster, yet a pill prescribed by a doctor carries a heavier stick. Naturally people want assurance, and to understand the current predicament of their bodies. We're fearful, inconvenienced, and downright whiny. The big picture of our lives—our relationships, satisfaction with our work, persistent stress, diet, physical exercise, time spent nurturing the spirit—rarely is weighed against the "germ of our current demise" or a chronic reckoning demanding our attention. We place our responsibilities at the feet of professionals and pay for expensive services rather than question our own reality. Not all physicians are reluctant to acknowledge the state of affairs that exists in doctors' offices across the country:

> It is estimated that 70 to 80 percent of the people who go to doctors have nothing wrong with them that wouldn't be cleared up by a vacation, a pay raise, or relief from everyday emotional stress. Only 10 percent require drugs or surgery to get well, and approximately 10 percent have diseases for which there is no known cure. Most illnesses run a benign course if left to what the Hippocratic physicians called the *healing power of nature.* The natural healing mechanisms of the body build in an 80 percent recovery rate from all illnesses regardless of medical intervention. . . . Harm done by overtreatment and overuse of technology may exceed the benefits of modern medical care, especially in hospitals. . . . Encounter medicine is able to cure and keep alive as many as 10 to 20 percent of the population who need curative therapy during their lifetimes, an achievement of inestimable value. . . . At issue is not the legitimate function of the physician, but the extent and character of physicians' practices. Too many medical practices are not of benefit to patients, or are not worth the cost.[2]

We are thankful for good doctors. Medical intervention proves itself whenever the surgeon repairs bones or removes stones, the internist uses antibiotics or insulin appropriately, or the pediatrician excludes a food that an enzyme-deficient infant cannot metabolize. Yet many situations call for more personal involvement and homegrown understanding. Interfering in the natural processes of the body can cause trouble. Iatrogenic (treatment-caused) harm is every doctor's worst nightmare. The listed side effects of pharmaceutical drugs should give patients pause to consider the additional health risks incurred to obtain a predicted benefit. Working humbly within these limitations makes physicians good at what they do. The mechanical repair of the human body can never be assured to the extent that the preponderance of medical malpractice suits might suggest. Doctors are as human as the rest of us.

Taking care of yourself and your family for the majority of everyday health needs is both plausible and sensible. Empowerment begins with knowledge. That 70 to 80 percent overdose of conventional health care certainly points to a livelihood long honored in Earth-centered communities. Herbalists can help people use plant remedies respectfully and intelligently. Going to medical school is not essential to be able to help people feel better. We have deeded the legal practice of medicine to an elite group on the basis of one type of training, much to our own confusion and chagrin. A significant chunk of our well-being will always depend on the intimacy we have with our whole selves and the green world outside our door.

Interest in an herbal approach to health is growing rapidly. However, this high regard for natural living is often accompanied by an allopathic perception of illness we've been raised to view as routine. We now take *this* herb for *that* condition. Modern medicine insists upon a physical explanation for each cause and effect. Symptoms are treated accordingly. Yet the whole of the matter often goes unresolved. Holistic plant medicine goes well beyond this kind of narrow-minded, simplistic thinking. Each individual has a different constitution. Different therapeutic strategies for seemingly similar conditions must take into account the biological, emotional, mental, and spiritual aspects of each individual. A good herbalist not only helps people become medically self-sufficient but also shares the journey into the big picture of who we are.

## TRADITIONAL HEALING WISDOM

People have long embraced the gifts of the plants as an everyday part of their lives. Today, Western culture views synthetic chemistry as scientifically superior to the offerings of the plant world. The pendulum of the twentieth century carried us from an in-depth study of plant medicines to an easy reliance on chemical drugs. Yet great worth endures in traditional ways.

Using plants as medicine predates written history. Anthropologists believe that people learned how to use plants for healing by trial and error and by watching birds and animals. The wild creatures certainly possess an instinct to seek out plants that are good to eat and filled with vital nutrition, while avoiding unerringly those that might be poisonous. Many traditional herbalists think that people have been equally blessed with an intuitive understanding of the gifts bestowed by the Creator. They believe that plant spirits (and keen taste buds) guided these attentive ancient peoples to find what they needed. No doubt some truth lies in each perception of the origins of herbal lore. Depth and presence are essential in accessing the teachings of the natural world.

Plant by plant, humans have added to a collective knowledge that has been handed down through the ages by word of mouth and later in written documents. Each cul-

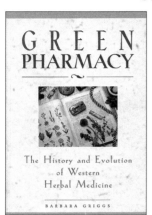

*Barbara Griggs provides a fascinating history of herbal medicine in* Green Pharmacy. *Clearly, these times are part of a much longer human journey to embrace the plants that heal.*

ture slowly evolved medical systems to describe their understanding of the energetics of the human body and the observed effects of their herbal medicines. Regardless of cultural understanding, where blood flowed, yarrow stanched it. When influenza threatened, garlic protected. Where bees stung, plantain soothed. Such plant remedies showed their effectiveness time and time again. That these discoveries were shared across the globe by cultures widely separated in place and time strongly supports a sense of inner knowing on the part of community healers. A hot water extract of *Hibiscus rosa-sinensis*, for example, has been used for fertility regulation and for menstrual problems among indigenous peoples in places thousands of miles apart—in Fiji, India, Indonesia, Kuwait, New Caledonia, Trinidad, and Vietnam. Extracts from this lovely flowering plant have since been shown to possess marked antiestrogenic activity.[3] This universal intertwining of plant and human biology will always provide potent medical impetus. Our genes know how to work with the phytochemicals in plants.

Here in North America, the aboriginal people had a multitude of uses for the plants of this vast continent. The Lakota, Cheyenne, Arapaho, and other tribes on the plains were the first to discover and use echinacea for its immune-stimulating ability. The Eastern woodland tribes would boil wild mint and inhale the steam to help relieve congested lungs and sinuses. The Apache, Hopi, and Navajo would rub powdered cayenne on arthritic joints to help block pain and reduce swelling. The Chippewa and other Great Lakes tribes boiled willow bark and drank the tea to reduce fevers and headaches. The Indian ways of using herbs were passed along to

eager settlers and pharmaceutical entrepreneurs needing knowledge of native botanical medicine. European herb lore and Native American plant wisdom came together, uniting many traditions under the banner of Western herbalism.

Various slants on understanding the human body and the effective uses of herbs are expressed in the medical customs of each generation. New perceptions of medical truth are constantly evolving. Certainly the past offers up nuggets of understanding that help guide our current meanderings as herbalists. In this regard, the influence of Western thinking over the past two centuries merits consideration.

The adherents of Thomsonian medicine in the early 1800s advocated the advice of a New Hampshire farmer-turned-healer. Samuel Thomson (1769–1843) found the heroic medicine of his time appallingly off-course. He believed that illness was caused by cold and relieved by heat. Herbs, particularly the purging influence of lobelia, and steam baths suited his healing philosophy. Bloodletting and mineral poisons did not. Adults were viewed as capable of caring for themselves and their families. The popularity of such "Indian doctoring" roused European academics to publish materia medicas that included America's native plants for the first time. Samuel Hahnemann (1755–1843) meanwhile had launched a system of medicine in Germany based on the principle that like cures like. Homeopathy proved to be yet another thorn in the side of the self-proclaimed "regular" physicians, who viewed the mysterious dilution of analogous remedies as so much humbuggery. The Eclectics arrived on the scene with a desire to reform medical practice by providing their fellow doctors with an empirically based rationale for herbal medicine. These careful clinical observers shied away from extravagant claims for herbs, focusing instead on confirmed effectiveness. Contrasting the relative uses of botanical remedies—noting failures as well as successes—gave Eclectic therapy its innovative thrust.[4] The physiomedicalists added yet another voice to the late-nineteenth-century clamor for natural medicine, the roots of which continue today in naturopathy and British medical herbalism. Their emphasis was on promoting nutrition of the tissues and excretion of waste by enhancing vitality through botanical remedies. Allopathy—modern doctoring as we know it—eventually carried the medical day through legislation aimed at eliminating the competition. Plain and simple, politics played a big role in determining who could practice medicine.

Today much of the world's population today continues to use herbs as their primary source of medicine. The World Health Organization (WHO) estimates that 80 percent of the world's people rely on herbs for their health. An unbroken chain of herbal knowledge has continued to be passed down in many cultures. The long-standing teachings of Chinese, Ayurvedic, and other Earth-centered medicines remain as valuable as ever. Yet for many of us in the Western world this chain has been broken. We have fooled ourselves into believing that synthetic medicine made in a lab by people wearing white coats has more worth than the humble dandelion in our backyards.

We need the perception and conscious intelligence of our ancestors to be embodied anew in every generation by women and men called to be healers. Those persons seeking and sharing knowledge about the plants are integral to a people's medicine.

They include the country doctor who is well versed in spending time with patients; the community herbalist who uses plant medicines for treating an array of dis-ease; a midwife who assists with home births; or a spiritual elder focusing healing intent in a traditional ceremony. We need not go back very far in time to find such everyday folk who speak to our hearts.

Tina Finneyfrock of Mountain Springs Herbals in New York shared this story of her first healing mentors: "My grandparents helped raise me. They were not well educated but they were very self-sufficient. My grandma went to school through sixth grade and my grandpa attended only through eighth grade. They didn't separate anything out as 'herbalism' or make a big deal out of 'living on the land.' Everything was integrated into their way of life. They didn't have special recipes; it was all just run of the mill for them. They made their own clothes, grew much of their food, and didn't go to doctors much. Everything they knew was brought down through the generations. They didn't know the scientific reasons for anything, as it was all anecdotal. The thing I learned the most from them was their way of being. Say I had diarrhea. Grandma would cut a green apple in half and scoop out the insides with a spoon and feed it to me when I was in bed. She didn't just give it to me and say 'eat it.' She sat with me and actually fed me. I learned from her that not only the remedy is healing but how you prepare and give it to someone."

The Wise Woman tradition nicely embodies the holistic process. Women—nurturing their families, taking time to listen to both plants and everyday concerns—are the ones who carry Earth wisdom forward. Men are good at creating medical systems and thinking they shape profound movements, but it is our mothers and grandmothers, gifted with plant knowledge, who make us feel better. "The Wise Woman Way is the oldest tradition of healing known on the planet, yet one that is rarely identified or talked about," says writer and herbalist Susun Weed. "It is an invisible tradition."

Women are the keepers of the hearth. The responsibilities of cooking, tending the herb garden, drying the herbs, making medicines, and brewing the brews traditionally have been met by their loving hands. Women tended to the birth of babies and the care of the sick in the homes of our extended families. The unique ones heeded a call to serve their wider communities. Few written accounts of these village herbalists exist. Yet we feel them deep within our bones and dream of them in our dreams. They inspire us with their personal strength, their wisdom about human nature, their intimacy with Earth, and a seemingly direct line to the Creator.

In our neck of the woods, a woman healer known as Granny Stalbard was born around 1730 and lived to be almost one hundred years old. She was known for traveling on foot or on an old horse, wearing a long plaid cloak, and bringing her bag of roots and herbs to anyone in need. She was one of the first white women to settle in Jefferson, New Hampshire, and learned the virtues of plant medicine from the Indians. One touching story tells how she staunched the flow of blood from a woodsman's ax wound by using a poultice of clover. Across the river, an herbalist known as Aunt Sarah was the one to call on in time of need. Born in a wigwam in Canada in the 1820s, she was the daughter of an Abenaki Indian chief. She lived most of her life around Lunenburg, Vermont, making sweetgrass baskets and gathering medicines. Aunt Sarah

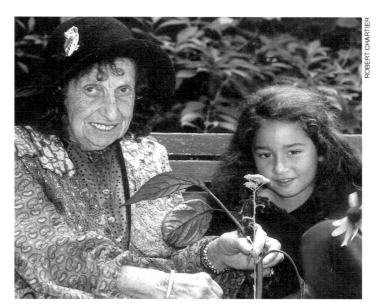

ROBERT CHARTIER

*Juliette de Baïracli Levy continues to inspire many of us with her healing wisdom and bright smile.*

experienced all of the major transitions that affected her native people over the course of her 108 winters. Through it all she learned to adapt and shared her healing gifts with people from all walks of life.

A contemporary village herbalist, Juliette de Baïracli Levy, chose to leave an affluent upbringing to live a simple, satisfying life. Juliette learned much of her herbal knowledge while living among the gypsies throughout the Mediterranean. Now in her nineties, this venerable elder touches us all with her teachings when she comes to herbal gatherings. Her book *Nature's Children* is a classic for looking up sensible remedies. "For me," says Juliette, "the art of herbal medicine is always pleasurable. It is a happy thing to be able to go out into the fields and gather herbs required for restoring to health those that I am asked to treat. It gives one a sense of achievement to be able to take the herb-collecting basket, and from the fields obtain the exact herbs required, knowing where to find them and further knowing which plants are the best for the individual case under treatment."[5]

People will always need good medicine. Accordingly, a process of trial and error has been going on for thousands of years, always directed at the same goal of making us well. Therapies that worked were passed down to subsequent generations; those that did not were forgotten. Plant remedies that survived this test of time, and especially those shared by different cultures from around the world, have tremendous validity. Coming to understand *how* these remedies work—the job of objective science—will never alter the fact that they *do* work.

## WHERE FOLKLORE AND SCIENCE MEET

A holistic view of Creation readily encompasses science. Yet today many people equate knowledge almost exclusively to a scientific viewpoint. Integrating empirical observation and spiritual intuition into the sum of what we know widens our view of this marvelously crafted world.

There's excitement in the air as we come to recognize both the science and the art of herbal medicine. Human wisdom builds continually, though we may not recognize all contributions at all times. A working knowledge of plant constituents and body chemistry provides depth to our understanding of how herbs work. Such information sheds light on the empirical results of centuries of medicinal plant use. Still, we must not lose sight of the fact that the cures and benefits of herbal lore came long before the "proof" the scientifically based crowd insists is solely relevant. Science can help to clarify the nuances of specific preparations. For example, it is useful to know that the blood-thinning ability of garlic is enhanced when it is macerated in a vegetable oil. Crushing the clove releases the allicin that breaks down

into ajoenes and dithiins.[6] On a purely inquisitive level, science attempts to understand the physical world in which we live. Herbalists acknowledge that science is a worthy part of our wisdom base, but we do not emphasize its importance above intuitive insight.

Human disagreements often come down to differences of language and faith. Most of us have difficulty seeing beyond our own strongly held beliefs. We can agree readily, however, that our very existence affirms a magnificent Creation best held in awe. A multitude of paths lead to the center of the circle, all of which touch on some elements of universal truth. Certainly a number of these incorporate science—some would even say science stands as its own belief system—but unmarked trails lead beyond our intellectual ken as well. People with varying points of view can begin to talk about these greater mysteries when we find a language able to reach beyond rational insistence. Physicians trained in modern allopathy, human anatomy and physiology, and pharmacology have added more than 40,000 words to their vocabulary. Herbalists don't necessarily encounter all these terms of modern medicine, but they can certainly share the basic information. The pyloric sphincter will always be the valvelike ring between the stomach and the duodenum, regardless of your belief system. Botanical Latin allows us to reference specific plant species regardless of common names that reflect regional variance. Healers, for the most part, ultimately share the gist of a working vocabulary. The rub lies in how we conceptualize the systems of the body and integrate vital life force with the medicines we each deem applicable.

How we think is much more than a question of language. "Herbs are really suited to broad patterns in the body," says Matthew Wood, a respected teacher on the herbal circuit. "They don't necessarily do the specific microscopic things that the scientists are looking for. Herbs often relate to general changes. This is why we can have well-documented herbs that do tremendous things, like St. John's wort and valerian, and yet scientists still can't figure out why they work. They aren't used to thinking the way nature thinks."

Our understanding of how herbs are used in healing continues to unfold. Today's herbalists can become divided philosophically between a rational view focused on identifiable phytochemical constituents and an empirical view that embraces varying combinations of folkloric tradition, eclectic medical observation, and plant energetics. Despite our sometimes divisive groping to understand plant alchemy, Western herbalists do share a holistic perspective when it comes to helping people heal. We look at how body systems have been affected by the totality of each person—mind, diet, environment, spirit—and then seek to promote health by addressing the underlying causes of illness. Herbs are used to strengthen the body's natural functions and to help bring about system balance.

"Folkloric herbalism reaches out and cares for humanity directly from the world of wonder," says James Green, director of the California School of Herbal Studies. "It is not difficult to understand why folkloric herbalism is ignored, as much as possible, by our Western rational science. Western science simply does not assimilate mystery very well. Its nature must know how; and it must know why. What it can't prove by its peculiar methods of investigation and manipulation, it tends to impulsively invalidate."[7]

Such rational disdain deserves a good look if we are to find mutual respect for each other. If an herb works time and time again, why debunk it? And yet in the eyes of a scientist, a thousand testimonials for a specific herbal preparation are no more evidence than a claim made by only one person. The so-called placebo effect raises hackles as well. It seems that confidence in a therapeutic approach has little validity just because someone gets well.

"Western medicine gave up the placebo effect in trying to quantify everything with double-blind studies," says David Winston of Herbalist & Alchemist, a manufacturer of highly respected herbal preparations. "It's not a bad idea to find out what really works and what is the placebo effect. But in trying to do this we decided the whole concept of placebo effect is a negative thing. If somebody comes to me and they are sick, they don't care why they get better. I don't care. All we care about is that they get better. It is true that 33 percent of the time if you do nothing, between placebo and self-limiting disease, people improve. In fact, one study shows that people get better because of placebo effect 60 percent of the time. The human mind is incredible."

Positive experience makes sense to us. Anyone who has had a successful chiropractic adjustment recognizes that manipulations of the spinal column do indeed effect a cure. A chiropractor adjusts bones to thereby adjust muscles and organs, leading to a reorganization of the whole body. And yet conventional medical theory regards chiropractic as so much bunk because its claims have not stood the usual tests of scientific validation. Quite simply, to a classically trained doctor with no particularly compelling treatment to recommend, that pain in your lower back is likely to go away eventually. The chiropractor who gains acceptance by taking time to talk with each patient offers an understandable prognosis, and gives hope. That you feel better after an adjustment is seen as mere coincidence. Effectiveness tied to hope seems to really get the rational blood boiling. This philosophical insistence on proving *reality really is real* comes with all the economic advantage of a stacked deck. Why go to a chiropractor—or an herbalist for that matter—if all that can be offered is hope?

Western culture at large has come to look upon scientists with the same veneration a traditional society might accord to its priest or shaman. Researchers' authority or methodology is often not questioned when word comes through the media that an herb proves too good to be true one day and then suspect the next. Many variables enter into everyday life that no therapeutic research can fully assay: Individuals differ in constitutional type, emotional history, and environmental upbringing. How herbs are pre-

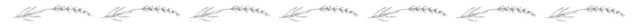

## *THE GERMAN COMMISSION E MONOGRAPHS*

T*HE GERMAN COMMISSION E Monographs* are widely viewed in media circles as an authoritative source of what works in herbal medicine. Varro Tyler, author of controversial herb books in his own right, claims the monographs "represent the most accurate information available in the entire world on the safety and efficacy of herbs and phytomedicines." So what exactly is this mighty therapeutic guide that the American Botanical Council (ABC) promotes at $165 a pop?

Experienced herbal practitioners write *herbals* to transmit their intimate knowledge about specific plants and their use. Committees create *monographs* that outline the scientifically sanctioned use of herbs in accordance with legal medical practices in a given coun-

try. The now defunct Commission E was established in 1978 to evaluate the safety and efficacy of herbs sold in Germany. Members of the health care profession and of the pharmaceutical industry participated. "Its Monographs," according to a critique by herbalist Jonathan Treasure, "are conservative, telegraphically short, and completely lacking any detail in botany, ethnobotany, or pharmacognosy. They have the minor benefit of considering some traditional usage, but they mostly reflect the specific situation in Germany, where, for example, injectable herbal preparations are commonly available." The highly touted English translation published by the ABC presents the German government's evaluations of 360 different herbs, with charts that let doctors look up

herb-drug interactions and safety warnings.

Advertisers for herbal supplements love to point out when their products are in accord with the monographs. For example, "Garlinase 4000 ® is the only one that equals the German Commission E daily recommendation of 4,000 mg of fresh garlic with just one tablet. The Commission E is recognized throughout the world as the model for regulating herbal products." That plug speaks volumes for who wants what in the herbal world. We'll take the fresh garlic, thank you.

"*The German Commission E Monographs* are equated by lots of people as the Truth. I find nothing wrong in it," concludes David Hoffmann, author of numerous noteworthy herbals, "but neither does it go very far."

pared and administered affects the patient-plant interaction. Isolated constituents in the plant rarely, if ever, have the same action as the whole plant. The energetic qualities of the herb often are not considered. Nuance proves subtle and immeasurable yet it often means everything: The soil that grows the plant, the potent moment of harvest, and the soulful intention in the heart of the harvester do matter. Ulterior motives behind any research can certainly determine desired outcomes. Contradictory results certainly happen.

"When you come right down to it, probably a majority of conventional medicines in our pharmacy today were not put to the standard of double-blind, placebo-controlled, randomized clinical trials," says Robert Rufsvold, M.D., a family practitioner at the New England Center for Integrative Health in Lyme, New Hampshire. "There's a tradition of empiricism in conventional medicine, too, and it's not necessarily a wrong one."

Any medical system is going to be either rational, empirical, or some combination of the two. A totally rational framework seeks an individualized differential diagnosis based upon a theoretical understanding of human physiology. A strictly empirical mind set, on the other hand, categorizes symptoms and diseases, takes note of what treatment has worked historically, and proceeds from there with a course of action. Remedies become a matter of routine based upon observed experience.

All of us can think anew. All of us can honor the teachings that have come before our time and through our own experiences as herbalists. There should be no wedge between people who want to help others feel better. Healers tend toward linear opposition when the broader perspective of an open-minded circle would keep us in better stead. Good medicine is both rational and empirical. An honest science can embrace mystery. Folklore only gets better when we try to understand why it works.

All of us enjoy knowing the facts about our favorite herbs that science can provide. The Cherokee, for instance, used yellowroot (*Xanthorhiza simplicissima*) for sore eyes. We now know that eye drops containing 0.2 percent berberine will alleviate conjunctivitis. They used yellowroot as a blood tonic and as a cancer remedy. Berberine has anti-cancer activity. Native peoples used yellowroot for cramps, hemorrhoids, nerves, sore mouths, and sore throat as well. The bitter berberine and other alkaloids present in this root have spasmolytic, anti-inflammatory, analgesic, antibiotic, and viricidal properties. The folklore worked long before science isolated and named the chemicals in the herb. Today we know so much more by putting the two together.

Ultimately, the debate over the scientific validity of herbal medicine will come down to who reaps the profits. The domestic herb industry argues for scientific respectability. The status accorded to pharmacological studies of plant constituents comes with a share of an encapsulated market. Any legislation to regulate of the sale of plant medicines will bolster corporate herbalism. Community herbalists and bioregional apothecaries, on the other hand, will continue to uphold tradition and the utterly wonderful availability of the healing plants for each and every one of us.

## LITTLE MEDICINE, BIG MEDICINE

The God-given ability of our bodies to heal on their own can be overlooked too easily in

*Text continues on page 14.*

# Matthew Wood

INDIAN PEOPLE learned about certain plants for medicine and food by watching the bear dig up roots, tear off barks, and collect berries with its claws. The bear is a totem animal for the native healer, bringing empowerment from the dream world. Bear medicines (osha, lomatium, and balsam root) are the first plants the bear seeks to eat each spring. The resins in these roots work on the lungs, heart, and liver. Native Americans believed the bear was taking care of the people by pointing out these remedies for the aeration, circulation, and metabolism of the body.

The herbal renaissance has a modern-day "bear" to heed in Matthew Wood. This Minnesota herbalist prods at the roots of healing traditions, seeking an integral understanding of body systems and plant energetics. "I spend a lot of time going through the old books," explains this eclectic explorer. "I see phrases that don't mean much today, like *keeping open the kidneys*, or *the condition of the skin*, or *keeping open the bowels*. I didn't initially get that this was a medical system." Little by little Matthew has come to realize that these expressions have meaning that tie together seemingly different approaches to therapeutics. An intensive teaching schedule has helped him articulate these fragments of lost healing wisdom into a congruent whole for other herbalists.

"Remember in the movie *Little Women*? The mother comes back to treat the daughter who's sick, takes down the covers, and says, 'We have to get the heat down to her feet.' She instantly knew what to do. These simple folk-medical ideas were the common property of doctors, mothers, grandmothers, healers, and herbalists in the nineteenth century," notes Matthew. "These medical sayings are still in our blood. Our ancestors want to speak. They healed and they know things . . . we can pick up hints from them and realize we do know about medicine after all."

Finding a language that meshes such folkloric perception with modern medical understanding is the challenge. "I recently made a big conceptual shift. The nineteenth-century botanical doctors refer to five different tissue states. Modern allopaths can get down to microscopic lesions, but the old doctors could only see general conditions of the body. Tissue overstimulation or irritation or heat would be one, contraction or spasm another, then relaxation. Those three are the basic biological response states that happen in living tissue. In addition, there's atrophy, or lack of nutrition, and then there's depression. These five tissue states correspond closely to causative agents long recognized in traditional medicine: hot, damp, dry, cold, and wind. This has knitted it all together for me. These five tissue states have analogies to old medical systems as well as roots in allopathy and nineteenth-century botanical medicine. It's simple, yet it takes in so much. I was not a fan of simplifying everything to four or five elements, till I understood these tissue states. Then, all of a sudden, *boom*. I began to read the nineteenth-century botanical literature with fresh eyes. Everything they did was defined in terms of these five tissue states, again and again and again. If you can define what you are looking at as one of these five states, and then understand what organ systems are involved, then you've got it. My work has gotten much more precise and clear and easy.

"I always felt from the beginning of studying herbal medicine that I didn't want to practice in a way that is boring, that is not uplifting to me. I don't want to be a doctor and just do mechanical diagnosis. Understanding what goes on in the body energetically cultivates my senses, my observational skills, and my mind to make deductions and put things together by intuition. This develops my own soul and spirit so that I am growing while my patients are growing. Otherwise it would be an imbalance."

Matthew considers himself a clinical herbalist of the Western tradition. This good-humored man prefers to get right down to the business at hand in his consultations. "I take their pulses, make note of indications in their tongue and skin, and hear what their doctor had to say. If it's a fairly acute, superficial condition, and I have the right remedies for it, I figure I won't see people again because their problem will be helped. But for a more subacute or chronic thing, I might need to see people two or three times over a half-year period. I don't get as much into lifestyle changes, eating, psychological factors, et cetera. I believe the herbs will change people."

Here is an herbalist renowned for his low-dose recommendations—one to three drops of a specified tincture. Matthew perceives that the plants work in our bodies on a much deeper level than the mechanical explanations offered by phytochemistry. His homeopathic application of herbal remedies can be puzzling, until you recognize this man's broad grounding in spiritual intent. "We need to understand the herbs as living beings, as personalities, as entities in themselves," he explains, "that we treat

with respect and that we can know and understand. I am a believer in a shamanistic interaction between medicine plants and people." A friend of Matthew's had eaten a poisonous mushroom, known as a death cap. When he got to her house, he gave her a few milk this-

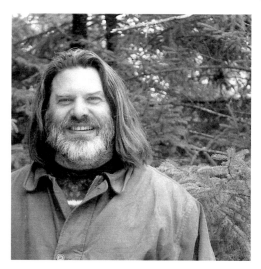

*I am a believer in a shamanistic interaction between medicine plants and people.* —Matthew Wood

tle seeds. The staff at the emergency room were not too hopeful for this friend's chances. Whether it involved an atypical antidote or spiritual trust, the woman walked home the next morning.

"Some of us arrogant types start out thinking we know it all. The herbalists who go around speaking at conferences tend to be people who have a lot of self-confidence. We need these kinds of trailblazers who've figured things out on their own. Speaking

for myself, I can say that when I knew a lot less, I thought I knew just about everything."

Matthew accepts that his views may be spurious to some. Certainly, like the native bear, he gives us much to ponder. His *Book of Herbal Wisdom* rates high in our collection of herbals, because it provides a thorough cross-referencing of many traditions. Physical indications and pulses are just a part of his tool bag. He calls simultaneously on intuition, psychic acuity, and past experience with plants and people to help him choose the best remedy.

Matthew always comes back to an understanding of general broad patterns. "Say you have an upset stomach that goes on and on. You go to the doctor, then come back again after another month. They give you a barium enema. It turns out you don't have cancer, so they say good-bye. You either have cancer or you have nothing they want to know about or can treat or help. The old medical books—and our herb books—say dyspepsia, ulcer, acidity, bilious distress, flatulence, bloating. We treat all these. Many of our simple herbs—the carminatives, like dill, fennel, angelica—are warming, drying, and help to dispel gas and bloating. This is just the wisdom of the ages, but it's ignored in modern medicine." ❧

an invasive medicine. The best gifts are often the simplest. Plant remedies offer a preferable option for many healing needs.

Plant medicines evoke a healing response rather than masking or attacking symptoms. Herbs bring nutrients to tissues and body systems. Some herbs work as irritants to stimulate the tissues, thus bringing more blood to the area so it can heal itself. Sometimes herbs soothe, calming inflammation. Herbs can be used in many chronic imbalances to help bring one back into balance.

For example, someone suffering from insomnia will benefit more from incorporating relaxing herbs such as skullcap and valerian than from reaching for an over-the-counter medication such as Nytol. A pharmaceutical drug such as Valium can become addictive and actually deprive you of restful sleep. If used long-term, Valium can cause depression and headaches, actually creating more problems than it first masked. Valerian and skullcap actually feed and nourish the nervous system rather than wreak havoc with it. Of course, working with one's diet and lifestyle is important as well.

Eating fresh wild greens and drinking tonic teas such as nettles and hawthorn is herbalism at its finest. Adding astragalus root, garlic, and shiitake mushrooms to our soups are simple ways to nurture good health. Herbal medicine is superior for long-term overall building of health. Nancy remembers teaching an "Introduction to Herbs" workshop sponsored by our local hospital. One of the nurses attending said later that the most important thing she learned was that herbs can be used to build overall health. This was a new concept for her.

Herbs offer an amazing adaptability. Most conventional drugs are expedient only for one or two indications. Herbs, on the other hand, have multiple and even divergent abilities. Garlic is used for a myriad of conditions such as hypertension, bacterial infections, and high cholesterol. An extraction of the leaves of the *Ginkgo biloba* tree is effective for improving blood circulation. Thus memory loss, chronic leg pain, ringing in the ears (tinnitus), and macular degeneration are all indications for ginkgo. This venerable herb also helps with autoimmune conditions, including some forms of hepatitis and asthma. Herbs go beyond working in a singular manner precisely because phytochemistry is so complex. Yarrow contains more than 120 different compounds, all in powerful balance with each other. These can potentiate, enhance, and mitigate each other's effects inside the human body. Thus such plant medicine can be seen as 120 separate medicines at work. The secret of plant alchemy lies in the synergistic interaction of the right compounds in the right body at the right time.

We have good reason to seek out gentler medicines. The *Journal of the American Medical Association* points out that almost half the patients who die in hospitals from iatrogenic causes meet their end taking prescription medication. This amounts to a significant 106,000 deaths each year.[8] The Food and Drug Administration (FDA) recalls approximately half the drugs approved over a ten-year period because of unacceptable side effects. Many side effects that are deemed acceptable (based upon a pharmaceutical risk-benefit analysis) might not be acceptable to the person taking the drug. The situation is compounded many times over by multiple prescriptions, with some people taking as many as a dozen medications at one time. Commonly used medications can make people drowsy, lethargic, nauseated, impotent, and fatigued. Rashes, ulcers, seizures, anemia, and jaundice can result. Conventional drugs certainly can save lives. Yet it is not unreasonable to consider alternatives in situations that are less life-threatening.

Fear of a debilitating stroke or heart attack plagues many people today. Narrowed blood vessels (hardening of the arteries) are common with a modern diet featuring altered fats, homogenized dairy products, and refined grains. One prescription given by doctors for stroke prevention is clopidogrel, first approved by the FDA in November 1997. This blood-thinning drug showed slightly more effectiveness than common aspirin in reducing the risk of atherosclerotic disease.[9] But now for the reckoning. The most frequently seen adverse effects in patients receiving clopidogrel were stomach upset, bleeding disorders, rash, and diarrhea. Gastrointestinal hemorrhage, however, occurred less for these patients than for patients on the aspirin therapy.

By way of contrast, let's look at some herbal approaches to dealing with cardiovascular health and stroke prevention. The focus shifts to treating the whole person, not just the disease. Diet, exercise, and stress reduction matter. Hawthorn is likely to be a key herb in such a person's healing formula. The tonic benefits for the heart of the leaves, flowers, and berries of *Crataegus* spp. are only gained from whole plant preparations ingested over a prolonged length of time. Hawthorn improves heart circulation through dilation of the coronary arteries by enhancing cell activity and nutrition. Most significantly, no contraindications or side effects have been noted for hawthorn.[10]

Food as medicine always comes to the fore when garlic takes center stage. The antiplatelet effect of *Allium sativum* has been confirmed in research.[11] Its blood-thinning ability helps prevent atherosclerosis. Fatty

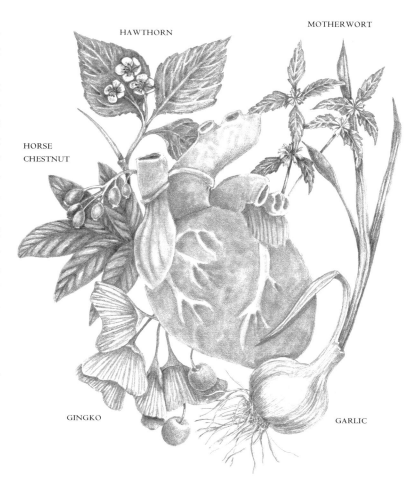

HAWTHORN

MOTHERWORT

HORSE CHESTNUT

GINGKO

GARLIC

*Herbs specific to cardiac health include hawthorn, horse chestnut, ginkgo, garlic, and motherwort.*

deposits on the linings of large and medium-sized arteries can cause blood clots. A subsequent blockage of the arteries that supply blood to the cardiac muscle can cause a heart attack, while a stroke can result if the clots lodge in arteries that supply blood to the brain. Allicin—a unique chemical in garlic that is well known for its strong antibiotic properties—inhibits clotting factors in the blood. Other vascular tonics are rich in plant constituents called flavones, found in herbs such as horse chestnut and ginkgo. All berries—in particular blueberries, strawberries, raspberries, and elderberries—when cooked contain more bio-available flavones, emphasizing once again that good medicine really can be as simple as good food. A high-vitamin diet has been shown to prevent, and even to reverse, atherosclerosis in humans.[12] Relaxing remedies such as linden blossom and motherwort are indicated whenever stress is a consideration. Absolutely key in this discussion is an herbalist's ability to customize a remedy formulated for each individual in a holistic context.

In any given health situation we each need to decide for ourselves the best things we can choose to support our own care. Allopathic medicine is best for severe pain, immediate crisis, and urgent life-threatening circumstances. Yet predictability in any matter can ultimately prove to be an illusion. A good doctor or herbalist will explain the rationale and expected outcome of a recommended therapy. That explanation will be steeped in the traditions and beliefs of the therapist. Holistic approaches come from holistic practitioners.

"Some systems are better for some situations or for some types of people," says our herbal mentor, Rosemary Gladstar. "If you tend to be a linear person, folklore herbalism will drive you crazy because there are no rules and everything is intuitive and perceptive and circular. But you can view herbalism from a strict biochemical dimension too." And indeed some people overlay herbalism with allopathic medical perception. Just as there are pharmaceutical drugs, there are herbal drugs. The major chemical constituents in the plant are viewed as having major impact on the body. Such herbal allopathy features that self-limiting dynamic in which a curative fix takes precedence over healing the whole. "All of which," Rosemary is quick to add, "takes away about 90 percent of what makes herbalism work."

Herbalists desire to promote health by taking into account the totality of the individual rather than just managing his or her disease. A person is not simply a machine with mechanical disorders that can be fixed by physical or chemical treatments. Herbs work with the body in treating underlying conditions. We make a conscious leap well beyond an immediate cure when we embrace holistic healing. Allopathic medicine focuses primarily on treatment of disease and suppression of symptoms, with less regard for cause. Acute circumstances often necessitate this approach. Suppression only works for so long, however, with chronic conditions and degenerative disease. A stronger pharmaceutical then becomes necessary, and the body becomes even more out of balance. Consider the thousands of diseases and remedies that the modern medical student needs to learn. John Christopher of the School of Natural Healing in Utah always liked to point out that herbalists, in contrast, have just one primary concern—a healthy body. We recognize that herbs work best proactively, to help maintain health from the get-go.

Antibiotics are a prime example of Big Medicine overdone. These miracle drugs have saved countless lives, but discretion in their use needs to become the better part of valor. One study showed that when doctors believe their patients want antibiotics, they prescribe them more than 75 percent of the time.[13] Antibiotics have been given for bronchitis, sinusitis, and viral infections, none of which can be cured antibiotically. One result has been resistant strains of bacteria, an ecological backlash.[14] Especially culpable are patients who do not complete the full bacterial purge of their bodies once an antibiotic regimen has commenced: Many stop taking their medicine once they start to feel better, thus allowing any remaining bacteria to rebound rapidly with improved resistance. And yet some people simply don't succumb to bacterial infection in the first place. Their immune systems protect their bodies successfully despite inevitable exposure to the same bacterial pathogens. We literally share our body with billions of bacteria that normally live in healthy symbiosis in and on our bodies. One to two pounds of "us" is bacteria, and it's a good thing. The friendly bacteria actually help fight off their pathogenic cousins and help our guts assimilate nutrients. Pharmaceutical antibiotics don't discriminate between friend and foe.

The talk fifty years ago was that these miracle drugs would provide humans with disease-free lives. Now we face superbugs of our own making, which the antibiotic marvel can no longer control. Supporting the immune system—specifically the thymus, spleen, lymphatic system, tonsils, liver, and bone marrow—with herbs such as ashwagandha and Siberian ginseng and foods heavy on the garlic and onions marks our best line of defense. Quite a number of herbs can help boost the body's fight against a bacterial onslaught. Chewing on a garlic clove is a far better alternative than dousing our gut with penicillin or streptomycin at the first sign of a sore throat or flu outbreak. *Herbal Antibiotics: Natural Alternatives for Treating Drug-Resistant Bacteria* is a must read for anyone contemplating a healthy coexistence with bacteria. "Perhaps," as its author Stephen Buhner so eloquently concludes, "it is fitting that the lowly bacteria will be the one to teach us humility."

Herbalists know that certain plants such as foxglove (*Digitalis* spp.) and belladonna provide strong, druglike medicine. Yet the majority of medicinal plants are milder, gentler-acting herbs. Rudolf Weiss, M.D., a founding figure of modern German phytotherapy and a clinician with decades of experience, has written that *gentle action* does not mean herbs such as chamomile or mint are more or less effective than stronger medicines. "One would not expect these plants to produce instant and powerful effects like those seen after an injection of digitalis or strophanthin," says Weiss. "These 'simple' medicinal plants do not as a rule have any appreciable toxic effects, and may therefore be safely taken over an extended period of time."[15] Herbs are congenial to who we are. Pharmaceutical chemistry can effect our cure, but rarely as mildly or efficaciously as herbs. We share biological roots with plants.

Let's talk about fevers. A rise in body temperature usually accompanies bacterial or viral infections. Physiologist Matthew Kluger and his associates at the University of Michigan Medical School have shown that the body resists infection by "running hotter." Interferon, an antiviral substance, is produced as a result.[16] Aspirin or other drugs aimed at this adaptive defense by our bodies to ward off invasive infection suppress more than the fever itself. The underlying situation that led to the fever has not been changed. Fevers that become too high can be dealt with through a combination of herbal teas such as catnip, elder, and peppermint, and tepid baths. Allopathic drugs can always be considered should a fever become potentially life-threatening. But mostly we want to let a fever run its course, to go with, rather than against, the body's attempt to heal itself. This can be a case where Little Medicine becomes no medicine at all.

Countless people take some responsibility for their cures at home. Over-the-counter medicines at drugstore chains provide a fix for the symptom at hand. Massive amounts of advertising dollars aimed at postnasal drip, searing headaches, hot flashes, and bad breath create much misunderstanding about how we might better care for ourselves. Natural product lines at these same stores do little to alter the attitude that an herbal supplement or two can bring a body back to par. Why change a hurting lifestyle if a little dab will do ya? The truth is, people want their medicine simple, with no personal need to act on dietary change, outlook, habits, or choices that create monumental stress. Claims on the label—or subtly introduced by other means to satisfy FDA oversight—reduce personal medicine to this lowest common denominator.

Local plant medicine, by contrast, is about the thoughtful use of the herbs in the context of a whole life. The use of ginkgo and vitamin E helps prevent memory loss. Milk thistle is an excellent herb to boost liver function. St. John's wort does temper mild depression. Hawthorn strengthens a weak heart. You can make such choices for yourself and your family. Word-of-mouth advice to do so will come from many channels. However, delving into the details, choosing therapies matched to individual constitutions, having a direct relationship with the plants—and ideally having a community herbalist friend available to help guide this discussion—brings the full empowerment of herbalism to the fore.

"As a botanist-physician, I believe that intelligent use of healing plants can make people more self-reliant in matters of health," says Dr. Andrew Weil of the University of Arizona College of Medicine. "In my own practice I use herbal preparations far more than pharmaceutical drugs. I have never yet produced a significant adverse reaction from giving patients plants.

More important, I have seen a great deal of benefit from their use as part of a comprehensive program of treatment."[17]

Good health encompasses a broad spectrum of wise habits: herbs, diet, exercise, meditation, a steady sense of purpose, the practice of loving-kindness. Attentive living lacks the profit margin on which our modern medical system has come to depend. Big Medicine is not cheap. Little Medicine often grows outside our back door.

## WE ARE WHAT WE EAT

Our bodies, in harmony with mind and spirit, have a natural ability to heal. Too many people dismiss this integral understanding of healing. They prefer to believe they are the victims of an outside cause instead of taking personal responsibility for their health. It's a cockeyed prescription, indeed, to recommend either plant medicines or pharmaceutical drugs without being sure that those in your care are already drinking plenty of pure water, breathing fresh air, getting enough sleep, and eating a healthy diet. Herbalism without such nutritional reckoning will ultimately fail the very people we want to help. Good food is the topic at hand.

Homegrown, organic food cannot be beat. The vibrancy and life force of freshly harvested fruits and vegetables brought to the table are tangible—they are lip-smacking delicious! If you are unable to produce your own food, buying from local organic farmers is the next best bet. Food grown nearby and picked at peak ripeness will be full of nutrients and flavor. Produce shipped halfway across the planet compromises the goods and the pleasure. In the last century most farm soils have been robbed of essential minerals. One Rodale report stated a 25 to

30 percent loss of mineral content in vegetables since 1975 alone.[18] Soluble nitrogen fertilizers simply do not build long-term vitality in the soils we ask to grow our food. Of course that affects our health. A slew of vitamin supplements are called on to provide what should be present in nourishing food grown in soil nurtured with manures and cover crops. Or, as JJ Hapala of the Farmer Cooperative Genome Project in Oregon likes to put it, "We used to eat one apple a day, now we need eight." The chemical fertilizers used in agriculture are more of a liability than we thought. We now raise crop varieties that consume petroleum as if it's a food resource. Organic agriculture, on the other hand, restores sustenance to the staff of life.

The chemical residues in conventionally grown food are said to be present in amounts too small to cause harm. The standards for acceptable levels of toxic agrichemicals in food are based on risks of acute toxicity. Unless you work on a farm, that possibility of exposure causing immediate harm is practically nonexistent. What's too often not considered are the risks of long-term cumulative damage to body defenses and healing ability. Cancer is on the rise, whether or not we want to argue about what twenty to forty years of consistent exposure to chemicals does to our bodies. Scientists and government officials don't consider the combined actions resulting from exposure to multiple toxins. Such synergistic chemicals have been shown to disrupt the human endocrine system. The unknowns engulf the known facts when we begin to contemplate our biology in this chemical soup of our own making. Organic agriculture again provides a leg up on a bad situation.

Eating from within our own bioregion assures the good habit of eating with the seasons. Don't overlook wild foods and more bitter tastes. "Many people are skeptical about the nutritive value of wild plants," says Doug Elliot, a naturalist from North Carolina, "even though these same people aren't so concerned about the sprayed and chemically processed foods they normally consume." Befriending the sour side of life bestows character. Spring greens of dandelion, chickweed, and baby dock (to name but three) are chock full of tonic power. Bitters stimulate digestion by encouraging the liver to produce bile. Adding arugula and cress to that summer salad might even make up for eating pale iceberg lettuce. Dark green kale, collards, and mustard greens are traditional fall foods with great virtue.

Small family farms are ideally situated to provide us with the healthiest meat, eggs, and milk. Farm animals raised happy make for a far better karma than the contaminated, devitalizing end faced in factory farms and feedlots. The growing demand for grass-fed beef and free-range poultry reflects a growing awareness of what confinement fattening does to meat. A rich egg has a deep yellow-orange yolk, produced by chickens left free to run in fields and gardens, scooping up insect pests and pecking at herbs. Fresh milk—unpasteurized and unhomogenized, thank you—retains all the enzymes and vitamin richness found in a sunny day. Old-fashioned butter suits because unadulterated fats are essential to a balanced diet based on nourishing foods.

This brings us most pertinently to nutrition researcher Sally Fallon. This feisty woman has taken on "politically correct nutrition" in all its guises. "Clearly something

*Your food shall be your medicine and your medicine shall be your food.*

—HIPPOCRATES
(460–377 B.C.E.)

is very wrong, even though many Americans have been conscientious about following orthodox dietary advice," she begins in her *Nourishing Traditions* cookbook. "They take exercise seriously; many have stopped smoking; consumption of fresh vegetables has increased; many have reduced their intake of salt; and a good portion of America has cut back on red meats and animal fats. But none of these measures has made a dent in the ever increasing toll of degenerative disease. We buy foods labeled low-fat, no cholesterol, reduced sodium, thinking they are good for us. Why, then, are we so sick?"

A good chunk of that answer centers on whole foods. Sally urges strict abstinence from sugar and very limited use of refined flour as good advice for everyone. These two products were virtually unknown in the human diet before 1600 and were never used in great quantities before the twentieth century. Average sugar intake in America has increased from 10 pounds per person per year in 1821 to 170 pounds per person today, representing more than one-fourth the average caloric intake. Another large portion of all calories comes from white flour and refined vegetable oils. "This means that less than half the diet must provide all the nutrients to a body that is under constant stress from its intake of sugar, white flour and rancid and hydrogenated vegetable oils," points out Sally. "Herein lies the root cause of the vast increase in degenerative diseases that plague modern America."[19]

Dr. Weston Price, a dentist, toured the globe during the 1930s to study the relation of nutrition to health and degeneration. He visited many peoples, from isolated Irish and Swiss, to Eskimos and Africans and Polynesians. All were eating a variety of traditional diets, always locally based. The majority of these people were healthy, with strong teeth, well into their later years. Their diets varied widely but the people were all eating whole, unprocessed foods. Without exception, once "civilized foods" were introduced into these societies, the people began experiencing health problems. Their teeth became crooked, got cavities, and many fell out. Bone structure diminished. Infertility, infectious disease, and degenerative conditions became more common. Our inheritance of vibrant health and physical perfection has gone the way of refined carbohydrates and devitalized fats.

A clarion bell should be ringing loud and clear. Today's typical diet fits nicely into industrialized precepts. People mostly depend on corporations to grow their fruits and vegetables. We see no evil when the care of farm animals amounts to a lower price per pound for their flesh. Wonder Bread lasts forever. Cheap sugar provides a sweetness that masks flavorless concoctions. Synthetic vitamins put into overprocessed foods imply that vitality can be recaptured. Milk makes a 500-mile round trip in the process of becoming considered "safe for human consumption." Test-tube flavors cost little compared to wholesome butter and honest garlic. Advertising makes words such as *fresh* and *natural* absolutely meaningless.

Perhaps an apple grower can cut to the quick here with some wise-guy humor. Michael does spray to grow fruit in our organic orchard here at the farm.[20] All materials registered for approved use, organic or otherwise, are held to the same accounting by the Environmental Protection Agency. The spray label needs to state clearly the percentage of active and inert ingredients in the mix. The so-called inerts need not be identified (proprietary secrets and all that rot), but you do get a sense of

The crucial role of diet in preventing illness points the way in taking responsibility for our own health. Ann Marie Colburn's Food and Healing *continues to be one of the more profound books on nutrition we have read.*

proportional reckoning. What if we did this with the foods offered in the grocery store? Certainly it would simplify that long list of unrecognizable ingredients. The *actives* would be the nourishing foods in a given can of soup, say, while the *inerts* could be bunched together as so many nutritionally useless, if not downright harmful, unknowns. The denatured grains, food additives, artificial colorings, refined sweeteners, heat-processed oils, and hydrogenated fats could all be summed directly on the front: "This dinner contains 87 percent inerts." Perhaps best of all, we'd lose this senseless preoccupation with low-fat, low-salt, low-worth advertising. People might start getting it through their heads that whole foods are the only real foods.

Why were heart attacks rare in the United States in 1900 but the leading cause of death by the late 1940s? Fully half of individuals suffering heart attacks today have none of the statistical risk factors generally implicated (high-fat diet, high blood cholesterol, smoking, diabetes, and hypertension).[21] The industrialization of food at the turn of the century must be the explanation. In particular three kinds of food were made universally available that had previously been only occasional treats: sugar, processed white flour, and refined vegetable oils and margarine. All are linked with heart attacks.

Our diets are very near and dear to our hearts. The gumption to make positive change is best brought about by awareness of how intimately health and nutrition are linked. *Food and Healing* by Annemarie Colbin is Nancy's current favorite for viewing the big picture. The information about the remarkable healing qualities of specific foods presented in this book complements herbal wisdom nicely. Andrew Weil recently added another gem, *Eating Well for Optimum Health*. We're absolutely intrigued by the integral perspectives Sally Fallon has brought to center stage in *Nourishing Traditions*. Read this book and you'll soon be setting yourself up to milk goats and learn entirely old ways to preserve foods through lacto-fermentation. The *Whole Foods Companion* by Dianne Onstad stands as our pantry encyclopedia to look up the nutritional value of each fruit, vegetable, grain, and legume, as well as culinary tips, health benefits, lore, and legends.

Food plays a major role in our health, but of course it is not the only underlying cause of disease. Elderly people who are in fine health, despite eating junk food and whatever else pleases, are testaments to other avenues to well-being and longevity. Breast-fed as babies, these people were then

## EATING SENSIBILITIES

- Enjoy your food. Prepare and eat it with thoughts of nourishment, beauty, and a spirit of gratefulness. The love and care we infuse into the food we prepare is life-giving as well.
- Eat whole foods in or as close to their natural state as possible. A good overall test of fresh food is the following: *If it won't sprout or rot, don't eat it!*
- Shop the perimeter of the grocery store. Here's where you generally find the fresh produce, dairy products, and less-processed foods. The foods you want have ingredients that all sound desirable to eat.
- Sit down. Chew your food well. Savor it. Eat to satisfaction, without overindulging.
- Remember, everything in moderation, including moderation. Strive to eat healthfully most of the time, but don't punish yourself with guilt if occasionally you don't follow your own guidelines. Being active helps balance out those occasional slip-ups.

raised on home-cooked food and were not given vaccines or antibiotics during childhood. They grew up *not* going to the doctor when they became sick. A warming cup of tea, perhaps a medicinal shot of sweet wine, followed by plenty of rest, got them back on their feet. At age ninety-one, Nancy's grandma certainly keeps showing the rest of the young'uns in this family there's something to be said for self-administered pluck.

A less-than-ideal diet cannot be the only cause of the diseases we see proliferating around us. Annemarie Colbin surmises that many of our problems stem from the medical drugs we take to treat or prevent illness. "If we avoid the inner pollution and disruption of drugs for minor illnesses," she writes, "we will be more resistant to outer pollution of unhealthy foods and unhealthy environmental chemicals. . . . The more time goes on, the worse it gets, and the more I

am firmly convinced that iatrogenic harm is the great unacknowledged, worldwide health tragedy of the twentieth century."[22] And that, friends, is why herbal medicine coupled with a whole foods diet makes such marvelous sense today.

## HERBAL UPROARS

Not surprisingly, as herbs become mainstream once again, issues such as licensing, standardization, government regulation, and unsustainable demand cloud the herbal horizon. Health concerns are deemed the domain of professionals. Government has the job of assuring the foods we purchase are pure and our medicines safe. We want, we buy—regardless of the environmental and social costs. Our disinclination to insist that individuals be responsible for their actions lies at the root of many of these so-called herbal uproars.

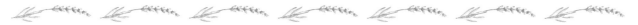

# PERSONAL RESPONSIBILITY

**M**ANY OF US never learned what it means to take the time to be well. *Dis-ease* invariably results, and then we look to doctors to patch up our negligence. The healing plants will change few outcomes if we perceive that someone else is responsible for what happens in our lives. Under conventional medicine, people "want to be taught, moved, treated, or guided rather than to learn, to heal, and to find their own way."* A heap of herbal supplements stacks up lightly

against the recognition that your outlook and daily respect for your body play a pivotal role in health. A good herbalist will prompt you to make sound lifestyle choices and can recommend nourishing teas and tonic herbs; but getting involved with one's health goes even deeper. The sum of mind, body, and spirit reflects how we accept life and the daily challenges to our inner serenity. A positive attitude does more good than any drug. Good relations with family,

friends, and community bring harmony to body systems as well. We may think we need a cure when all we actually desire is care—both for ourselves and flowing profusely in return. The responsibility for health lies foremost within each of us. Affairs of the spirit might seem too simple to explain a chronic ailment, but they often are at the crux of the matter.

————
* Ivan Illich, *Medical Nemesis: The Expropriation of Health* (New York: Bantam, 1976), p. 210.

## Licensing/Certification

Choosing a healer who resonates with love and community approval is one way to be responsible about your own health. However, the freedom to choose therapies one deems most helpful and in accord with personal beliefs is not a constitutional right in this country. The right to practice medicine is deeded by law to the doctoring profession in all states but Oklahoma and comes rife with problems. Herbalists need to take a long, hard look at any call to emulate this same legal structure. The interest in licensing expressed by some in the herbal community stems from three lines of reasoning.

The first situation involves a novice herbalist, fresh from a brief one-weekend-a-month "apprenticeship" program, who sets up shop and declares her certified ability to provide clinical consultation on herbal medicine. Just because such a person says she is an herbalist does not necessarily make her knowledgeable, conscientious, or capable. The same could be said of carpenters, teachers, and candlestick makers. The ease of not taking responsibility or even acknowledging that being an herbalist involves years of training and active engagement with both the plants and people, can be addressed by licensing requirements. One really radical alternative is to expect all people to be knowledgeable, conscientious, and capable. The ethic of personal responsibility covers solid ground.

"I am not in favor of licensing herbalists because of what has happened with midwives and the home birth movement," says Tina Finneyfrock, a community herbalist in central New York. "Licensing does not ensure good care or devoted practitioners. Still, for every good and knowledgeable herbalist, there are four not yet ready. Some with their hearts in the right place but not

*The only way to prevent quackery is to diffuse a knowledge of medicine among the people, and also to point out to them the proper course to pursue to prevent being sick.*

—Benjamin Colby, *A Guide to Health,* 1848

knowledgeable enough; and then some who are opportunists."

Faye Burtch, an herbal healer and licensed massage therapist in State College, Pennsylvania, heartily believes in the regulation of massage therapy, but licensing herbalists is another matter in her eyes. "You can do a lot with muscle, but if you don't have proper training in anatomy and physiology, improper manipulation can cause greater damage. People need to understand the limits of their knowledge. But if herbalists try to regulate each other on the basis of formal education, we'll stop good people already practicing in their communities." Faye points out that mainstream medicine is in intellectual hands, and that denying tradition will take away the good plant medicines now available to all. "People should study for years before they announce to the world that they are now herbalists. Spend five to ten years helping your family and friends, then hang your shingle. Start too early and you can give herbalism a bad name."

The advantages granted medical professionalism are tempting. By restricting the practice of the unqualified, those who do meet minimum educational, clinical, and testing requirements are left with a greater portion of the health care marketplace. Thomas Preston, M.D., captured this sentiment well in a revealing book called *The Clay Pedestal:* "Doctors, who are as honest as any other professional group, indulge in unconscionable self-enrichment, however it may be rationalized as supporting the best medical system in the world."[23]

More to the point, qualifying herbalists would receive a noticeable boost of approval from a public accustomed to having the government decide who can be professionally responsible for individual health care needs. Licensure would need to be granted by state legislatures on the basis of protecting the consumer, for otherwise government cannot activate its acknowledged right to protect the health, safety, and welfare of the people. The days of struggle to make a successful living as an herbalist might become less of a struggle. Understandably some see possibility here, not by cornering the market, but by simply being allowed in the door. Joyce Wardwell in Michigan thinks the only way herbalists will get societal recognition is through licensing. "Perhaps I feel this way because of the legal climate in my state," Joyce says. "I spend a lot of time explaining to people that I am not telling them what to do, but just sharing information. I tread very lightly." Being ordained as legitimate by licensing invites any qualified herbalist to open a community-based consulting practice with far less fear of medical inquisition.

Yet we need to understand how professionalism really changes healing custom. Milton Friedman and others have noted that after licensure the practice of medicine becomes resistant to change and innovation. Prices rise quite high. And, most telling, the level of competence is not greater than before licensure.[24] "Licensure advocates can fail to distinguish between attendance in classes totaling a certain number of hours in certain subjects and a true and deep grasp of the herbal vocation," adds herbalist Stephen Buhner. "Quantity is not quality, never has been, never will be. Some physicians are living proof of this." Stephen, the grandson of a former United States Surgeon General, sees the dynamics reported above already at work in the short history of licensed massage, psychotherapy, and midwifery. Herbalism, with its rich history of diversity and indigenous tradition, is likely to change under licensure into one primary form that could never reflect its total essence. That prognosis may well be grim.

Last, on a very practical note, professional licensure would enable herbalists to receive health insurance reimbursement. Many people see insurance as their financial means to health care, thus clearing any hesitation about being able to pay qualifying herbalists or doctors. Insurance companies would then be vested in defining which herbal therapies are deemed rational. All herbal pharmaceuticals covered would certainly be standardized in accordance with proven purpose. Such lab-sanctioned drugs are much more profitable than plants that anyone (gasp!) can harvest for homegrown (gasp!) healing intent. Worthy goals do get changed by the means of obtaining them. The whole concept of insurance for disproportionately priced health care will get more scrutiny later in this book.

We each pick and choose among—or reject—these rationales in our desire for mainstream acceptance of herbalism. Thomas Jefferson proposed that the original Bill of Rights guarantee the right to choose any kind of medical treatment an individual wished. The Founding Fathers missed the boat on this one. *The pursuit of life, liberty, and holistic healing* offers a shining alternative to a licensing framework for medical practice. King Henry VIII signed a proclamation (which stands as English law to this day) allowing people to practice any kind of medicine they wanted in Great Britain. The onus lies with the people to decide for themselves who is a fitting health care provider.

A significant number of practicing herbalists consider certification by a self-regulating body to be a far better alternative to government licensure. The American Herbalists Guild (AHG) seeks to achieve the legal right for herbalists to practice without the risk of being charged with practicing medicine without a license. Professional members of the Guild currently use the title "Herbalist, AHG" (or simply AHG for short) after their names. This title represents the approval of the only peer-reviewed professional organization for clinical and traditional herbalists in the United States. The criteria for professional membership includes a working knowledge of at least 150 plants, a theoretical foundation in therapeutics, a system of differential diagnosis, and training in the basic sciences of anatomy, physiology, and pathology. Applicants list their training, clinical experience, and motivations for seeking professional membership. Essay questions delve into treatment protocols for numerous conditions such as rheumatoid arthritis and hypothyroidism. Three letters of recommendation from recognized clinical herbalists and other licensed health professionals (with acceptable herbal qualifications) are required.

Aviva Romm serves as executive director for the American Herbalists Guild: "We don't want to create a hierarchy in the herbal community where people who are in the Guild or meet a certain standard or credential are the only ones licensed and legal.

# THE HERBALIST'S CHARTER OF KING HENRY VIII

*An Act That Persons, Being No Common Surgeons, May Administer Outward Medicines*

Bᴇ ɪᴛ ᴏʀᴅᴀɪɴᴇᴅ, established, and enacted, by Authority of this present Parliament, That at all Time from henceforth it shall be lawful to every Person being the King's subject, having Knowledge and Experience of the Nature of Herbs, Roots, and Waters, or of the Operation of the same, by Speculation or Practice, within any part of the Realm of England, or within any other of the King's Dominions, to practice, use, and minister in and to any Outward Gore, Uncome Wound, Apostemations, Outward Swelling or Disease, any Herb or Herbs, Oyntments, Baths, Pultes, and Amplasters, according to their Cunning, Experience, and Knowledge in any of the Diseases, Sores, and Maladies before said, . . . without suit, vexation, trouble, penalty, or loss of their goods; the foresaid Statute in the foresaid Third Year of the King's most gracious Reign, or any other Act, Ordinance, or Statute to the contrary heretofore made in anywise, notwithstanding.

---

Others, such as Rosemary Gladstar, Susun Weed, or Jeannine Parvati—who are brilliant at what they do, but don't want to be affiliated with that type of thinking—would be excluded. Anything that passes on a legal level has to be totally inclusive." The Guild has taken a formal stand that it will not support any regulation that creates exclusivity for herbalists. Jeopardizing the freedom of anybody who doesn't want to be licensed is not an AHG goal.

"We are creating standards for someone who wants to practice in a hospital or a doctor's office," says Aviva, "or for someone who wants to get insurance reimbursement for their clients. There are herbalists who really want to interface with the medical community and not just do backwoods/community herbalism. That is where the Guild is coming from, to create some kind of understandable framework that institutions can recognize to bring herbalism into those institutions but still maintain the grassroots integrity of herbal medicine."

That is not an easy thing to do. The debate goes back and forth constantly. The standards being set establish solely what makes an AHG herbalist. A recent proposal for a two-tiered system of membership in the Guild would recognize a national registry for applicants who have met the Guild's education guidelines and completed a core competency test. "Registered Herbalist" would be trademarked for such members. These herbalists would then be eligible to sit for the certification exam being developed with the Botanical Medicine Academy (BMA). Board certification within the BMA and a proposed registered trademark of "Certified Clinical Herbalist" would then be conferred. Behind all of this lies recognition for certain educational paths and therapeutic choices that not all practitioners will consider to be the only options. Other herbalists can be just as good, kind-hearted, and knowledgeable without any guild designation behind their names.

"There has always been a place in all cultures and times for folk practitioners and those who practice outside the established practice of their day," says Missouri herbalist Bob Liebert. "This is where many important discoveries and new modes of healing have occurred. In shamanic cultures it is the individual who steps outside the norm of daily life into the spiritual realm to discover the new and powerful. Here in the Ozarks there have been several cases of the authorities trying to crack down on 'yarb doctors,' only to have the whole community show up at the trial and hound the authorities into backing off. Something like the American Herbalists Guild can be good as long as they continue to consider the tried-and-true experience of the local community herbalist as being as valuable as courses offered in a naturopathic college taken by someone who would have no idea what a plant even looks like."

"We need to be respectful of our craft," says Deb Soule of Avena Institute in Maine. "Lay midwives, and they aren't licensed, have organized very well state by state. Some of them have gone to school, others have apprenticed. Herbalists need their own integrity too." Networking with other herbalists within one's bioregion certainly expands healing horizons and brings treatment protocols into the light of divergent opinion. Yet the crux of the matter remains who approves who? Open membership organizations create the opportunity to dialogue and learn from each other but don't satisfy those who feel the need to establish base criteria to belong. A professional organization such as the American Herbalists Guild can be promoted to expand livelihood prospects for its members.

There is room for both approaches as long as we don't confuse professionalism with expertise. Opening up medicine to all holistic healers so people can choose should remain the one overarching goal. The AHG was established in 1989 to grab the licensing bull by the horns. Standards based upon peer review are a worthy alternative to the legislation of professional mores. Community herbalism can thrive in its own right as well, encouraged and celebrated by all of us who choose an Earth-centered path toward well-being.

And what if mandatory licensure happens? "Most people I know that are true herbalists are generally anarchists," concludes Mimi Kamp, an artist/botanist/ healer in Naco, Arizona. "And so herbalism will go underground. People who want this type of healing will find us."

"I'm not so bothered about the whole legal, political issue anymore," adds Rosemary Gladstar. "Things gain strength underground. We have to have a tremendous trust in the larger cycles of life. Herbalism became almost illegal to practice from the 1940s on, yet here we are again. Stronger and clearer and more revolutionary."

## Standardization

Philosophy enters deeply into the debate on standardizing herbal preparations. People oriented toward a scientific point of view feel the need to quantify healing possibilities by knowing the concentration of the chosen active principle (constituent) used to achieve results. Others view synergy and spirit as working in ways not fully understood but certainly observed with whole plant remedies that embrace healing, often in more ways than one.

Standardization generally refers to chemical extraction of the constituent deemed to be active. Two assumptions come immediately to the fore. Does one ingredient alone reflect the curative power in a given plant medicine? And does this ingredient become more potent in a concentrated extract than in the whole herb itself? Few herbs are actually standardized to a relatively pure isolate. Turmeric standardized to 95 percent curcumin has been manipulated to up the normal ante of 3 to 4 percent of this spice constituent. Other popular standardized herbs include milk thistle with 80 percent silymarin, ginkgo with 24 percent flavoglycosides, saw palmetto with 90 percent free fatty acids, kava kava with 40 percent

kavalactones, and grape seed with 95 percent polyphenols. A single constituent is usually present under 12 percent in nature.[25] A strong solvent (such as hexane, methyl chloride, acetone, or benzene) with an affinity for the designated constituent is used to achieve the desired concentration, often in conjunction with a different solvent to precipitate out constituents deemed to be superfluous. Under such a regime, the complicated interactive chemistries of such herbs are destroyed. The valid medicinal use remaining accepts both the limits of the concentrated isolate and the possibility of side effects. Such phytopharmaceuticals are more akin to allopathic drugs than the original whole plant remedy.

A subtler form of standardization is admittedly more benign. Lab technicians check to ensure that targeted constituent levels (usually based on the upper end of naturally occurring percentages) of an herb product are achieved. High-performance liquid chromatography, or HPLC, is used to ascertain the consistency of a marker ingredient in each batch. That marker may be the deemed active constituent or possibly another constituent unique to the herb. Hypericin in St. John's wort, for instance, naturally reaches a 0.3 to 0.5 percent level in this herb. An assumption is made that a standardized extract of St. John's wort with 0.5 percent hypericin reflects a better-quality preparation. Plants vary, of course, as does each growing season, each soil, and the exposure of the sun at each growing site. We hasten to add that each person taking a given herb remedy varies considerably as well. This kind of testing helps a consumer concerned that a commercial product indeed contains the listed herb, but that's about it. An herbal extract testing low may be mixed with a batch of the same herb that has an especially high marker to achieve the stated consistency. Or it may be sold down the line to a large company that does not promote standardization or local herb connections.

Whole herbs come with life force intact. The subtle constituent balance herbalists have trusted for millennia is put in arrears in a standardization process that focuses on a single isolate. Such borderline pharmaceuticals have the potential to give herbs a bad name through misapprehended side effects or just inactivity. A good example is salicylic acid, chemically extracted from willow bark to make aspirin. This ubiquitous drug has been found to have side effects in some people, including internal bleeding, leaky gut syndrome, and in some instances, death. Herbal preparations of willow help reduce pain without this concentrated risk. The wide-ranging benefits that make up the gestalt of the whole herb are lost in a narrow science that promotes plant medicine only if it is guaranteed by laboratory technique.

"It is nevertheless true, with most gentle phytopharmaceuticals, that there is no standardized active principle that solely or largely determines the drug action. The gentle phytopharmaceuticals demonstrate in particular that with plant remedies one very often has a comprehensive complex of active principles, with individual components interacting with others, so that only the complex as a whole will produce the therapeutic action." So begins Rudolf Fritz Weiss, M.D., in his highly respected book, *Herbal Medicine*, originally written to explain the relevancy of plant remedies in clinical medical practice.[26] Learning to take medicinal plants for what they are, rather than seeking to isolate pure constituents, challenges the reductionist basis of the scientific process. Proofs run far simpler when synergy does not need to be accounted for. Synergy refers to the actions of two or more substances to achieve an effect of which each is individually incapable. The notion that we need to standardize herbal preparations to achieve specified therapeutic effects essentially scoffs at the notion that herbal potency lies in synergistic alchemy. Science does not yet have a way to assess synergy. Concentrating the levels of so-called active constituents in an herbal remedy allows science to proceed.

But let's go for the jugular here. Herbal medicine has been called the medicine of the people precisely because the plants and the traditional knowledge of how to use them are accessible to rich and poor alike. The assertion that quality lies in a standardized preparation breaks the essential link of every person to plants that heal. How can a home herbalist possibly guarantee the concentration of hypericin in St. John's wort, for instance, at 0.5 percent by volume?[27]

The marketing hype spread by some companies that standardized extracts are "safer and more effective" is untrue. "Claims for the clinical superiority of standardized products are unethical commercialism and an attempt to dupe the public in the name of science," says Northwest herbalist Jonathan Treasure. "The starting quality of the herb used in the extraction process is far more relevant to quality of the final product than any laboratory manipulation or 'correction' during manufacture. Many companies offering standardized product start with crude herb purchased by third-party brokers in the international marketplace, the provenance and quality of which is inevitably beyond their direct control. The adage, garbage in, garbage out, is pertinent."[28]

As an example, no one chemical or chemical group has been found to be solely responsible for echinacea's ability to stimulate the immune system. "Measuring the quality of an echinacea preparation based on total phenolic compounds is like judging the quality of an automobile based on its iron content," according to Rudolf Bauer, professor of pharmaceutical biology at Heinrich Heine University in Düsseldorf, Germany. Manufacturers generally standardize echinacea products to either echinacoside, phenolic acids, or alkylamides. *E. purpurea* does not contain the echinacoside (stated as having mildly antibacterial action in a 1950 study) found in *E. angustifolia* and other species, so the "standard" switched more recently to total phenolic compounds.[29] Phenols are a large group of compounds, not all of which have an isolated medical use. The concentration of any and all phenols in a standardized extract of echinacea assumes an across-the-board approach to biological activity. That numbing sensation on your tongue when you take an echinacea tincture can be attributed to the alkylamides, some of which have been shown to be immunostimulatory. Yet the debate over which chemical standard best defines the potency of echinacea has one outstanding resolution: Put your trust in the whole plant remedy.

Jean's Greens in Norway, New York, combines the whole unprocessed herb with an extracted version of itself. Milk thistle, saw palmetto, Siberian ginseng, and kava kava are offered as herbal dietary supplement capsules featuring the favored constituent of the day. The inference that science somehow makes herbal medicine more potent can be hard to dispute when the public is bombarded by standardization logic. Reductionist thinking carries the day

in modern culture. Perhaps combining the two—making the case for whole plant remedies as well as active constituent levels—reaches some of the people some of the time. Clever marketing helps if it pricks public consciousness into comprehending the whole truth.

We end this discussion with just a few more unstandardized salvos. "Herbalism is about holistic healing, about Gaia," says Mimi Kamp. "Squeezing our plants into isolated elements is not herbalism." "A standardized extract," says Joyce Wardwell, "is a poor substitute for a complex interaction and vitality found in whole herb preparations, especially if people further empower themselves by gathering their own medicine. But then I prefer driving a whole car rather than sitting astride a running engine." Southwest herbalist Michael Moore sums this all up with characteristic clarity: "The active principle is the whole plant."

### Food and Drug Administration

Getting a proper handle on the U.S. Food and Drug Administration—its mission, its purpose, its worth—requires some perspective across the board. This government agency is charged with regulating many of the substances that people eat, drink, or otherwise consume. "Are herbs food or drugs?" has always been the big question for the FDA in determining a regulatory approach to herbal medicine. The Dietary Supplement Health and Education Act passed by Congress in 1994 settled the argument by calling herbs food supplements. Most herbs can be sold in the United States, and no exacting guidelines exist regarding what manufacturing process must be used to make a product. The rub lies in making specific health claims for an herb or herbal remedy on the packaging label.

That specificity brings us to two contrary views for encouraging herb use. The herb supplement industry works to push the bounds of labeling allowance. The claim that an over-the-counter remedy can *promotes regularity* passes muster, while declaring that a product *alleviates constipation* is language reserved for approved drugs. The American Herbal Products Association provides an infrastructure for the herb industry to negotiate with the FDA about proper adherence to good manufacturing practices, compliance with honest labeling and advertising practices, and the acknowledgment of how herbs can be used. More than a third of Americans currently take a dietary supplement of one kind or another. Business is booming and money is being made. Regulatory oversight seems fitting here. However, promoting specific herb use on the pill bottle's label removes people from a holistic understanding of how a plant medicine might best serve them.

Community herbalism is more about a direct relationship between people and plants. Health claims for a particular herb don't need to be made as much as shared among families. Earth-centered livelihoods exist quite nicely within the current latitude granted to the direct sale of herbs. We can sell any herb we grow. Tinctures and formulations can be offered within the circle of community. Brewing tea is a high and vital right.

Regulatory presence can and does protect people from egregious mishandling of the foods we eat and limits the number of unsafe pharmaceutical drugs available.[30] And yet the FDA does not require genetically engineered foods to be tested or specially labeled. The stretching of this variable mind-set into herbal medicine often seems controversial, as we shall see below. Ultimately, personal responsibility and trust based on intimacy protect the herbal product user far better than centralized oversight. Used as a tool in the name of safety, regulation can spell the end for the little guy. We have seen this happen in agriculture with the closing of small local dairies, farm butchering operations, and cider mills, made unprofitable by the mandatory rules aimed at much larger operations. Neighborhood apothecaries and herbalists currently have leeway to make products and market them locally. What now seems to be frustrating FDA interference may one day be seen as the good old days if the herb industry works adroitly to close loose gaps. *Small is beautiful* is our idea of a good regulation.

Let's consider the case of comfrey. Comfrey is on the FDA's list of dangerously toxic herbs to avoid for internal use. Pyrrolizidine alkaloids were first isolated in this common plant by a Japanese scientist in 1968. Because these alkaloids are linked to certain cancers and cause liver damage, government bodies felt compelled to act. Practically overnight comfrey went from being a tried-and-true herb to being considered hepatoxic. But in the eyes of herbalists long respectful of *Symphytum officinale* (the genus name comes from the Latin word meaning "to heal") it remains a proven medicine. Taken internally, comfrey is prized for its demulcent, nutritive, expectorant, and hepatonic properties. Externally, it is an extraordinary wound healer. Pennsylvania herbalist Faye Burtch bristles when asked about the government's dangerous drug classification for internal use of comfrey: "The FDA concentrated on one chemical constituent of that plant. Of course it will be toxic when given to an animal in a concentrated form. The whole plant has a balance which an experienced herbalist can use safely. No one takes a whole bottle of aspirin for a headache or mainlines a chemical constituent of a single plant."

Everything we've been told about "killer comfrey" in the mainstream media has been misguided. The *Journal of American Medicine* conducted a worldwide search and found only three possible cases (out of millions of people using comfrey) who developed liver problems that may have been related to excessive comfrey consumption.[31] "Putting this in perspective," says medical herbalist David Hoffmann, "we see 10,000 people have died in the United States from nonsteroidal anti-inflammatory drugs taken in conjunction with kidney disease. Yet these other drugs are shown to be 'safe' biochemically." The risk analysis on which such FDA assessments are based reflects a belief in the efficacy of pharmaceuticals on the one hand and a doubting Thomas approach to herbs on the other. If the pharmaceutical industry were subject to the same scrutiny now demanded of herbs, no drugs would be on the market at all. In Japan, where the controversy began, comfrey continues to be the recommended treatment for cirrhosis of the liver. Some herbalists here now suggest a more judicious approach to internal use, in moderate amounts and not for more than two one-week periods per year.[32] Some herbal apothecaries, already nervous over compliance with FDA labeling laws, voluntarily keep such controversial herbs off their shelves rather than risk lawsuits. The ripple effects from government agency decrees do reach us in various ways. Perhaps comfrey will help heal herbalism in the end. The legal risk of selling symphytum products for internal use will leave no alternative but

to encourage people to grow this powerful herb for themselves. The bill of fare will continue to be local plants for local people.

"Every state is different," Jean Argus points out, "depending on the FDA agents in your area." A business with gross volume under $250,000 usually won't receive inspection unless a complaint is lodged. Jean's Greens got inspected during the plantain recall in the mid-1990s. A shipment of plantain leaf bound from Hungary to Germany and eventually to the United States turned out to be heart-stopping digitalis. "An inspector came unannounced, flashing her badge, all suited up in high heels. She wrote down everything that was said, never looking at the herbs. Then came the report, requiring my signature. I didn't want to sign without certain corrections." More meetings followed, and as Jean and the inspector got to know each other, a rapport developed. "Our dialogue became a friendly exchange. She let me know what her bosses would look closest at, that the biggest concern was with making health claims in our literature. After that I began calling everything an *herbal dietary supplement*. And while the 'cancer' word is still in our literature, I'm careful not to put it on any product."

The last time the FDA came to Jean's Greens was to oversee the destruction of a batch of Easy Transition Tea. Safrole, an essential oil distilled from sassafras, had proved cancerous in laboratory animals given large doses. Sassafras roots have been the target of a government purge ever since. Soft drink manufacturers stopped using sassafras in traditional root beer by 1960, substituting artificial flavors. Part of an Appalachian healing tradition, when applied externally, this root serves as a salve for skin problems, and taken as a tea it can be used to bring on sweats and cleanse colds and flus at an early stage. "There was no point in my telling them oil of sassafras is not soluble in water, and therefore, those lab tests don't apply to a tea infusion," Jean laments. She offered to compost the tea, but—given that the FDA boss had no idea what composting was— concern would have lingered that the sassafras tea would somehow have been reused. Those herbalists can be so tricky! The bureaucratic ruling on this venerable root still stands: Sassafras products must be labeled "for external use only."

"Them yerbs, they ain't goin' hurt you, even if they don't do no good. But those FDA drugs, they'll hurt you more often than they'll help. But I'm not in the business for the money. I'm in it to help people," said Alabama herbalist Tommie Bass back in the 1980s.[33] A passel of politics and economic interests gets wrapped up in a governmental effort to regulate our food and drugs. The FDA serves a good purpose on occasion, but when the dust finally settles, we pray it won't fall on the plants now growing humbly alongside this particular regulatory road.

## Sustainable Demand

"I wish herbs were not used incorrectly, that people understood what exactly each herb can do. It's like electricity: We think we have plenty so we waste so much of it. Ours is a commodity-oriented culture, sucking up everything it can. No one wants to change their lifestyle," observes Don Babineau, the craftsman behind the Woodland Essence homestead in upstate New York. "Take goldenseal, for example. Ninety percent of the 35,000 pounds harvested each year gets used incorrectly. It's in so many formulas

that it doesn't need to be. Ginseng is the same."

"More and more people want good health, but how many are willing to change their lifestyle?" asks herbal partner Kate Gilday, echoing the heart of the issue. "Magic happens when we start respecting herbs and our own bodies."

Many people walk this planet today. A culture conscious of its earthly roots perhaps would not have the problems we do. Herbs processed into bottles are a product to be consumed, not a plant to be revered and honored. Well-being magazines promote natural health; advertising stirs further interest. Rumor has it that goldenseal will mask drug use on a drug detection test— absolutely false!—and be of use with viral infections. We have a friend who regularly puts echinacea tincture in her morning cup of coffee. The message has gotten through about boosting the immune system, but not the how and why of it. The popularity of wild plants such as black cohosh, lomatium, and lady's slipper endanger a fragility that won't support market interest for long. Widely touted herbs put into so-called nutraceutical drinks and foods are there more for name recognition than for any useful therapeutic effect.

Public willingness to accept the gifts of herbal healing is growing. We now need to blow away the advertising chaff and recognize the seeds of possibility given to our culture to plant and nourish. We will talk much in the pages ahead about organic cultivation and ethical wildcrafting. Eco-herbalism encompasses the big picture view of walking in balance on this beautiful planet. We applaud the good work of United Plant Savers (UpS) (see page 307) and others in addressing the serious loss of plant habitat. Answers to big questions are indeed coming. Our path to sustainability will fall short, however, if we fail to distinguish between those times when we truly need to call upon an herbal remedy and more frivolous occasions.

Could you pass the ginseng chips now, please?

## MEANWHILE, BACK IN OUR COMMUNITIES . . .

Learning to live locally will provide answers to most of our outstanding ecological and social crises. Gentle plant medicines certainly can be available at low cost. What's needed are knowledgeable herbalists who can help bring the vital relationship between people and plants to the fore. We have lost the Earth-centered heritage that once flowed between generations and within families. The herbs have become a seemingly inaccessible mystery rather than the ready gift intended. The healing dynamic between people and plants will be reclaimed as we come to understand healthy lifestyles for both ourselves and Earth. This reclamation will come on the individual level, one-to-one, in ways that touch souls for the good. Healers have their work cut out for them in many ways. *A home herbalist in every family and a practicing herbalist in every community* is a vision worth underscoring.

We believe in local herbalists using local herbs to help local people achieve good health. Community herbalists support their neighbors with everything from traditional flu remedies to a gentle prodding toward a holistic lifestyle. They teach home herbalists how to use plants as both food and medicine for their families. The community herbalist may be found keeping a ready supply of tinctures, tea herbs, and roots on hand, often growing or wildcrafting the desired plant medicines themselves. Local economic connections are cultivated with regional growers to assure a sustainable and truly healing agriculture. Helping out can be as simple as taking time to listen and bringing by a warm loaf of whole grain bread in stressful times. In-depth herbal knowledge—what we call medicine—is enhanced by a glad flow of love and concern for the individual.

"We encourage the kind of networking that helps people to heal themselves," says Maine community herbalist Deb Soule. "Our services are provided through an apothecary, often set up in our homes, where plant medicines are made available. We work as both educators and consultants, or at least as a resource to other health care providers. Doctors have been set up to [supposedly] know everything. Herbalists come in with knowledge of food and holistic nutrition. . . . And this comes back to our role as educators: helping people understand how to eat, how to rest in the winter, how to work at something they enjoy.

"I think of a community herbalist being there to serve the community from birth when the babies are first born until death. We bring valuable information and experience to people to help them in healing ways in all aspects of their lives. Community herbalism is much more than having a practice," says Kate Gilday of Woodland Essence. "It is very multidimensional. It can feel like you are wearing a lot of different hats, but it has this common thread running through it—to be really healthy and be able to give. . . . Honoring the Earth, and honoring the plants themselves: My calling is to

*Text continues on page 36.*

# Aviva Romm

I BELIEVE EVERYBODY can be an herbalist and a midwife," asserts Aviva Romm. "My perception of midwifery and herbalism has always been that it is really a people's medicine. Everyone can do it. During exceptional times when it gets beyond your skill level or what you are comfortable with, when something is truly complicated, then, yes, you seek help from someone who is more experienced. Teaching people how to do home health care is my main goal. Even with pregnancy, I try to get the point across that I (as the midwife) am not doing someone else's birth. Prenatal care is not just what they get from me; prenatal care is what they give to themselves."

Aviva now practices as an herbalist and midwife near Atlanta, Georgia. She wears many other hats as a mother of four home-schooled children, a wife, and the author of four books. She offers regular clinic hours in an office at her home. "My practice is very integrated. I do things that stretch into other realms: working with an HIV patient with a chronic cough or a man with prostate problems, though that's more of an idiosyncratic client for me.

Most of my practice is moms and kids. I will also work with a dad if he has something going on during the course of a pregnancy." People often start out in a primary relationship with Aviva as their midwife and then she ends up doing extended family care, sometimes for years. "This enriches my practice in every way. People learn how to use herbs for health, nutrition, and healing once I start out helping them with their birth."

Her determined views on the accessibility of good health care accentuate a deep vein of thoughtfulness and genuine caring. Aviva speaks from the heart while encompassing the broad picture of herbalism in America today. "Some people ask me how much of my practice is midwifery and how much of it is herbs. I don't really separate the two. I do approach my care as a practitioner as a midwife. An herbalist can practice just like any allopathic doctor—I say that knowing there are some very heartfelt allopathic doctors out there, and many, many holistic herbalists. But it's pretty hard to be a midwife and not practice as a midwife. The midwifery model honors the integrity of the client and is

educational. I enter into a relationship with my clients rather than require power over them. I bring that to my care as an herbalist. So it doesn't matter if I am treating some man for prostate trouble, or some woman well out of her childbearing years who has high blood pressure and constipation, that may have nothing to do with obstetrics and gynecology or children's health. My approach is still that of a midwife. I am there with that person to honor their space. It's not so much which herbs you use, but how you use them."

Aviva enters daily the debate over licensure of herbalists on behalf of the American Herbalists Guild. "Anytime anything becomes more popular it becomes a little bit trivialized. Fifteen or twenty years ago the people who were becoming herbalists were the people living on the land, and herbal medicine was part of a way of life. Many of us were hippies and political activists, listening to reggae and growing organic food. Some of the people coming into it now see herbalism solely as a way to make a living—it isn't a way of life for them. They think, 'Oh, there is big money in herbal medicine. I am going to go to six months of weekend workshops and set myself up as a medical herbalist.' They don't realize being a community herbalist and dealing with issues that are in the realm of their experience must come first. Many of us in the Guild have come to see the value of a standard if someone is going to put themselves out there as a clinical herbalist.

"I definitely am a total grassroots, rebellious, radical midwife/herbalist. The etymology of *radical* means "root," so to me I have a root practice. I have no problem saying that I do primary care and

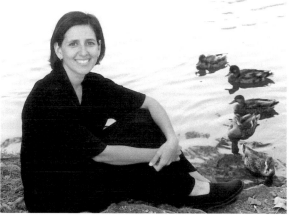

all kinds of things that we are not supposed to say we do, because I do them. Why should someone have to go to the doctor if they don't want to just because an herbalist is not supposed to do something? I have no problem taking stitches out of somebody's wound if they are ready to come out." Not surprisingly, this self-educated and apprenticed midwife practiced outside the law for more than a decade in Georgia, where attending home births as a direct-entry midwife is not yet clearly

legal. People who push the edges of a system slanted toward professional exclusivity help make health care an affordable human right.

"I have had good relationships with obstetricians and family physicians wherever I have practiced. I have been very fortunate in this way. It does help to speak the language. I think for herbalists, if they are going to practice in a medical realm, it helps to have enough knowledge to look competent in that realm." Aviva does

*My perception of midwifery and herbalism has always been that it is really a people's medicine.*
—AVIVA ROMM

understand medical concepts and terminology that are sometimes intimidating to others. Her goal as a writer is to make accessible what the medical profession makes inaccessible through jargon. *Natural Healing for Babies and Children* and *The Natural Pregnancy Book* are indispensable reading for parents and parents-to-be looking for a graceful understanding of early family health.

"My basic approach to my midwifery practice is that birth works. Pregnancy works. Our

bodies know how to do it. I don't see the need for women to take tons of herbs during their pregnancy, any more than I think they should be taking anything else during pregnancy. I don't usually recommend many herbs during the first trimester, unless they are having a lot of discomfort or nausea that they just can't cope with. I will recommend some of the nutritive herbs in the second trimester, just something like a simple tea with raspberry, nettles, oat straw, and maybe red clover. Then, if somebody does have health problems, I will not hesitate to use any number of botanical remedies that are appropriate for them. It is interwoven, but it is not automatic. Just because someone comes to see me, it is not a given that they are going to walk out with gobs of herbs."

Mother, healer, woman—Aviva thrives on being a midwife/herbalist: "I just love working with people and watching them blossom with empowerment to take care of their own health or birth their babies. I have the opportunity to see so many different people from so many walks of life. The way they live their lives and their philosophies gives me a broad exposure to human beings. There is a tremendous satisfaction in watching somebody accomplish something and knowing I had a part in their happiness and healing." ℘

bring plants and people together in whatever ways, whether it's a walk, or talking about something, or teaching."

We all have healing abilities that go hand in hand with being human. The majority of our greatest needs cannot be met with professionalism and technology. Times do come when we might need a doctor, when an invasive medical procedure is an individual's best choice on the road to recovery. Yet accepting the high-end system of medicine does not mean we need to ditch traditional roles and Earth-centered understanding. True health flows from loving relationships, good food, time spent in Nature, daily hugs, inner peace, meaningful work, and breathing thankfully of the richness of this life. Community herbalists can help reestablish these vital connections. And, when illness comes, these are the people who help reveal the healing bounty offered by the plants growing outside our doors.

Years of experience and training for the herbalist usually precede any consulting practice where individuals in the community at large come to seek out specific health advice for chronic ailments and degenerative disease. Herbalists can gain their initial education in an accredited program or by a more folkloric route. Traditional healing wisdom can prove as valid as certified medical training. Ultimately, it is the direct experience of helping people cope with all manner of dis-ease and observing how the plants facilitate healing—again and again— that establishes the abilities that count. The setting in which you direct these abilities often determines how you choose to describe yourself as an herbalist.

Traditionally minded herbalists like the word *herbalist* to capture the whole of this sensitive "who's who" discussion. We will each discover tiers of knowledge and practical experience throughout our lives. The herbal path is more a continuous journey than an achieved destination. Our real import will always lie with our ability to help people, not with the verbal designation we each think fits best.

"I use the term 'practicing herbalist,'" says Margi Flint in describing her take on the name game. "That feels really honest to me. There is something really humbling about realizing we are always just practicing. My herbal path is like a big swell in the ocean. I get to a point where I'm really gliding along and then I hit a point where I'm learning continuously. Then comes that point at the top of the swell and I fall off! You need to be constantly reminded about what you don't know." Margi's experience in teaching herbal medicine at Tufts Medical School (see page 134) and working with doctors gives her reason to make a point about one of the terms on our list. "I think if you say you are a medical herbalist, you really should have an M.D."

"When people say they are folkloric herbalists, they don't tend to incorporate medical jargon into their practice. They are more apt to say 'this is what the grandmothers did, this is what people did traditionally,'" says midwife/herbalist Aviva Romm. Perhaps you have a boil. Tradition points to a plantain, chickweed, or burdock poultice to help. A clinical herbalist might recommend exactly the same thing. The difference lies in the setting and more often the approach. "The one will say, 'Come over for tea, we'll talk about your boil.' The clinical herbalist sees people on a regular basis in their office," points out Aviva, "kind of like a family physician. Now you have someone who says, 'Come into my office. I have this training to evaluate your condition.' She may even lance the boil and drain it for you."

All herbalists ultimately serve their communities and complement medical physicians. Just getting people to realize we each have responsibility for our own health is a big step. "Anyone can learn to keep himself relatively healthy most of the time and to recognize and correct most deviations from health without consulting professional practitioners, whether orthodox or

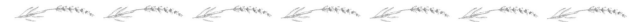

# COMING TO TERMS WITH OUR HERBAL ABILITIES

QUANDARIES ABOUND with the words herbalists choose to define themselves. The suggestions here provide a shared framework for us to offer as an herbal community. Just because one person uses the term one way does not mean that someone else understands it the same way. The call for professional standards stems from experienced practitioners, who want novice herbalists to understand better what we should be when we make our claims to the world at large. There are no ratings in all this, just slants to what we each do.

**Certified herbalist:** After completing a two-week course, or a seven-month intensive, or a degree program in herbalism, one receives a certificate. Quite frankly, any significance given to certification will remain nebulous without a consensual agreement among participating herbalists as to core requirements. Many traditional herbalists will continue

to view certification as one of many paths to herbal knowledge.

**Clinical herbalist:** Those herbalists seeing patients as the mainstay of their herbal practice. Obtaining the skills necessary to discern an individual's overall health and to ascertain which herbs and formulations are needed to help correct disease and imbalance involves years of supervised training. Many community herbalists have clinical experience, though few arrange to see a large number of clients.

**Community herbalist:** Those herbalists serving the community in which they live. Practicing herbalists help neighboring families understand a holistic lifestyle and the everyday use of herbs, offer specific advice about traditional uses of plant remedies, work with other health-care practitioners, grow and wildcraft regional herbs, prepare plant medicines, and teach workshops and course intensives on all aspects of the herbal healing art.

**Folkloric herbalist:** Those herbalists appreciative of empirical tradition and a direct relationship with the plant world.

**Herbalist:** All who use, revere, and share the healing gifts of our green friends.

**Home herbalist:** Anyone using herbs as both food and medicine for their families in their daily lives.

**Medical herbalist:** Those herbalists appreciative of a rational understanding of herbs in a holistic healing context. Many use this term interchangeably with *clinical herbalist.*

**Master herbalist:** A term that best comes from our peers, in recognition of a deep understanding of plants and their profound healing effects on our bodies and psyches. Honoring the master of any craft bestows heartfelt admiration for a lifetime of experienced wisdom. Modesty will always precede true mastery.

unorthodox," says noted author Dr. Andrew Weil. "Most of what I know about keeping myself in good health I did not learn in my training as a medical doctor. I learned it from observation of myself and others, from intuition and thought, and from my own experience."[34] Learning to take responsibility for one's own health begins with viewing healing as an innate capacity of the body. The people available to help—doctors, herbalists, or loving moms—facilitate that healing journey.

## NOTES

1. The average visitation time actually spent with a family physician continues to be pared down as the business agenda of profitable health care carries the day. The need for intimacy and holistic care falls to the wayside in any healing relationship based foremost on monetary considerations. Neither patient nor physician benefits in the ways that matter most in this arrangement.

2. Thomas Preston, M.D., *The Clay Pedestal* (Seattle: Madrona, 1981), 114–15.

3. Norman R. Farnsworth, "Rational approaches to the search for and discovery of new drugs from plants," paper presented at the first Latin-American and Caribbean Symposium on Naturally Occurring Pharmacological Agents, Havana, Cuba, June 23–28, 1980, 7–8.

4. A thrust that's still very much alive for us today in books such as *King's American Dispensatory*. We'll scope out these Eclectic classics in the herbal library section of chapter 3.

5. Juliette de Baïracli Levy, *Herbal Handbook for Farm and Stable* (Emmaus, Pa.: Rodale, 1952, 1976), 19–20.

6. The ajoenes and dithiins are the strongest known blood-thinning constituents of garlic. Thus macerated oils are considered best for stroke or heart attack patients. Consult with a physician if blood-thinning drugs are already in use. Ajoene, not present in significant amounts in raw garlic or in other garlic preparations, is considered to be a potent blood thinner. See Paul Bergner, *The Healing Power of Garlic* (Rocklin, Calif.: Prima Publishing, 1996) for a fascinating in-depth look at both the tradition and science of this wonderful bulb.

7. Michael Tierra, ed., *American Herbalism: Essays on Herbs and Herbalism by Members of the American Herbalists Guild* (Freedom, Calif.: Crossing Press, 1992), 38.

8. Barbara Starfield, M.D., "Is U.S. Health Really the Best in the World?" *Journal of the American Medical Association*, Vol. 284, No. 4 (July 26, 2000), 484.

9. Seven out of ten people with atherosclerotic disease were helped with either pharmaceutical in controlled testing. Clopidrogrel showed slightly more effectiveness in reducing the risk of a major clinical event, particularly for patients with peripheral artery disease and myocardial infarction patients for whom aspirin treatment was contraindicated. See *Medical Sciences Bulletin*, "An Internet-Enhanced Journal of Pharmacology and Therapeutics," http://pharminfo.com/pubs/msb/clopid243.html.

10. David Hoffmann, *An Elder's Herbal* (Rochester, Vt.: Healing Arts Press, 1993), 56.

11. Simon Mills and Kerry Bone, *Principles and Practice of Phytotherapy* (London: Churchill Livingstone, 2000), 199.

12. E. W. McDonagh, D.O., "Vitamins versus Drugs," *Acres USA*, Vol. 30, No. 10 (October 2000), 37.

13. R. M. Hamm, R. J. Hicks, and D. A. Bemben, *Journal of Family Practice*, Vol. 43, No. 1 (July 1996), 56–62.

14. The regular use of antibiotics in raising farm animals contributes greatly to the buildup of resistant strains of bacteria. Humans are ultimately not immune to a cheap food system based on close confinement, contaminated animal feed, and antibiotic-protected tissue growth.

15. Rudolf Fritz Weiss, *Herbal Medicine*, translated from the 6th German edition (Beaconsfield, England: Beaconsfield Publishers, 1988), 1.

16. Dana Ullman, M.P.H., "Don't Suppress Your Symptoms," *Herbs for Health*, Vol. 4, No. 6 (January/February 2000), 74.

17. Andrew Weil, M.D., review comments on *Medicinal Plants of the Desert and Canyon West*, by Michael Moore (Santa Fe: Museum of New Mexico Press, 1989).

18. Macrobiotic nutritionist Alex Jack points out in the October 2000 issue of *Garden Design* magazine that the nutrient values of several vegetables have dropped by as much as half in the past

twenty years. Based on averages for a dozen vegetables checked, calcium levels had fallen by 27 percent, iron by 37 percent, vitamin A by 21 percent, and Vitamin C by 30 percent.

19. Sally Fallon, *Nourishing Traditions* (Washington, D.C.: New Trends, 1999), 23.

20. Kaolin clay, elemental sulfur, and *Bacillus thuringiensis* (a disease organism specific to moth larvae) are commonly used in organic orchards.

21. Paul Bergner, editorial in *Medical Herbalism*, Vol. 9: No. 2 (summer 1997), 4.

22. Annemarie Colbin, *Food and Healing* (New York: Ballantine, 1996), xxv.

23. Preston, *The Clay Pedestal*, 143.

24. Stephen Buhner detailed this information in an appeal to herbalists not to pursue licensure in response to an article appearing in the spring 1997 edition of *Medical Herbalism*. See *Medical Herbalism*, Vol. 9, No. 2 (summer 1997).

25. Bob Brucia, "Standardization," *Herbal Views* (The American Herb Association, Vol. 13, No. 1, 1997), 3.

26. Weiss, *Herbal Medicine*, 1.

27. Hypericin is demonstrably not responsible for the antidepressant effects for which this herb has been standardized. Recent research suggests that another compound, hyperforin, is the most likely candidate for the active antidepressant principle. And this says nothing about the compounds responsible for the many other actions of St. John's wort, which is far more than an herbal antidepressant.

28. Jonathan's Herbal Bookworm Web site is truly a treasure of impassioned opinion on all things herbal. Check out www.pond.net/~herbmed/bookworm.html for book reviews and more. The passage quoted here was taken from the critique "Deconstructing Varro Tyler's *Honest Herbal*."

29. Stephen Foster, "The Latest on Echinacea," *Herbs for Health* Vol. 6, No. 4 (January/February 2000), 8–9.

30. A drug approved by the FDA can still be misused by doctors. An antibiotic prescribed for viral pneumonia won't be of any use. Yet because patients expect and demand treatment, voilà!

31. None of the three cases conclusively point to comfrey as the culprit. In 1984 there was a case of veno-occlusive liver disease in a forty-nine-year-old woman who had been taking comfrey-pepsin tablets for four months. Another woman reportedly drank as many as ten cups of comfrey tea a day and a handful of tablets and developed veno-occlusive liver disease. The third reported case involved a twenty-three-year-old New Zealand man who died of liver failure reportedly due to veno-occlusive liver disease. He was said to have eaten four or five steamed comfrey leaves every day for a week or two before he died. For additional information see Rosemary Gladstar, "The Comfrey Controversy," *Journal of the Northeast Herbal Association* (spring, 1992).

32. Christopher Hobbs, *Herbal Remedies for Dummies* (Foster City, Calif.: IDG Books, 1998), 22.

33. John Crellin and Jane Philpott, *Trying to Give Ease: Tommie Bass and the Story of Herbal Medicine* (Durham, N.C.: Duke University Press, 1989).

34. Andrew Weil, M.D. *Health and Healing* (Boston: Houghton Mifflin, 1983, 1998), 273.

# CHAPTER TWO
# The Gamut of Herbal Possibility

ECHINACEA
*Echinacea purpurea*

Brother-in-law Kevin, a good all-American skeptic, asked me a reasonable question: "Are you an herbalist now? What is an herbalist anyway?" ❧ Well, yes, I am an herbalist. I have always been fond of Rosemary Gladstar's definition: "An herbalist is a person who loves herbs with all their heart and uses them every day for food and medicine. A professional herbalist is just one who does it more and longer." ❧ The power of the plants is vast. "What is an herbalist?" is a big question. People want to know who they can consult as a reliable source of information about herbs and health. The herbs we use for medicine need to come from knowledgeable growers and wildcrafters who gather the right plants at the right time. Our medicines need to be prepared for maximum effectiveness and with maximum love. Passing on herbal wisdom to each other and the next generation is important work. Tending to the spirit touches the very core of what the plants share with us. ❧ People have always picked herbs from the wilds or from their gardens to use them for food or medicine. Nature offers a whole range of medicines to those who know how to use them, from the nurturing tonic herbs to plants capable of stopping hearts in a few moments. ❧ The community herbalist has a firm foundation in the use of locally available herbs. We have experienced the healing power of these herbs firsthand in a variety of situations and can share this knowledge with others. People in our communities gradually seek us out, asking for herbal and health-related advice. Traditionally we are called to help with such common ailments as a colicky baby, morning sickness, and fertility problems. Requests for help come from loved ones suffering from insomnia, urinary tract infection, sore throats, and flu. As *we become more experienced, we educate people to work with more complicated conditions and help clients use herbs to complement other medical treatments. We often train home herbalists to nourish and heal their families. Depending on our passions and gifts, we devote more or less time to one of the many paths of herbalism: consulting, growing, medicine making, running an apothecary, teaching, or spiritual work. We likely do a bit of it all. We are active in our communities. We give introductory talks and conduct herb walks; we build community gardens, start free clinics, and make house calls; we encourage people to start community supported agriculture ventures (CSAs) with farmers; we initiate food co-ops, and organize holistic health fairs. ℘*

*So, Kevin, that's what an herbalist does.* —N.P. ℘

THE GIFTS HERBALISTS have to offer our communities definitely need to be shared—the healing plants lead here by sterling example—and we eventually find ways for our communities to support us in turn. Some herbalists create a working niche in one area; others blend many arenas of talent to find this tenable balance. We never really compete against each other. People are drawn to the right person for their situation, just as the right plant beckons when we listen. The herbal gamut includes us all.

"Some of us really love to help as a practitioner," says Kate Gilday. "We love sitting with people and listening to their stories and suggesting to them changes they can make or herbs that they can take. Some really love to do research, they just really want to zone in and find out all of the chemistry and history of something and then share this knowledge to help others. There are people that are amazing gardeners—their gift is in creating gardens, not only in their own homes, but perhaps working with others to develop urban community gardens, or teaching gardens, in the woods or at libraries. Teaching is a great way to make an impact. So use your skills to reach out to your communities in whatever ways that you feel you can. I love doing a little of this and a little of that."

## THE HERBALIST AS PRACTITIONER

Diagnosing a patient condition and prescribing therapeutic remedies are things no law-abiding herbalist can do. Many speak instead of comparable patient histories and traditional uses of plants in order to assist people seeking herbal advice. Choosing acceptable vernacular indicates that we are not practicing medicine without a physician's license. What we are doing is helping people to feel better.

Why is it that some herbalists' biggest fear is practicing without a license, and others don't even seem to take notice? Consulting lies at the heart of sharing our knowledge about plant medicine and being able to care for individuals in our communities. A healthy respect for authority does not mean we have to abandon this calling.[1] Medical legitimacy, of course, is in the eye of the beholder. Doctors, having obtained the legal right to ordain who can practice medicine, can be expected to guard their lucrative turf. Other health care practitioners tend to step carefully on the sidelines. Integrative medicine might prove ultimately to be one vehicle for opening up the right to practice. Yet the ultimate thrust for practitioner legitimacy lies in citizens being granted the medical right to choose any healer (licensed or not) that suits their personal needs and belief systems. For the practicing herbalist, tolerating legal semantics and not calling attention to the humble art of helping people heal themselves works surprisingly well.

"Herbalists in this country have more freedom than most herbalists do in the rest of the developed world," asserts Rosemary Gladstar. "Things are perfect as they are now. There's a lot of advantages to not being legal. You can't charge a lot, you can't advertise. All the things that make healing a business."

Just as the culture at large needs to embrace individual responsibility, practicing herbalists need to be aware of the great responsibility we owe people who come to our doors. We can't be afraid of what we know—our power lies in trusting this inner knowing—but we also need to acknowledge what we don't know. It's fine to say, "Let me read up on this and discuss it with my colleagues, then I will get back to you." Being able to say *I don't know* is powerful. Integrity flows from such humility. Acknowledging one's own vulnerability is the very best way to acknowledge the same in clients.

Village herbalists connect people to good resources. Directing folks to other practitioners who hold a holistic view of the healing process can be just as vital a service as sharing herbal knowledge. "A layperson is not going to go to medical school," observes Deb Soule, a highly respected teacher of community herbalism in mid-coast Maine. "So it's important to know our limits so we can refer out." Herbalists aren't trained to be primary health care providers. We should encourage a person with really bad chronic headaches, for instance, to rule out the possibility of a more serious condition. Feverfew as a headache remedy won't help if a brain tumor lies behind that migraine.

The journey toward practical application of herbs begins with ourselves. What better body than our own to first explore the wonderful interaction of plant chemistry and spirit? We constantly learn as herbalists from our own sickness and well-being. We probe, we question. Which herbs work better here? What is best for the short term? What is best for the long term? Following a health plan for yourself provides insight into devising therapeutic programs for others. The plants we come to know intimately are sources of medicine we can honor and share. We should never give an herb to anyone if we have not tried it out ourselves, because herbalists serve as an intermediary between plants and people on the basis of direct experience. Memorizing every herb for every situation is not necessary. And yet, over time—be patient and ever so receptive about this—we will know many different uses of plants and will encounter many experiences of human imbalance and recovery.

One of the most healing things we can do for anyone is simply to listen. Being uncritical helps us become better listeners. Many herbalists find getting people to keep a *diet diary* (where everything eaten over the course of a week is revealingly recorded) is most useful in helping them sit up and take notice of unhealthy patterns. In time we develop knowing patterns of our own as we delve into similar conditions again and again. Identifying stress points becomes really important, for instance, whenever dealing with someone who has a chronic problem. We call upon nervine and adaptogen herbs often in addressing degenerative disease. Helping someone improve his diet and embrace bitter tastes generally serves as the kick-off a body needs to heal. Herbalists are needed precisely because we excel at these sorts of things. "What herbal medicine does well, Western medicine is weak in," says David Winston. "And what Western medicine does well, herbal medicine is weak in. We are not competing: We are actually complementing."

Only the Creator and the patient can take credit for the healing process. Our primary role is to maintain a vision of a healthy future for our clients, to cultivate hope and spiritual well-being. Reestablishing a connection to Mother Earth enables people to breathe in her peace as they let go of past pain. More often than not the plants become guides for this journey to the source. Botanical remedies are but one aspect of the power inherent in herbalism. The same can be said for the role of herbalist-healer.

Physicians examine patients through physiologic and pharmacologic testing of tissue. Each specific disease is seen as stemming from a biological reason that can be treated mechanically. The subsequent cure can be effected through manipulation of the physical body, whether by chemical or surgical means. Herbalists reject many of these methods as falling short of the mark. Holistic practitioners take into account the mind, body, and spirit in the healing process. Our view on disease and therapeutic approach supersede any rigid practice: Ultimately the body will direct its own healing. A cure can be part of this, and we do indeed celebrate the resolution of symptoms. Yet healing goes further, just as our consideration of each client's situation seeks broader connections.

"Battlefield medicine is expensive," points out Ryan Drum. "That's largely what's being practiced, a medicine always in crisis and on the battlefield. That type of energy becomes the war on disease, the war on pathology. But what happens when we pause to consider the therapeutic value of a pathology? The body did this on its own. Is it maybe better to not intervene? Or to help the person get through it themselves? Most modern medicine is *diagnose and fix* as opposed to *diagnose and see what's actually going on with the person*."

Blindly relying on any authority figure in health matters is not good. Empowering people is fundamental to the work of herbalism. Just as the body knows the business

*Text continues on page 45.*

## AN ATYPICAL DISCLAIMER

HERB BOOKS these days cannot go without some statement disclaiming any and all responsibility for passing as medical advice. Our publisher has been astute enough to cover our collective behinds in the front of this book. Yet one can't help but admire someone who speaks right to the heart of the matter.

> Any opinion contrary to expressed or voiced authority is by some people considered heterodoxy, akin to scientific agnosticism. But we are irregulars. An ostracized people, a minority section in medicine. But by this very fact I hope we are liberated from phases of mental bondage forbidden him bound by the code of ethics that restricts mental expansion. We believe we have the right to walk into fields hitherto untrodden, to think, to reason, to expound theories new and strange and proclaim reasons for our opinions, be they what they may. No man can to us say, "I am authority," and by that self-sufficient assertion deny others the right to individual thought. No one, in our opinion, has reached infinity of thought.
>
> —JOHN URI LLOYD (*American Journal of Pharmacy*, April 1922)

# Deb Soule

PEOPLE FROM Maine have a broad footing in self-sufficiency. Perhaps it's only natural that Deb Soule in Rockport, Maine, delights in all aspects of being a community herbalist. Hers is a Zen soul, inwardly quite strong in what she believes, mightily rooted to the living Earth. Deb thrives on helping people strengthen local connections, bringing about thoughtful balance in the workplace, and empowering women to take charge of their health. She has one of those forever young faces with a bright twinkle in her eye that invites you to find out what she knows. Deb's essence, of course, draws from her relationship to the plants.

The arched gates at Avena Botanicals welcome garden visitors into a deep embrace of beauty. Gravel paths slope gently past vibrant beds of *flowering everything* toward a ceremonial center. Sweeping walls of native bedrock lead past this raised circle to a cedar arbor walkway. Greek mullein candelabras hum with the daydreams of a hundred bumblebees. Trellised codonopsis partially hide a statue of Tara, a Buddhist bodhisattva, held entranced by towering blooms of black cohosh near the forest's edge. And yet this palette continues on, radiating up the hill where production beds of St. John's wort, yarrow, and plantain speak as much for art as they do bulk harvesting intent. Waves of nourishing oats stretch to the edge of this herbal vale. Here, at the crest of the sky, red clover blossoms beckon wildflower fairies and children alike.

Deb created this astounding garden with the help of many women friends. A gardener who can integrate beauty, ceremony, and apothecary purpose certainly understands something about celestial harmony. "I'm drawn to the spirituality of biodynamic gardening practices. The influence of the moon and planets resonates with me. Of course," Deb acknowledges, "you need to be a good organic farmer to start with before you can understand and practice biodynamics. There's something about spending this time, putting energy and intention into the garden, that works."

Deb and the other gardeners at Avena work five days a week, with the apothecary open Tuesday, Wednesday, and Thursday. "We purposely set up to work at making medicines three days a week so everyone in our women's circle can have their own lives," Deb explains. "Fifteen years ago I started off alone, with people saying I wasn't going to make it, that they couldn't find my products in the stores." Now five women share the mixing of formulas, bottle the tinctures, do the shipping, and handle a busy

*I'm drawn to the spirituality of biodynamic gardening practices. The influence of the moon and planets resonates with me.*

—DEB SOULE

office routine. Avena's herbal products are carried throughout northern New England. "Still," Deb muses, "I do think once we're done paying the mortgage, the regional scope of the apothecary will probably shrink."

Such a scaling down will come about precisely because these women focus first on the needs of their immediate community. Growing and making plant medicines is what led Deb to share the magic of herbs with others for nourishment and healing. Now this community herbalist helps local health care flourish in further ways. Midcoast Maine has become more tolerant of healing alternatives in part because of her networking efforts. Some medical doctors have begun working with homeopathic practitioners and herbalists. Nurse practitioners and women doctors particularly are the ones asking for more information about herbs.

"What is lacking for most herbalists is figuring out how to

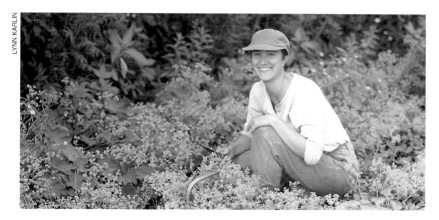

LYNN KARLIN

see people. I like the idea of working in collaboration with a licensed practitioner. An herbalist would not have the job to diagnose, but, rather, bring in the herbs that are supportive." Deb mostly sees clients in the fall and winter, after the intensity of the

growing and harvesting season has passed. Starting a women's clinic that will integrate all types of healing modalities is an ongoing goal. "We need to think creatively yet carefully within this legal system. Working with a licensed nurse practitioner who wants to

open a women's center is one idea. I like the grassroots approach to making connections. People will find out who's open-minded about health care in any community. Personally, I don't want to replicate the medical model now in place. I'm trained in a really different

system than family doctors and other conventionally trained providers. We each have a certain set of skills. We can help each other see health in broader ways."

Teaching others about herbal remedies comes readily to this inspired visionary. "The tradition of herbalism is not about going to school, but learning directly from the plants and experience," says Deb. "Our best guide is where our knowledge base has been and is going." Avena Institute offers plant-centered learning experiences through foundation and intermediate medicinal herb courses. Garden visitors are welcome on Wednesday and Saturday afternoons, with guided herb walks scheduled throughout the growing months. Deb is currently developing a three-year program to train community herbalists that will encompass all the facets of connected caring she brings to the fore. Her book, *A Woman's Book of Herbs*, demonstrates amply how vital such a program will be. ❧

of healing, each person can discern his or her best course of action given the right information. A healer needs to respect and honor individual choice. One practitioner is not going to be right for everybody. "Word gets around in the community as to who is good," says Deb Soule. "People who feel drawn to go to another herbalist should, by all means, just as I know others will come here."

"Almost always the first time I see someone I am just using nourishing and tonic

herbs," says Kate Gilday. "Mostly I want to help their systems to equal out before I give them something else. Some people never call back, about 20 percent of my clients. They were probably just not ready to make the commitment to their own health care. Some people don't want to make changes, especially in their diet. I ask people to stop—or if that is too hard, just to limit— one thing and ask them to start another that is good for them. Usually I ask them to reduce red meat and begin eating leafy greens. The plan needs to be a workable program for them. I explain that herbs often take a while to work, that people really need to stick with it."

That first session with a person is best kept simple and practical. Suggest one tea and one tincture at most. Give diet tips and lots of love. "I avoid the heavy stuff in the first session," advises Christopher Hobbs, a fourth-generation herbalist. "You want it to be empowering and positive and to build your relationship with them. Ultimately it is the love that is healing."

## THE HERBALIST AS GROWER

Some of us begin our journey in plant medicine by learning which herbal remedies help a particular condition. Others resonate first with a special herb, seeking out a broad understanding of how one plant can avail time and time again. Such inclinations enrich how we each verge upon herbal knowledge. A *plant person* may find that providing herbs to *people-focused herbalists* is the perfect calling.

We work hard to make a living growing and gathering herbs. A life in the presence of plants offers rewards that need to be viewed as more than an hourly wage. All farming is like that. The only up-front certainty here is lots of blessed time spent outdoors. Being one's own master in the field will never provide an overly cushy bank account. Livelihood hinges entirely on the ability to get each crop harvested and marketed successfully. Don't underrate the second half of that statement. Networking with practicing herbalists and building a high-quality reputation requires consistent effort and personable savvy. Our connections with the people we serve make all the difference. Offering a wide array of medicinal plants calls for more know-how and

management, but breadth is essential in reaching a large circle of supporters whose commitment in return makes a local medicine farm possible.

The nuance and beauty of each herb and tree intrigues us no end. Each day has a rhythm and a flow that suits the pace of the unfolding year. Staying centered in the task at hand—rather than being overwhelmed by the whole—allows this to happen. Our agrarian lives took a turn for the better with the decision to focus on medicinal plants. Fresh vegetables require an intensity that the drying process with healing herbs eases, namely having to market at the same time you harvest. We live far from the madding crowd: Bustling farmers' markets and large CSAs[2] require a vaster population base than we find in our hometown. A bioregional medicine farm gains far greater outreach by shipping dried herb when orders are placed. The wild plants add considerably to our harvest potential, with no effort on our part beyond responsible gathering.

Herbalists enthralled by the idea of growing and wildcrafting plant medicines to sell have two advantages over organic vegetable growers who are simply shifting to a more promising crop. Here at our farm, Nancy knows when plants are at peak potency and how best to preserve each herb. This big picture view of how quality herbs work in the human body cannot be overemphasized. We touch the right depths when we both understand how to use a green medicine and experience the living plant. An herbalist/grower can point out readily alternate uses for each plant medicine, and emphasize particular farm herbs that can be used in place of at-risk wild herbs. For instance, lovage (*Levisticum officinale*) root is an aromatic stimulant, diaphoretic, emmenagogue, and

*Text continues on page 48.*

# OSHA, THE NEXT GENERATION

ABIDING RESPECT for the healing gifts of a plant goes hand in hand with an abiding respect for that plant as a living entity. Loss of habitat and overharvesting have put certain herbs at the top of United Plant Savers' At-Risk plant list (see page 308) for good reason. Some concerned herbalists no longer wildcraft plants such as osha (*Ligusticum porteri*), which an ever demanding market quickly could decimate. But herbalists who live in the mountainous West—where this root herb seems abundant—wonder if we really need to strike it from our collective materia medica.

So far Osha has proved impossible to cultivate. This member of the parsley family is a stickler for wildness, growing only at elevations of 9,000 feet or higher. Wildcrafters gathering osha could help its regeneration, however, by understanding more about its life cycle. Richard McDonald of Desert Bloom Herbs in New Mexico shared the following insights he learned from Shawn Sigstedt, a man who has studied different species of *Ligusticum* around the world.

"We can obtain a 96 percent germination rate from osha seed. A person can actually regenerate more than the amount they dig, very easily. The trick is to make sure the seeds are ready to fall off the plant. The seeds cannot be green, but need to be brown and dry. Some of the seeds from the umbel probably will have fallen off already. By holding the stem just below the umbel, and then gently breaking off the brittle stalk below with the other hand, a person can usually collect the entire umbel without losing too many seeds. After a soft flat 'step' has been prepared on the hillside (where the seeds will be planted), the individual umbelettes are gently broken off the main umbel. These have five to seven seeds each and are placed upside down on the earthen step, looking much like mini tipis. The oil duct of the seed needs to be in an upside-down position for optimum germination. Space these out rather closely, since osha plants like to grow together, intertwining their roots into a large mass. All the planting steps should be carefully covered with light soil and decaying leaves, but not too deeply, perhaps one half to one inch is best. Then, as an added precaution, I try to protect the newly seeded area with branches, small logs, or whatever is nearby to prevent animals from smashing the new seedlings as they sprout. I tell people to collect osha only in the fall season, when the seeds are ready to plant.

"My firm belief is that unless people adhere to this technique, they should just leave osha alone. Or buy it from those of us who really are concerned with the status of the stands and are willing to spend just as much, if not more time replanting this marvelous herb as we do collecting the live roots."

*Umbel seed head of osha*

diuretic. The Chinese name for lovage translates to "European dong quai," because many of the female toning qualities of *Angelica sinensis* are found in lovage as well. Native peoples of the Mountain West use osha (*Ligusticum porterii*) for similar purpose. Hispanics call lovage the "osha of the garden."[3] Which of these plant species grows readily in northern New Hampshire? Which medicine can herb farmers promote bioregionally? An herbalist can point out such advantageous connections by including educational inserts when mailing out a yearly price list to farm customers.

Ecological niche should be stressed as well as medicinal niche in choosing herbs to grow. Simulating a microclimate and soil type for non-native species requires more work than *growing the right plant for this place*. Medicinal farming gets exciting when we realize how we can work much more in accord with Nature than we do with domesticated food crops. We will explore just how much plant sense makes human sense in chapter 6. Harvesting dandelions that pop up among the garlic and onion beds in the waning months of summer may be more profitable than the bulb crops themselves. We are learning to let the plants guide our growing.

Organic certification of a medicine farm is not requisite in a bioregionally oriented economy. Thanks to diluted federal standards, what was once a legitimate marketing "badge of honor" for a small family-scaled farm now suits corporate-scaled agriculture more. Certification is not what makes us organic. Foods and medicines grown with love and holistic savvy don't require purchased approval. A radical leap in consciousness would take us well beyond this perceived need for third-party confirmation of farmer integrity. Herbs grown for healing intent

should, of course, be nurtured on untainted soil. But DDT residues and the like contaminate every pocket of this precious Earth already. Organic agriculture is not about ignoring the woefully misunderstood ramifications of chemical agriculture; rather it is about moving ahead sanely despite ignominious mistakes made in the past. Isn't it time the human race insists on existential sanity as a starting point and not merely a certifiable alternative? We've come to view organic farm practices as a given here on our land. We don't use pesticides or herbicides; we don't salt our ground with soluble fertilizers to inflate short-term profits. Let's take this all a step deeper and talk about what we do.

Our lives depend on the soil. The bacteria and other microorganisms that decompose organic matter make possible the creation of new organic matter. Plants grow. Animals eat. The health of the entire system hinges on proper nutrient cycling, which in turn supports immune function.

Organic agriculture, to a large extent, is curative soil practice. We recognize the cycles of a living soil and choose gentler ways to tread sacred ground. This is all to the good, yet farming can be much more than obeying bureaucratic prerogative to use natural remedies in an allopathic manner. True healing encompasses spirit. Our culture must find the spiritual discernment necessary to establish viable small farms. Farm animals need love and sunshine, not production quotas that legitimize keeping "organic cows" under a roof and "organic chickens" cooped up to lay the healthier egg. We rely on our animals in turn to contribute their grazing and manure to the overall health of the land. The emphasis in procuring our food needs to shift from constantly cutting production costs to investing in sustainable diversity.

The healing plants have not been domesticated to the degree that food crops have been bred and genetically altered. Merging the wild element into agriculture strikes a chord with Nature that deepens our role in the scheme of things. Permaculture and biodynamic agriculture take vital steps toward embracing a wise view of soil stewardship. We will constantly allude to these underlying agrarian philosophies in discussing herb growing throughout this book. The notion of integrating permanent crops into a dynamic farm system that works with both biological forces and cosmic influence strikes us as thoroughly sound.

Robert Wooding grew up on a family farm in Virginia. Southern Virginia Herbals was born in 1976 when the healing plants found Rob pondering how to survive on land that formerly sustained tobacco and cattle. He began by planting ginseng and goldenseal in the woods and soon discovered that he could harvest more than fifty medicinal plants growing wild on his property. Today the arable half of the farm produces several acres each of red clover, oats, and alfalfa, as well as smaller amounts of fifteen other medicinal herbs. Balance and intimacy are as important to him as organic production. "There's lots of research showing the biodynamic preparations recommended by Rudolf Steiner enhance fertility and that crops do better," says Rob. "The practice of biodynamics is not only viable on a business level, but it enhances the energetics of the crops you are trying to sell. Most importantly, you are doing something that's good for the earth and working in relation with the big picture."

Organic guidelines as established by national certification standards are merely toddler steps toward the salvation of agriculture. There are valid marketing reasons to becoming certified—contract sales require it—but we should never forget that the goal of USDA certification is to make inroads for industrial agriculture into a lucrative consumer market. The ethics of animal care, regard for the living soil above all else, and nurturing intimacy of spirit and community are not a part of certification status.

"We are certified organic by NOFA [Northeast Organic Farm Association] NY," says grower Matthias Reisen, "but with reluctance. Certification makes sales possible to herb companies that require this stamp of approval. But we've kept the word 'certified' off our Healing Spirits label." The argument against certification comes down to lessening bureaucratic structure whenever and wherever we can. A local farm serving an intimate market does not need third-party inspection to assure customers of its integrity. People who know each other know what the other is about. Customers can always get honest answers direct from the horse's mouth.

Everyone can and should make time to gather healing herbs of their own. The energy of the plant flows most strongly when we have this direct relationship. Not many of us have a childhood connection with plant medicine passed down from the previous generation. The impetus to start comes in many ways. A Potawatomi medicine man came by to see the organic gardens of Ocoee Miller: "He told me, 'Ocoee, you have so much here. The land provides your shelter, your heat, your food. Now you need to learn how it can provide your medicine as well.' Not long after that a pharmacist friend offered some seeds, saying 'Ocoee, you live the lifestyle. You need to grow this plant [echinacea]. You'll find out how to use it.' And that's how I got started growing the healing herbs. Paths open before us when the time is ripe." This family-oriented

*Humanity has only two choices: either to start once again, in every field of endeavor, to learn from the whole of nature, from the relationships within the whole cosmos, or to allow both nature and human life to degenerate and die off.*

—RUDOLF STEINER,
*Agriculture*

herbalist now offers workshops in the Lawrence, Kansas, area to encourage others to take those first delightful steps with plant medicine.

Apprenticing on a medicine farm reveals what the grower's path might entail. Monica Rude of Desert Woman Botanicals hits the nail on the head by asking her apprentices at the start, "Have you ever worked before? I mean, really worked?" Most people have no idea how much physical labor it takes to farm. The apprenticeship experience provides the opportunity to become more realistic about one's dreams of being an herb grower and getting rich quick. Being with the plants, taking care of them, rubbing up against them, looking at them while weeding or mulching—simply experiencing

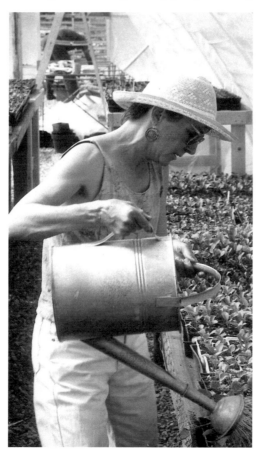

*Monica Rude thrives in the herbal mecca she has created at Desert Woman Botanicals in Gila, New Mexico.*

them—can be an incredible, life-changing encounter. Monica spends time with apprentices in her herb lab making tinctures and sun-infused oils for salves. "We talk about product development, good manufacturing practices, labeling, and marketing techniques. The value-added part of my farm business is more profitable than selling straight bulk herbs. Many growers have found they have to do a combination of the two to stay in business." The chance to learn firsthand starts with asking an herbalist/grower if this opportunity is available. Apprenticeships work well when teaching intent is matched with a responsible influx of energy into the farm. Not all growers are good teachers, nor are all apprentices dedicated to the field. Crafting a living on the land requires plenty of self-initiative and Earth-inspired devotion.

## THE HERBALIST AS MEDICINE MAKER

Herbal pharmacists use the good herb to make the medicine. Extracted tinctures, formulated capsules, and medicinal tea blends enhance the healing potential for an array of human conditions. Our vision of local medicine recognizes that not all folks are going to make their own herbal remedies. The next ideal goes one more step up the chain: knowledgeable community herbalists at work making herbal preparations for extended families and neighborhoods from the highest-quality, freshest herbs available locally. Bioregional companies serve a good purpose in meeting the demands of larger markets.

The ancient tradition of using herbs for healing gave rise to the current tradition of modern pharmaceuticals. We suffered two losses in the switch. The first—the natural remedies versus synthetic drugs debate—animates the herbal renaissance. Many of us, on the other hand, are not so aware of what the diminution of the pharmacist's role has meant. The science of compounding and dispensing medication, herbal or otherwise, is a healing art as well. Pharmacology began to develop as a profession separate from medicine in the early eighteenth century. Accordingly, collaboration between physicians and the people making medicine increasingly became an economic double play. Today, despite their considerable skill, pharmacists are thought of primarily as people who sell us drugs.

The art of medicine making cries out for connection all around. Power lies in approaching all our endeavors from a holistic framework. A drug viewed as working primarily through chemical potency on the human body does that and little more. We observe empirical results and thereby rationally deduce both the indications and contraindications for that drug. Patients have been known to have great expectations, to the point that human will—call it the placebo effect if you wish—imbues a medicine with inexplicable oomph. Spirit, for many, introduces more intangible mystique. Prayer garners the attention of scientific study as a factor in healing now. Can it be that medicine ultimately serves us best when all the parties involved are attentive to the physical, volitional, and spiritual attributes of the cure?

Herbalists have always had a hand in gathering and preparing the plant medicines given to the people in their care. When we harvest herbs for a specific individual, prepare a remedy with that person "held up to the light" as we work, and offer our love along with the medicine, something magical takes place. Similarly, the preparation process can be infused with a spirit of caring for folks who might need the medicine at a later time. Bioregional herb companies can bring a vital spiritual component into their relationships with growers and the process of making medicine in a lab.

"I think the attitudes that you have when you are making something is transferred into what you are making," shares David Winston of Herbalist & Alchemist. "The people in our lab certainly know what they are doing and are very attuned with the plants. We hand-garble every herb shipment [some companies just throw everything into a grinder] and hand-pick seeds and anything else that might adulterate the product. Some herbs coming in are not always identified correctly. For example, one day the manager had me check a shipment of couch grass that looked very nice, but didn't seem quite right. I called up the supplier, who was a well-known wildcrafter, and said, 'This isn't couch grass; if you send me some of the flowers I can key it out.' It turned out to be Johnson grass. He responded that it had to be couch grass because it's what he'd been supplying everybody else with. Having the right herb that was gathered at the right time and in the right way is important. How you then prepare the medicine and your attitude in doing that makes the medicine even better."

Small companies such as David's are fighting to maintain sensory testing (identification of purchased herbs by sight, smell, and taste) as an allowable part of good manufacturing processes. Larger companies are trying to make microscopic and chromatographic tests mandatory on incoming raw materials, which of course can be necessary for powdered plants coming from a questionable source. We have reason to be concerned whenever government regulation makes the costs of doing business affordable only to big corporations.

Our understanding of herbal potency can certainly be furthered by laboratory analysis. But standardization (see page 27) of one active constituent does not need to be the one stupefying goal in applying scientific methods to medicine-making techniques. Legitimate questions abound that we as growers, gatherers, and preparers of plant medicines cannot necessarily intuit. For instance, there are more than one hundred species of hawthorn. Do certain species yield leaves and berries of greater medicinal content than others? Are fresh preparations of certain herbs absolutely necessary to achieve intended results? Experience has shown that shepherd's purse (*Capsella bursa-pastoris*) loses hemostatic and diuretic value once dried. Are losses resulting from drying other herbs more subtle, but still relevant? Or are some herbs actually preferable dried? The berberine tinctures from Oregon grape root and goldenseal, for instance, are best made from the dried herb. Alcohol is better than water at extracting some constituents, but which alcohol? Some swear by a double extraction of echinacea. The leaves and flowers are tinctured first, then strained, with the potent root added to the same menstruum once the plant dies back in the fall. Others say an alcohol solvent can only absorb so much, that it's better to make separate extractions and then blend the final medicine. Who's right? The list of highly intriguing questions goes on and on. We'll examine more such nuances of medicine-making in chapter 7, but one point stands out clearly: Medicine makers need broad and deep knowledge.

Of course, one can become unruly when battered by too much technical concern. Our knowing friend Matthew Wood speaks for those of us inclined to forge ahead regardless: "Medicine should taste like the herb, and everything else—proportions, weights, and measures—be damned."

## THE NEIGHBORHOOD APOTHECARY

Few of us ever keep a supply of every herb on hand. Herbal apothecaries, whether in the heart of town or a mail-order away, meet our specific requests as the need arises. Determining the freshness and quality of bulk herbs and medicinal products can be hard without first knowing the reputation of the gatherer and the medicine maker. Many people rely on the good judgment of the apothecary instead. Chain stores exist solely to sell us marketable goods: The people there do not know what herbal products are for, nor do they understand how to best use herbs. A grassroots herb store, on the other hand, more often than not has a venerable community herbalist at the helm.

Walk down the main street in Silver City, New Mexico, and you know you've come to an herbal mecca. Desert Bloom Herbs beckons first, and one block farther up awaits Bear Creek Herbs. Jars of wildcrafted and locally grown herbs line the walls of both stores. All tinctures and salves are made on the premises; not a single national brand name is to be found in either store. The people living around this small mining town just south of the Gila National Forest are obviously receptive to plant medicines.

Purple Shutter Herbs in Burlington, Vermont, emphasizes locally grown and gathered herbs on its store shelves. Regional herb farms share in herbalist Laura Brown's good intent by checking off which medicinal crops on her preseason list they will have available. These two- to twenty-pound orders for different herbs—split among the different farms to keep everyone going—keeps local dollars invested in northern New England farms and businesses. Quite simply, it's a consciousness we all need to cultivate.

"Herbalism in the public eye too often gets reduced to being about tinctures in bottles," says Faye Burtch. "Let me show you what a down-to-earth herbalist can offer their community from their home."

Faye's apothecary in State College, Pennsylvania, centers around a worktable where jars of dried herb have recently been pulled off the shelves for customizing a tea blend for a massage client. This herbalist prefers crafting remedies specific to each individual she works with rather than offering general formulas and tonics. Gallon jars of each herb are wrapped with tan tissue paper to lessen the deterioration caused by light. "Smell this wild bergamot," beams Faye, as she puts the green fragrant leaf in Michael's hand. "Can you feel its energy?" Grain alcohol tinctures fill a second set of shelves. The expected red of a good St. John's wort extract appears an even darker maroon. Faye explains, "I don't hesitate to follow my intuitions about making medicines. The books say that the good volatiles of St. John's wort are in the flowering tops. Yet I've observed the effect of hypericum seed on depression. The plant tops in this jar were already browning when I harvested, meaning that some of the flowers had already set seed, and this results in a darker color."

Two upright freezers line yet another wall of this cellar apothecary, wedged between additional shelves of vinegar extracts and dried roots. Frozen poultices of comfrey leaf, celandine, and calendula blossoms are available to be thawed for winter treatments when the plants themselves rest dormant below ground. Faye finds poultices preserved fresh by freez-ing to be more powerful than reconstituted dry herb. Refrigeration adds yet again to this out-of-season potential for freshness. One fridge hums away, keeping infused oils chilled, while another stores dug roots of black cohosh, dandelion, burdock, poke, and comfrey in optimal condition. "Winter is the time for roots in food and medicine," says Faye, ever diligent about using the living plant when possible. "I can make very specific formulations from all this. The energetics of the different plants can be matched to the energetics of each person." Mason jars of elderberry rob (you'll find the recipe in *A Modern Herbal* by Maude Grieve) preserve the goodness of elder in a traditional honey-ginger syrup. A lone *Vitex* (chaste tree) plant reaches toward the light of a basement window, its green leaves an unceasing testament to the healing vibrations filling this room.

People are bound to ask for health advice wherever herbs are available. Jean Argus of Jean's Greens stresses that she is not a practitioner, that she is more comfortable offering tonic herbs and proven formulas in her mail-order catalog. "People can delve deeper into plant medicines on their own," she tells such callers, while happily offering to help research their particular condition. "Once informed, if they want certain herbs, we're happy to supply them. I do recommend people work closely with a practitioner in trying any new formulation." One man asked her to custom-mix capsules of senna and cascara sagrada—"a combination that would be most uncomfortable to anyone taking it unless they had been constipated for weeks!"—which Jean felt was an idea inspired by rabid book-learning but lacking in clinical experience. She graciously declined the order.

*Text continues on page 55.*

# HERBS FOR OUR ANIMAL FRIENDS

Aʟʟ ᴛʜᴇ ᴘʀɪɴᴄɪᴘʟᴇs of holistic living that we urge for human folk certainly apply to our pets and farm animals as well. Diets for many domesticated animals are atrocious. The unsavory ingredients in commercial pet food come cheap, but at a great price: reduced vitality and shortened lives for the animals we love. Farm animals raised to industrial precepts are kept propped up with antibiotics and growth hormones to produce meat and milk from manipulated feeds. Veterinarians dole out medications after the fact simply because of how the majority of animals are treated.

These creatures in our care deserve a far better life. Grazing animals need good pasture as much as sunshine and fresh water. They have an instinctual appetite for certain plants at certain times, seeking out the broad-leaved herbs, flowering tips, and lush grasses encouraged by rotational pasture management. Good hay is going to include dandelion and nettle among the fescue and timothy. Grains, vegetables, and wholesome meats are easy to prepare for our animal companions once we understand how vitally their health depends on our taking this time.

Animals can become ill or injured despite devoted attention.

Bypassing the immune system with corticosteroid drugs, antibiotics, and vaccines—in addition to poor diet—often lies at the heart of chronic problems. Herbal remedies for fleas, arthritis, internal parasites, urinary tract infections, and the like can be used with great success if we address the underlying situation. Homeopathy in particular is catching on with those farmers who insist on healthier animals and lower vet bills. The *Herbal Handbook for Farm and Stable* by Juliette de Baïracli Levy brings holistic understanding to animal care.

A similarly broad view makes *All You Ever Wanted to Know About Herbs for Pets* much more than a prescriptive guide to herbal medicine. Greg Tilford and Mary Wulff-Tilford of Animals' Apawthecary (a company that produces low-alcohol herbal extracts for animals) cover the gamut of natural pet care in this book. The Tilfords address which

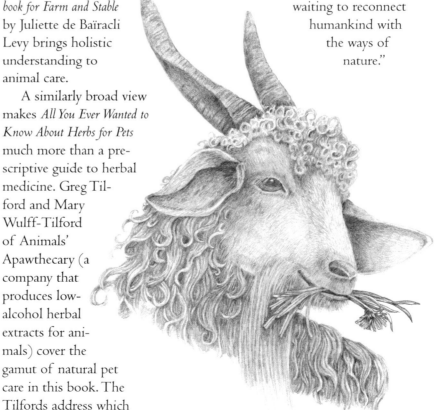

herb to use, how much, how often, and possible side effects.

"From the moment a puppy, kitten, baby bird, or other companion enters a human life, a special bond with nature begins," write Greg and Mary. "From this bond we can learn innocence, compassion, respect, unconditional love, and the tragedy of time wasted. And, most important of all, we can finally realize that despite centuries of our abuses, animals and plants remain quietly waiting to reconnect humankind with the ways of nature."

The advice of an herbal practitioner can be found at Jean's Greens by appointment. Kate Gilday sees clients one day a week in a room above the bustle of this upstate New York herb shop. People who come to see Kate can obtain very quickly any herbal recommendations downstairs as they leave. "Jean blends custom teas for my clients as needed," affirms Kate. "I was finding that I was going in too many directions and trying to do too many things. Now I write up a tea formula or a capsule formula [Kate offers her own tinctures.] and Jean makes it up." This wonderful combination of effort works both ways. Local people become aware of all this mail-order apothecary offers, while some of that inevitable pressure to consult is off Jean's hard-working shoulders.

A cooperative space arrangement with the natural foods market holds great potential for increasing the local portion of Teeter Creek Herbs' business. Bob Liebert is on hand in his apothecary nook on certain days each week to help folks decide which herbs might do them the most good. "We've been supporting our family covering all the bases. Doing more retail business will help us get away from wholesale," muses Bob, an herbalist who is all too aware of tight business margins. "To be honest, it's hard convincing other stores to carry local products rather than national brands. Our opportunity lies in people realizing those cheaper herbs in Wal-Mart aren't so good." Jean's Healthway continues to sell the Teeter Creek product line when Bob isn't at the store, which is a real advantage for an herbalist with a farm to tend. "Other than some of the older Ozarkers, who remember 'yarb doctors,' I think modern folks don't know what to make of me. Herbalists are kind of scary," chuckles Bob. "I've gained a lot more acceptance from my neighbors by

opening an herb shop here in town. My practice is in matching the right herb with the right person. I also seem to do a lot of psychological/emotional/spiritual counseling on the side."

Such a collaborative approach has merit for community herbalists. Running a full-fledged business—paying store rent, committing to regular hours, advertising, and all other aspects of retail marketing—is not necessarily the heart and soul of what we might want to do as herbal practitioners. Teaming up with a natural foods store brings two community health partners together. "Jean Farbin [owner of the store in Ava] has done an amazing job over the last twenty years of educating people about health in this part of Missouri," Bob Liebert points out. "Now that we've joined forces, she sends folks to me with herb questions and I send them back to her for good things to eat and a supplement or two. We're really making an impact on the health of the community here."

Certain ethical decisions need to be made in any community herb store. Women come in occasionally, for instance, asking for herbs to induce an abortion. "I have provided information in the past after talking to the woman at great length and then had many sleepless nights wondering if I did the right thing," shares one anonymous herbalist. "What if the woman changed her mind and just took enough to damage the baby? What if she hemorrhaged at home and had no help? We no longer give out any recommendations for this. I actually feel it is better for the woman to have a clinical abortion if she is determined to go through with one. Herbal abortions are horrible, you have to make yourself so sick." Another store deals constantly with miners asking for herbs to help them pass a drug test. Recommending herbs for this reason is not what most of us are about. Promoting good health is the bottom line that counts.

## THE HERBALIST AS TEACHER

Herbal wisdom needs to be passed on to each generation. This link was nearly broken during the past century of allopathic medicine in North America. But the pulse of the people's medicine never stopped beating. Good folks kept at the good work of healing others with plant medicines, humbly and ably. The old books waited, holding the bones of knowledge left to us by our great-grandparents. Oral traditions were passed on to a dwindling few, but that was enough. The tree in the middle of the garden has leafed out once again. Herbal medicine is in demand. What's desperately needed now is a proper understanding of what we can receive from the plants and offer in return.

Home herbalists and community herbalists alike need to be inspired and given opportunities to deepen their understanding of herbs and constitutional healing.

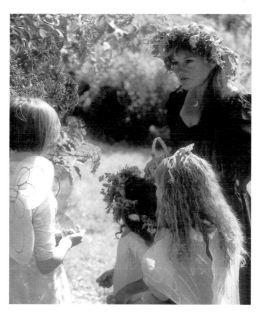

*Magic takes place in the garden whenever we invite the fairies for tea.*

Herbal teachers effect powerful change, especially when we teach children at a young age that they are their own healers—that they can go out and pick an herb, or sit by the stream and be healed. People have a deeply set notion that they can't make their own medicine. Working with the young seems particularly hopeful, because this kind of ingrained dependence can be chucked out the window from the start. Self-reliance goes hand in hand with personal responsibility in getting people to walk knowingly on herbal ground.

That brings us to Earth awareness and the whole eco-herbalism movement. Just as the Lorax spoke for the truffala trees in Dr. Seuss's proverbial tale, the plants need spokespeople to make the case for ecological sanity and wise relations among species. A living relationship with the plants that heal cannot be bought in the drugstore. Our job as herbal teachers goes well beyond looking at ways of healing our own. Expanding consciousness has always been the integral mark of any successful teacher, herbal or otherwise.

A natural ability to relay information and bring a subject to life exists in all of us to some extent. We'll look at specific tried-and-true techniques for teaching confidently to different levels of students in chapter 8, "Spreading the Word." The ardor to teach others about herbs and holistic living requires an ongoing commitment to molding ourselves into good teachers as well as herbalists. Some of the best training to be had lies in watching other herbalists teach. Gatherings are a great place to further our abilities. Attending a beginner-level class to observe another teacher's techniques and interactions with students can provide good ideas for our own introductory classes. The ability to relax, tell fun tales that bring those cherished smiles, and make our teaching a multisensory event as opposed to a humdrum lecture comes easier when we see how others go about the very same task.

At times we need to be patient with our students. Eagerness to learn about plant medicines does not necessarily come paired with holistic consciousness and consideration for others. "There are two dreadful things that I encounter in beginning and advanced students," notes Ryan Drum. "Herbs are associated with sickness by people who are in distress. It's difficult, unless you have a very secure core, to encounter pathology and pain and unhappiness on a regular basis [outside the classroom let alone while teaching] because of one's own sense of mortality." Individual students do sometimes try to make their personal situations paramount while we're teaching. Encouraging a private consultation at another time can be a courteous way to reclaim the setting for everybody else.

"The accompanying distress for me as a teacher," continues Ryan, "comes from certain questions like, What herb do I use for paranoia? What herb should I use for hangnails, Dr. Drum? Students want a mechanical solution to a physiological, potentially spiritual/emotional presentation. They like to have the good parent herb to fix their problem." The real magic of herbs lies in nourishing good health, of course, and far less in offering an allopathic alternative for symptom relief. Perspective matters here. What we teach is meant to make that message clear.

Herbal teachers can make a legitimate income from this good work. Our culture accepts the idea of paying for a learning experience, if not willingly, then at least creatively. "When someone asks me to give a talk, like a garden club," notes Joyce Wardwell, "I tell them I charge $300 plus expenses. If I have to stay overnight you have to put me up somewhere. Well, they can't afford that. Do I turn them down and miss an opportunity to share with people? I offer to bring my products along to sell. If I sell $300 worth of products, I waive a speaker fee, but if I sell $150 worth, they pay me a $150 speakers fee. They still need to pay my expenses."

"I'll tell you a horrible but true story. I was invited to teach at the Open Center in New York City," shares herbalist Susun Weed. "They were charging $50 or $60 for a three-hour talk on menopause. It seemed so expensive to me, so I arranged for a women's bookstore in New York to have me give a free talk on menopause that same afternoon. Three women came to the free talk and 125 came to the expensive talk."

"I have a new policy: My teaching does not come for free," asserts Faye Burtch. Often she has been asked to give workshops gratis for accredited classes at the university in her town. The requests usually come from professor friends who earn far heftier salaries than she does. "Most people can pay something. They won't value a workshop if it's not worth anything. I now charge $50 an hour no matter what I do," adds Faye. Teaching is an energy exchange, and money serves to see that the exchange goes both ways.

Teaching for free certainly has its place, but these stories emphasize how our culture assigns value. All herbalists are teachers at the one-on-one level when helping another

*Text continues on page 59.*

*Herbal education begins with changing our consciousness.*
—PAM MONTGOMERY

# Mimi Kamp

MIMI KAMP of Naco, Arizona, is one of the guardians of the sacred Southwest. She knows the plants of her bioregion intimately and feels a strong responsibility to protect them. She is cautious in giving out information that could lead to overharvesting. "Back East there is so much green, so much growth and renewal, where our West is a different scene. Bare earth and drought make us aware of the preciousness of plants. We must be wise in choosing what plants to use." Her own body—tall, wiry, and seemingly as fragile—emanates an abiding respect for this vulnerable desert world.

This gentle soul has worked as an herbalist for more than thirty years—consulting, teaching, making medicines, gardening—and is currently working with a Mexican *curandero* and his wife in both Bisbee, Arizona, and in Mexico. "I'm making a terrible living doing lots of different herbal things. Tinctures are the most efficient way to extract plant chemistry and to assimilate it into the body for healing. Yet I like to tell people to experience plants directly. I want to turn people on to plants and to something deep within themselves." She is a self-taught botanist, a trained artist, and a spiritual ally of plants. Her botanical drawings reflect her intimate connection to herbs and they grace many of Michael Moore's books.

Walking with Mimi in the desert is a delight. We come from lush New England, where we have plenty of rainfall and a profusion of summer greenery. Stepping into a desert area during a severe drought is more than a little shocking. Crossing a

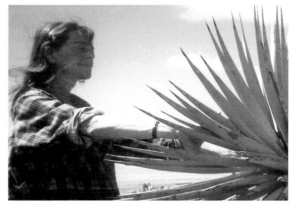

*Bare earth and drought make us aware of the preciousness of plants.*

—MIMI KAMP

road and going under a barbed-wire fence into the desert is like stepping into Mimi's living room and being introduced to her beloved family. She knows and shares botanical information about every plant—details about its structure and how it survives in this harsh environment. The side teeth pointing upward on the sofof leaf and downward on the agave leaf provide exemplary lessons about introspection. "You can run your hand easily along agave this way, but in the reverse direction you are caught, clawed. The energy follows the spines. Sofof guides us outward; agave takes us deep within." The barren soil beneath our feet hides tubers and seeds that await the generous rain to release a long-held promise. Such patience attests to an eternal rhythm. Here in the desert, with holy plants beneath the bright blue sky, we soothe that constant urgency with which we've come to view our own human lives.

Mimi really shines in her spirit connections with the green world. "If you need therapy but can't afford therapists, you can do it with plants. Pay attention to which plants draw you. Your frequency is likely the same frequency as the plant." People tend to pick her brain for medicinal information and botanical facts, but sometimes she just asks them to sit with a plant to learn of its energy. The squat rainbow cactus draws one into inner male/female places, often evoking memory and healing of childhood experience. Saguaro's plant medicine finds expression along a continuum that changes and evolves for what is needed. The ocotillo appears so stark while it awaits moisture to release its leaves. Mimi relates how a vision of its branches came to her when witnessing

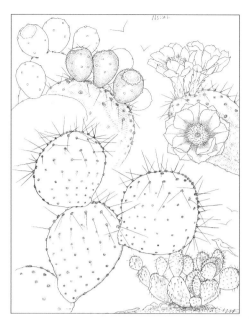

bodywork on a woman with bad arthritic pain. She administered three drops of ocotillo tincture. Those present felt an unmistakable vibration move up the woman's spine. "The response was too quick for the herb to be working physically to improve lymphatic circulation. This was on the energy level," says Mimi. Plant spirit medicine flowed as swiftly as the ocotillo responds to a desert rain. ℘

*Mimi's drawings reflect her intimate friendship with the green world.*

person get well. We share remedies and offer encouraging advice whether or not part of our living comes from formal teaching about herbs. Creating class opportunities around other aspects of a green livelihood sometimes can make great sense.

"We placed an ad for farm apprentices in an Albuquerque newspaper. A hundred calls came, but all from people wanting advice on how to grow herbs in their yards and make medicine," says Monica Rude. Opportunity was knocking: Desert Woman now holds urban workshops on the cultivation of medicinal herbs for backyard gardeners. The workshops are offered when spring bedding plants are ready to sell. The five-hour drive one way from an isolated farm is a long distance to go, but then again, the truck returns empty every time. "We gross a couple thousand dollars on these trips, because I try to squeeze in several plant sales and classes over a few days," sums up this herbal teacher/nurse/grower/medicine maker.

## TENDING TO THE SPIRIT

The tradition of plant spirit medicine reaches back beyond the millennia. Spirit medicine comes direct from the Creator, not through tradition or study. It cannot be handed down. This connection with our source is direct. Humans in touch with the natural world are alive to the spirit that permeates all being. Admittedly, inner knowing can take many forms. Different cultures express it in many ways. That Creation might have messages for us, as shamans and traditional peoples have long ascertained, is a far-out concept in these "enlightened times" of stock market obsession and genetic manipulation. Today it seems that few recognize how the purpose of life actually centers on spiritual awareness and love. It is possible, when we slow down enough to listen, the plants and the four-leggeds, the winged creatures and the fishes, the rock beings, and the smallest of the bacteria are communicating essential intelligence to the great mystery we call life. Listening within can direct us to wisdom that often transcends

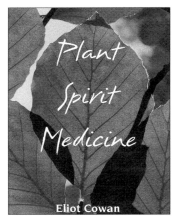

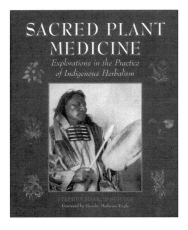

Sacred Plant
Medicine *by*
*Stephen Buhner and*
Plant Spirit
Medicine *by Elliot*
*Cowan touch on the*
*spiritual depths that*
*underlie herbalism.*
*The plants are*
*willing partners in*
*our personal*
*journeys to be well.*

what we think we understand about medicine and the marvel of each human body.

Practice and everyday use hone any skill, and this includes stilling ourselves to sense deeper realms. Two recent books have done much to open herbal ears to the direct teachings of the plants. *Plant Spirit Medicine* by Elliot Cowan and *Sacred Plant Medicine* by Stephen Buhner bring to the fore the realization that the plants are here to give completely to us. Ours is a shared existence, a shared biology, a shared spirit. This psychic approach to healing draws forth an inner knowing to reveal possibilities that otherwise might be lost from view. The mind-set necessary to be in a sacred relationship with plants does not come readily to the Western perspective. And yet anyone—anyone—can find ways to be in harmony with the natural world. To find that visionary inspiration and the revelation of Earth wisdom, we begin simply by asking the plants for their help.

"I found that the Earth cannot understand language, that most powerful of human inventions. Embedded in the body of ceremony is the language that Earth understands," writes Stephen Buhner in *Sacred Plant Medicine.*[4] People create ceremony to encourage spirit, whether individually or

collectively. All cultures have their customs and rituals that are alive to the present moment. Some are directed toward specific healing purpose, others evoke human participation in the greater circle of the seasons, and still others quietly acknowledge spiritual awe. Sometimes just thinking about life or healing is not enough. We need to fan the flames of physical reality and focus good intention in order for spirit to open our hearts. Ceremony possesses a living essence that helps us to trust in a power greater than ourselves. Ritual prayer, song, and dance allow us to forget our skepticism and remember that we too belong to Earth. And then we become engulfed in infinite blessing.

"Ceremony is a way of bringing the spirit of the divine into consciousness," explains Pam Montgomery, a plant spirit practitioner in Danby, Vermont. "It takes spirit from that realm of otherworldliness into our very being. Ceremony consciously acknowledges that there is spirit in everyday life. Rituals with the plants is another way to consciously acknowledge the magic behind the green. That harvest offering of tobacco or cornmeal or crystals, whatever it is, needs to be important to you. If it has no meaning to you, it's empty. One of the things that I do is give a piece of my hair. I've realized my hair gets a lot of attention, usually positive. It's a part of myself that holds that positive energy. To give my hair as an offering means something to me, and it holds that admiring energy. My admiration for the plant is passed on in this exchange. Bringing ceremony and ritual into our work with the plants makes for medicine that is more powerful than if you don't. Part of our evolution at this point in time is bringing ourselves into partnership with plants and the world around us. As different types of conditions come up for people, the plants evolve to meet those needs. Plants have the ability to work in one particular way on one person at one time, and in another way for another person at another time."

"I believe rational explanations are destroying medicine today, as well as our society at large," explains Dr. Lewis Mehl-Madrona about lessons he's learned from Native American ceremony. "To be healed, we need to believe in the possibility of healing, and in a greater world, and in higher powers than our own. We should not trivialize spiritual experiences, saying, 'It's just this, it's only that.' It is a grave and sometimes fatal mistake to insist that every experience have an explanation that avoids the spirit. We cannot live without spirit. It is arrogant and in a sense dishonest—dishonest because scientific thinkers are not so much trying to explain as trying to explain *away* the miraculous."[5]

Lewis talks powerfully about the sweat lodge and other intentional ceremonies in his book, *Coyote Medicine*. Drawing in family and community to express love for a person in need focuses everyone's healing intent. Improvisation keeps any ceremony vital and relevant to those on hand. Creating harmony within the circle of community—and clearly relishing a oneness with the Earth Mother—can bring our bodies into vital healing resonance.

"If we change our minds and grow our spirits, our physical body follows along. Number one, we do this by ceremony," points out David Winston. "Ceremony was given to each person by spirit. That is why we all have different ceremonies. In order for ceremony to be meaningful it has to be connected to your life. If you work in an office and stare at a computer all day, it may be hard for you to decide what your ceremony should be. But if you grow herbs for a living, then your ceremonies will be around growing and harvesting. If you are a singer, then your ceremony is certainly going to have music. Whatever it is that you do in your life, your ceremony should involve that. Second, ceremony has to connect you to the Great Life. All of the Cherokee ceremony revolves around the cycles of life: full moons, no moons, solstices, equinoxes, sunrises, sunsets, women's moon cycles. Ceremonies connect us to something bigger than ourselves. We need

## THE GIFT OF CEREMONY

*David Winston kindly shared this Cherokee teaching about ceremony.*

WE BELIEVE THAT when people first came into this world we were originally just two-legged animals. But eventually we were given a gift. All species have at least one gift, and in our case it is the cortex, the ability to think and to reason and to solve problems. This came with the two-edged sword of self-awareness and ego. Anyway, we originally got our gift and it became apparent to the plants and the animals that we weren't really mature enough to handle our gift.

They could see these two-leggeds were going to cause mischief and trouble in the world. They looked at us and sort of shook their heads and said, "What are we going to do with these guys?" It was kind of like giving a kid a loaded gun. So they came to us, at some point far in the distant past, to every people in the world, bringing yet another gift, and said, "Here. This is for you."

What they brought were their ceremonies, and these ceremonies were designed to connect us and thus keep us out of our own heads. Ceremony is designed to help us to remember that we are not individuals, but rather that we are part of a Great Life. We are part of something bigger than ourselves.

---

*The elders believe that herbs have vibratory effects on man's soul as well as a metabolic effect on the body. The medicine men and women must first perform a feat to purify themselves before they go out to pick herbs. When they pick herbs, they enter the plant world, a kingdom all of its own, a regal kingdom. They wear their finest clothing and best jewelry. Then they talk to the herbs; they tell the herbs the name of the person needing their healing power. They tell the plant why they are going to use it. They plead for the assistance of the plant, that way they are recognizing the spirit energy of that plant.*

—Phyllis Hogan, *The Herb Quarterly*, winter 1989

to give our lives to service. When I give away to other people's lives, I will be given back what I need. Our basic needs are food, water, homes, community, *and* ceremony."[6]

It's a big leap for some people to contemplate plant spirit medicine. The notion that we can communicate with the plant spirits

## NOTES

1. Questioning authority can be just as healthy as abiding by the rules of the game.
2. People purchase a share of the harvest of a Community Supported Agriculture farm at the start of the planting season. Such a shared agriculture addresses cash flow and marketing unknowns, allowing the farmer to focus exclusively on growing good food for CSA members committed to good eating. See *Sharing the Harvest* by Elizabeth Henderson (White River Junction, Vt.: Chelsea Green, 1999) for an inspiring look at CSAs.

and vice versa is hard to swallow for someone on the straight and narrow. Physical reality seems safely manifest compared to the unknown vastness underlying spiritual reality. Shamanistic thinking stretches beyond those conceptions of what's rational and what's empirical. But the chemical constituents of a plant are not separate from the spirit of the plant. "A separation has been created in modern-day herbalism," notes Pam Montgomery, "but we really can't separate spirit from physical reality. The same is true of what happens in our bodies. We can't separate our spirit or emotions or any other aspect of ourselves from the whole. How a plant's chemical constituents work on the body is an integral part of how the spirit of the plant works for the spirit of the person."

Mind, body, spirit. The dominion of herbalism lies within the whole of our selves and the whole of the plants. Each of us has gifts that touch upon different aspects of the inimitable whole. Curing depends on biophysical remedies. Both folklore and science serve this function, but healing encompasses something more. Caring opens all these doors. And then spirit rushes in every time.

3. Steven Foster, *Herbal Renaissance* (Salt Lake City: Gibbs-Smith, 1993), 140.
4. Stephen Buhner, *Sacred Plant Medicine* (Boulder, Colo.: Roberts Rinehart, 1996), 103.
5. Lewis Mehl-Madrona, M.D., *Coyote Medicine* (New York: Fireside, 1997), 119
6. David Winston speech at the 4th International Herb Symposium at Wheaton College in Norton, Massachusetts, in June 1998.

# CHAPTER THREE
# *Learning Your Path*

VALERIAN
*Valerian officinalis*

*I*'ve had this sense of urgency that I really need to catch up to where a woman in her thirties and forties should be in learning about herbal medicine. ❧ Two understandings about this inner prompting come to mind. Many of us are being called at this time by the plants themselves. We may not even know why we are studying so hard, but we trust there will be a need to share healing skills as life continues to evolve and change. Our consciousness about Earth and spirit are awakening rapidly while at the same time our material culture seems so empty. In contrast, the gifts of the plant world seem so full and vibrant. Helping people discover healthy possibility for themselves is an integral job of every herbalist. I want to be ready as times change. ❧ My other motive for hastening onward centers on my daughter. I'm determined to restore that wonderful pool of knowledge about the plants and healing that older women have always made available to the next generation. Nobody was able to share such herbal wisdom when I was growing up, as so much already had been forgotten. By observing what my sweet girl knows already, I realize now how much I missed. Grace has been brought up with the healing plants. She doesn't have to retrain her mind to accept the possibility that the medicines she needs are right outside. If she is listening, she may get messages from the plants. She knows how to make a tea, a vinegar tincture, and an infused oil. She understands what is safe and tasty to graze on in the gardens and in the fields. She understands that taking echinacea and doing a rosemary steam will *help her body heal more quickly when she has a cold. These things are interwoven in an Earth-connected life between mothers and fathers and their children. My learning may have been late in some respects, but the calling ahead is clear.* —N.P.

P URSUING HERBAL WISDOM is indeed a lifetime journey. Our education truly begins when we start to know the plants directly. Gatherings, schools, and apprenticeships with a chosen mentor all follow from there. Learning comes at a pace that matches our readiness to understand and the needs we feel called to meet for our families and communities. Ultimately, personal experience makes the best teacher. We perceive the finer points of herbal nuance in working with the plants as spirit guides and in making medicines. Holistic insight into the human condition requires practice and more practice.

So be patient. Every day offers a vital teaching, no matter how much we think we already know.

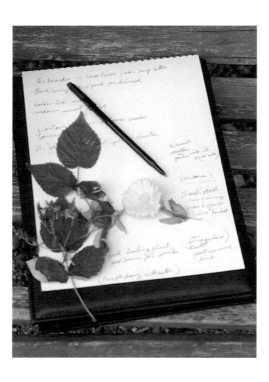

*Begin learning about a plant with an artist's eye. Recording visual impressions and intuitive feelings helps many herbalists get to know a new friend.*

## MEETING THE PLANTS

Nature insists that we slow down, listen, and observe. Beauty and stillness fill us when we stop our incessant human chatter. Deep in our being we know we've come to this place before, that we too belong in the natural world. We might start with a botanical approach to learning about the plants, with a field guide in hand. We might be walking along with a plant person simply to hear the lore behind each herbal friend. We may be working in rich soil, rooted in a gardener's passion bigger than ourselves. Regardless of where we are, the notes of the song begin. A melody calls to us. Where once we trod swiftly by a mass of green, now we see individual plants we know well. Miniature landscapes open before our eyes. And all the daunting information about these plants we felt we'd never be able to grasp miraculously begins to take hold. Botany falls into place as surely as an understanding of energetic qualities and medicinal use.

Facts are not what bring us to know the plants. When we meet a new person we learn her name, observe the color of her eyes, and ask where she lives. But these details don't mean you really know that person. Long lists of facts become rather meaningless without the bond of friendship. The same holds true for our relationship with plants. Spirit and enthusiasm are what's required to meet the plants.

"I love all the plants and want to know them all," says 7Song, an herbalist particularly known for his botanical zeal. "I have a huge library, and most of the books are on botany. It is not just knowing the plants for medicine: When I see a plant, I want to know all about it." Here is a man whose goal is to learn the scientific name of every plant on Earth. 7Song gathers most of the three hundred herbs in his regular materia medica, purchasing only about twenty of them. Such wide-ranging knowledge flows foremost from a genuine love for plants.

Or, to put this connection another way: "My path as an herbalist is one of not much formal training," notes Cascade Anderson Geller, who has been on the fac-ulty of all three naturopathic colleges in the United States, "which is fine, because it provided me with the need to learn from ancient beings—the plants."

### The Name Game

Names allow us to distinguish individuals and family groups. In the eighteenth century the Swedish naturalist Carolus Linnaeus pioneered the standardized naming system for plants and animals that we call *binomial nomenclature*. His system grew into the rules now set down in the International

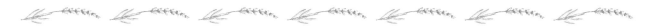

## ARE HERBS SAFE?

H ERBS ARE in the headlines everywhere. Our mothers clip and send us articles from women's magazines and local newspapers with the latest herbal information. They and their friends want to know what they can use safely. Will they have good results with ginkgo for their memory? Or horse chestnut for varicose veins? So much information is available, but not all of it is holistic or trustworthy.

Opinions run the gamut from "Herbs are natural so therefore completely safe" to "Combining herbs with any pharmaceutical can be very dangerous." Experienced herbalists know that neither statement is true. Some herbs are exceptionally safe and can be used in almost any situation without risk. Milky oats, rose hips, dandelion, and nettles, for example,

should be incorporated into our daily foods and sipped as health-building teas. Other herbs are potentially dangerous and should only be used in specific circumstances, with great care, by experienced practitioners. Laypeople should get advice when using poke root, lobelia, and ephedra. Few herbalists ever work with possibly fatal herbs such as digitalis, belladonna, and mandrake.

The common use of herbs around the world and throughout history has a safer track record than that of conventional medicine and over-the-counter drugs in the past 100 years. Herbs used in traditional ways are less toxic and have fewer side effects. Deaths caused by nonerror prescription medication—which according to a conservative *JAMA* estimate in July 2000 amount to 106,000 per year in the United States alone

(see page 14)—are given short shrift in any mainstream discussion that questions the safety of herbs. Conveniently overlooking such facts indicates a deliberate bias against Earth medicines.

Herbalist Michael Tierra has countered successfully the suggestion that feverfew is contraindicated with ibuprofen, for instance, noting that ibuprofen alone is responsible for 9,000 deaths a year from gastrointestinal bleeding. The reasoning goes that, because feverfew has actions similar to ibuprofen (yet another assumption), people shouldn't take feverfew with ibuprofen for their headaches. This kind of backward thinking seems to lead to a recommendation to take ibuprofen alone . . . hmmm, now what did we just hear about that option?

Both the popular and medical

Code of Botanical Nomenclature. The Latin agreed upon in this code allows us to be sure we're talking about the same plant. Many common names of plants vary from region to region. A plant that normally has one botanical name in Latin may have a dozen common names. We recognize *Achillea millefolium* as yarrow, but would we be sure if our herbal talk referred to "old man's pepper" or "nose bleed" or "thousand weed"? Latin was chosen to name plants officially because it was the lingua franca of scientists and scholars, even if we sometimes don't

have a clue how to pronounce this now-dead dialect. Common names are fine to use, and often help us remember a particular plant or one of its properties. A yarrow poultice helps stop bleeding, for example, thereby making the names "staunchweed" or "bloodwort" quite apt. The botanical name becomes critical when recommending herbs to others for medication.

Every plant's unique scientific name comes in two parts. The first part is the genus, and it is always capitalized. The second part is the species, which makes for a

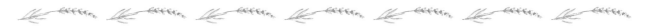

media have become fixated on the potential interactions between prescription drugs and herbs. The usual assumption behind such published warnings is that the herb somehow diminishes the effectiveness of the drug . . . a curious position to those of us who tend to use herbs to nurture and tonify, and who might wonder if the drug somehow diminishes the effectiveness of the herb. Most herbs do not interfere with the action of chemical drugs. A few herbs have been shown in clinical studies to reduce the drug effect. St. John's wort, for instance, reduces the pharmaceutical benefit of indinavir (a common HIV protease inhibitor) as a treatment for AIDS. Yet other herbs, combined with drug therapy, increase pharmaceutical efficacy and lessen adverse effects. Ginger increases gut absorption,

thereby increasing the bioavailability of many drugs. Qualified practitioners might recommend milk thistle extracts to help protect the liver from the toxic side effects of cisplatin chemotherapy. Researchers willing to delve into *polypharmacy*—the combined use of herbs, herb and drug together, or multiple drugs—are recognizing synergy as a worthy focus of exploration. Still, some physicians maintain that the underreporting of herbal adverse drug reactions (ADRs) gives a false impression that plant-derived medicines are indeed safer. Arousing generalized suspicion about herbs furthers the call for repressive regulation, and indeed, in some European countries certain popular herbs can be prescribed only by medical doctors.

Contraindications should be considered by herbalists seeking

to build health in people who have chosen an allopathic protocol. Every good herbal lists situations—such as pregnancy—in which certain herbs are not advised. The three-volume series *Adverse Effects of Herbal Drugs*, edited by P. A. De Smet (published by the Royal Dutch Association for the Advancement of Pharmacy), provides a comprehensive overview of botanical adversity. Possible adverse reactions of specific herbs and constituents are listed alongside the expected therapeutic benefit. Jonathan Treasure now offers access to information about specific herb-drug interactions on his Herbal Bookworm Web site. A counter look by this herbalist at the nutrient deficiencies contraindicated by certain drugs offers some refreshing balance to the debate.

specific identification within the genus. Both parts are italicized to indicate the Latin. This binomial is like people's first and last names, only the order is reversed. Our family unit is categorized within the genus *Phillips,* with three distinct species identified as *gracie, nancy,* and *michael.*

Latin nomenclature becomes familiar to all of us in time. Names seen in books again and again begin to stand out. Labeling herbs and tinctures with both the botanical and the common names drives the lesson home. Materia medicas arranged by common name invariably include the Latin as an adjunct. Some herbalists adhere strictly to the Latin name first. This may be frustrating initially, but their books nudge us into familiarity with a naming system we eventually will use. Such binomial indexes are usually accompanied by a cross-referenced listing that provides the common name.

Truthfully, until these names are pounded into one's consciousness, no real rhyme or reason exists for grasping the meaning of Latin for those unfamiliar with the language. It helps to know that some common names, such as valerian—*Valerian officinalis*—are derived from the Latin. Here's a case where the species name, *officinalis* (sometimes *officinale*), happens to ring a bell, too. It means "of the workshop," and alludes to the medieval apothecary shop. The name signifies that any such plant was once prized by herbal pharmacists as the official species to use for medicine. Thus lemon balm is *Melissa officinalis* and the dandelion is *Taraxacum officinale.* Other species names provide similar clues. Geographic origin is indicated by *canadensis, europaeus,* or *chinensis.* Do you see a connection for Greek mullein in *Verbascum olympicum*? Color names its hue: *alba* or *album* indicates white, *nigra*

indicates black, *purpurea* indicates purple, and so forth.

Sometimes the scientific names change. The nomenclature follows what seems to be a straightforward hierarchy of order within the plant kingdom. Genus and species are actually the tail end of a classification system that links taxonomic relationships as a means of distinguishing this order. Opinions among botanists are not set in stone, however. The herb feverfew presents one such example: If you encounter *Chysanthemum parthenium* in one herbal and *Tanacetum parthenium* in another, the feverfew plant is still one and the same. Such nitpicking can be traced to the naming source when an abbreviation of the botanist's name suggesting the change follows the Latin. Understand that now and then your confusion may actually be someone else's confusion! Some botanists propose an entirely new system of classification that would acknowledge a plant's relationship to the ecosystem in which it lives. The idea is that the current Latin nomenclature—based on shared traits among species rather than on interrelationships—creates an illusion that one component of the ecosystem can exist independent of the environment in which it is embedded.

Perhaps someday each plant with a dozen or more scientific names will be known best by its one simple common name.

## Identifying Plants

Under the current naming system, plants named by genus and species are assigned to a family grouping. Thomas Elpel makes wonderful sense of this family order and offers a quick way to identify plants in his book *Botany in a Day.* He begins by having his readers look for patterns in plants. The aster, bean, rose, celery, and mustard

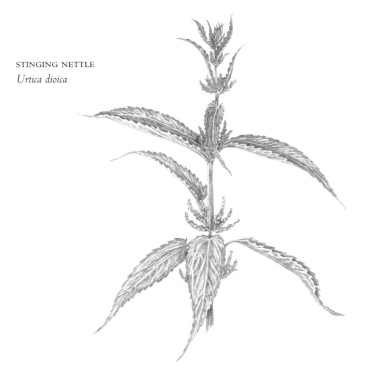

STINGING NETTLE
*Urtica dioica*

families are recommended as especially good groupings with which to start. After reading about these plant families and their characteristics, one can then go for a walk and look for plants that fit the classified patterns. The point is not to concern oneself with individual plant names just yet, but rather to make the same connections among various related plants that botanists made in the first place. Tom's overview of the evolution of plants helps tremendously in understanding how these patterns came to be.

Let's say we choose to take a closer look at the Urticaceae family. Members of the nettle family share an unmistakable trait: The hairs on the underside of the leaves function like little hypodermic needles that inject stinging formic acid into your skin when you brush against them. The other key traits that identify this family are squarish stalks with opposite leaves. Worldwide there are 45 genera and 550 species belonging to the Urticaceae family. Armed with this

knowledge, you possess the clues to look at a plant and reasonably deem whether it indeed belongs to the nettle family.

Bit by bit more family groupings and their identifying traits become part of our working knowledge. Individual species within a family can be identified more readily in field guides by searching through drawings or photos of plants within that family. Such guides approach plant identification in one of three ways. Some are organized alphabetically, which requires a lot of page flipping to find the right picture! Others are keyed by the color of the flower and guide the reader through a list of petal traits and leaf arrangements. *Newcomb's Wildflower Guide* is a good example of this style. Ultimately, books organized according to plant families best serve the herbalist because they abet from the start our learning of basic botany principles.

The process of "keying out" plants is explained in field guides. Basically, plants are arranged by visual features or sometimes by habitat. Flower types are either irregular or come with seven or more regular parts. Wildflowers may possess no apparent leaves, basal leaves only, alternate leaves, or opposite leaves. Shrubs and vines have their own distinctions. Leaf types come entire, toothed, lobed, or divided. Learning general botany terms along the way will help in using these guides. A *raceme,* for example, is a type of inflorescence, elongated and unbranched, with stalked flowers arranged along a central stem. The flowers mature from the bottom upward, as one delightfully finds on lily-of-the-valley every spring. The goal is to arrive confidently at a plant's identification by focusing on its appropriate features through an ever dwindling list of possibilities. Once a plant has been matched to an illustration, the specific botanical information describing that plant can be confirmed.

Herbalism is very much about familiarity with all aspects of a plant. Naturally enough, this includes tasting to experience the plant's healing potency. One worthy rule every medicinal field botanist should heed concerns positive identification: *Do not ingest any plant until you are absolutely sure of its identity.* Some very innocuous looking plants (such as Queen Anne's lace) bear close resemblance to some very poisonous ones (poison hemlock). Be certain.

## Herbariums

Another great way to become more knowledgeable about plants is to create your own herbarium. Such a collection of plants or plant parts—picked, pressed, dried, and then mounted for permanent display—becomes a standard reference collection we can share with others. Best of all, the process of creating such an herbarium commits us to a detailed observation of each herb. An intact and complete plant, including the flowers and seedpods and possibly the roots, makes the ideal specimen. Choose an individual plant that seems representative of a healthy population (but don't collect if only a few plants are present). Ask permission from the plant before you begin respectfully to snip or dig. Take along a field notebook on these collection forays to record all relevant observations about species identity, location, elevation, habitat, and soil type. Specimens can be put in paper bags, each carefully numbered to correlate to the field observations. A field press (two cardboard sheets and a rubber band will do) may be needed to transport fragile plants such as goldthread.

Most plants can be dried successfully in a simple homemade plant press. Two pieces of plywood, approximately 12 × 18 inches each, with holes drilled in all four corners for ⁵⁄₁₆ × 3-inch carriage bolts, provides the pressing power. Use wing nuts on the bolts, as these tighten readily by hand. Corrugated cardboard cut to the same size as the plywood (and aligned with the bolt holes) serves as ventilating layers between the plant specimens. The trick here is to align the open edge of the corrugation with the short side of the press to allow the moisture to escape more quickly. Each specimen will be placed between newspaper, with blotter paper between that and the cardboard ventilators. Several layers of plants can be pressed at the same time. A makeshift dryer can be created by stacking bricks or books to reach above either side of a small lamp. Lay the press on the brick or book towers, forming a bridge across the lamp. A 40-watt bulb produces a gentle rising heat. The faster a specimen dries, the more true the colors will

*Becoming fluent in botanical terminology helps tremendously in using a keyed guide to plant identification.*

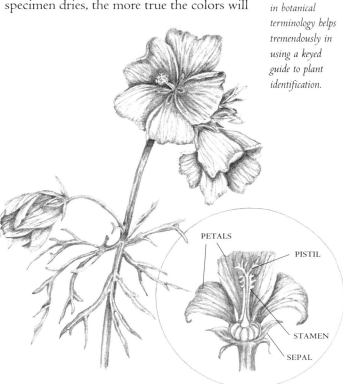

PETALS

PISTIL

STAMEN

SEPAL

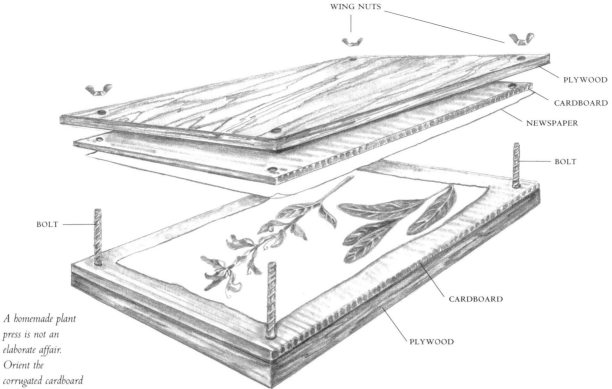

WING NUTS

PLYWOOD

CARDBOARD

NEWSPAPER

BOLT

BOLT

CARDBOARD

PLYWOOD

*A homemade plant press is not an elaborate affair. Orient the corrugated cardboard layers to carry moisture out along the short side of the press. Quicker drying helps preserve the vivid color of the fresh plant.*

remain. For really moist specimens, an additional layer of newspaper (between the blotters and the ventilators) can be changed every day to hasten the process. The press needs to be tightened each morning. The drying time can range from a few days to a week, depending on the moisture content and the size of the specimen.

When the drying process is complete, each plant gets mounted onto a sheet of acid-free rag paper with white glue. Heavy metal washers can help hold down the dried plant until the glue dries. A label applied in the lower right-hand corner fully identifies each specimen. Scientific and common names, locality, overstory and understory species, traditional uses and medicinal actions, name of collector, and date collected are the kinds of information to display. These sheets are then kept in herbarium storage boxes, filed alphabetically by family,

genus, and species. Placing this box in a plastic bag helps keep out herbarium-gnashing insects. A ring binder works equally well if plant specimens can be fit onto notebook-size paper. Honest-to-goodness herbarium paper and boxes (see our source list) can set off such an herb collection nicely.

We simplify the herbarium-making process for kids participating in our summertime Nature and Spirit camp: Fresh plant parts are held in place on file cards by clear contact paper. The children write the common name of each plant and one medicinal use directly on the card. A green leaf or two, and a blossom if available, will dry surprisingly well beneath the creased plastic.

## Doctrine of Signatures

People have long been aware of yet another set of patterns in plants. The ancient *doctrine of signatures* helps some of us comprehend the personality and virtues of certain plants. This theory suggests that each plant resembles the disease or organ for which it has medicinal value. We enter into very subjective territory when we interpret such signatures, and this has led quite a few herbalists to disregard this view of plants. The value of this approach, however, lies in helping us to remember what otherwise seems overwhelming.

For example, the lungwort lichens (*Lobaria* spp.) come recommended for chest disorders. These plants contain antibiotic chemicals effective against the bacteria that cause tuberculosis and many other lung infections. The pouched, lunglike appearance of these lichens would suggest this connection. The flower of self-heal (*Prunella vulgaris*) looks like a throat, and indeed a tea from the leaf of this plant has long been used as a gargle for sore throats. Plants that grow in wet locations often relate to the kidneys and other organ systems that handle dampness in the body. Gravel root (*Eupatorium purpureum*), found in swampy thickets, has been used traditionally to eliminate stones in the urinary tract and treat urinary incontinence in children. Brilliant blue flowers almost always indicate a calming influence: Lobelia, skullcap, and blue vervain each help ease spasms or cramps. A plant's "signature," in effect, provides us with an insightful clue to its medicinal properties.

One learns to see these similarities between plants and people as one experiences how the herbs are used. The doctrine of signatures takes on fuller meaning when we entrust this observation to our intuition and imagination. One of Matthew Wood's favorite herbs, agrimony, bristles with stiff hairs standing on end, which corresponds to its use as a great remedy for tension of any kind. Time guides us to a personal understanding of what the plants have been suggesting all along.

## Medicine Power

We're not sure why the medicinal qualities of a plant develop. Some have a bitter taste, a repulsive smell, or a poisonous compound to prevent insects and other animals from eating them. But such repellents and poisons are not always offensive or toxic to every organism in every situation.

"Plants may develop mechanisms with their chemical constituents for all kinds of reasons," says Rosemary Gladstar. "People think the chemical pathways a plant develops are for the plant's own use. But that's not really true. Scientific studies have shown that many of the chemicals in plants aren't vital to their own biochemical work. These are often the most powerful medicinal compounds as well. One thought is that maybe they have developed those pathways over thousands of years for other purposes. Perhaps selected by humans, perhaps other forces are at work."

*Text continues on page 74.*

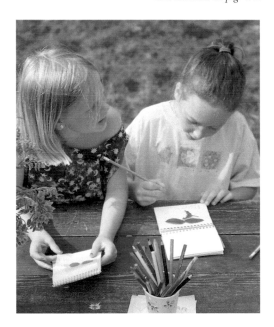

*Plant identification books are a big hit at our Nature & Spirit Camp. A fresh sprig dries fairly well under clear contact paper, and the children can write down the plant's name and a traditional use on the side.*

# Ryan Drum

THE WONDER of herbalism is in the details. Working with the plants intimates an understanding of how they grow and recognizing the potent moment of harvest. A healer constantly explores the depths of medical acumen and human insight. We enjoy such journeys into herbal nuance with Ryan Drum as our guide. Long known as one of our preeminent wildcrafters on the West Coast—his good name is practically synonymous with kelp extraordinaire—Ryan brings to light details that enliven our sense of plant magic and environmental sanity. We caught up with our friend at Waldron Island to pose some questions.

### Where did your journey into the nuance of herbs begin?

As a young man, I had a pretty harsh training in analytical chemistry. I would often be concerned with parts per billion of iron or some other element, both in assessing water supplies and when I worked for Shell Oil. This wasn't just nuance, but the ultimate in minutiae and the limits of what we could test. I did fieldwork in the ecology of one particular group of algae in an entire river system over five hundred miles long. I looked at their cell biology on a level no one had ever done before, as electron microscopy had not existed previously. I was working at fifty thousand to one hundred thousand magnification, way beyond what we could have imagined viewing previously. I saw that what was happening at the molecular level affected what happened at the gross community level. Certain small differences in how some critters grew enabled them to produce one hundred tons an acre of wet biomass, just because they figured out one particular aspect of hanging on to stuff. Their "glue" was better. They outcompeted other species.

### And these kinds of small differences on the molecular level no doubt enter into our interaction with plant medicines?

Most certainly. When I began studying herbal medicine through ethnobotany, I noticed an intense ritualization of behavior in the folks harvesting the plants over thousands of years. The harvesting of certain tree barks only when the morning sun hits the tree comes to mind. The all-night chemistry that has been going on in the plant is most active where there's the most heat. This is just the law of cold-blooded reality: The temperature is hotter where the morning sun hits. In the overhead sun time, the forest canopy precludes light striking anything but leaves. This presents a very narrow window of opportunity, both in terms of light and biochemistry. In dozens of different cultures, there are specific rules about harvesting the bark on a particular side of the tree in the early morning. Never later in the day. What an amazing thing to realize, that that would be the most active site of conversion.

### So these people intuited the chemistry that would make for the best medicine?

Primitive folks practiced an intense attention to detail because their lives depended on it. We don't connect with this anymore as the pharmacy and the allopathic prescription medicines are one hundred percent available to us. These hover around saying, "We'll fix you, we'll save you." That intensity of chemistry has replaced the intensity of doing things correctly in a natural relationship with the source of the medicine.

I see the loss of nuance as a loss of sharing the healing journey with plants. We ask for an allopathic response rather than giving of ourselves in an energetic way and in a thinking way. We need to be conscious to do the right things in detail, not just in identification. "Got thick blood, take red clover," instead of thinking about all the details of the red clover's life and how that can best fit in with our lives, and acting accordingly.

*The changes we've brought upon ourselves go beyond this loss of intimacy with the plant world. How does our global lifestyle affect human biology?*

We have a cultural, mechanical situation presented by pathologies that are virtually unknown in the primitive lifestyle. The material reality of vehicles that will go 100 miles an hour didn't exist. Vehicles that will fall out of the sky with 360 bodies in them didn't exist. Microbial exposure to the entire planet has increased. Previously, such exposure might have been a hundred square miles at the most. One became extremely companionable over the generations with everything that was in the environment, adjusting and adapting to things where you were. Now we have to develop immune systems that adapt responsiveness to an entire planet instead of just a small area.

*Given this global microbial exposure, can local herbs help?*

There are exclusive cultural events that preclude the success of herbal medicine, especially in North America, on the molecular level. The receptivity to herbal medicine starts with your grandmother,

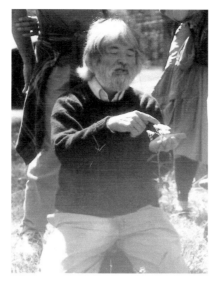

*Our hope lies in having a living relationship with the plants we use for medicine.*

—RYAN DRUM

your maternal grandmother. When you as an egg are formed in your mother, that's when the molecules in the environment that are taken in to make you up are determined. If your mother is eating foods from South America, Iceland, Mexico, you're not living locally. The indigenous model is autochthonous: You arise from the soil where you are from, if not for hundreds of generations, then at least for two or three. You and the soil and the plants are one being. You are not strangers to each other. Part of the success of indigenous medicine is that there are no strangers. The molecules involved have been around each other all the time. Herbal medi-

cine is optimally effective when we are a part of the soil that makes up the herb. Your waste, your stool, your urine feeds the plant. The plant in turn has a vested interest in taking care of you—as a community event, not as a selfish event.

This helps explain secondary metabolites that seem to have no function in the plant, such as epidermal growth factor. As far as we know, this has no function in the plant itself. Yet we can really use epidermal growth factor, it helps us topically. People use the spit poultice of plantain as a topical treatment for wounds. This perennial plant is long lived, hundreds of years if left undisturbed. Certain of the plantains will thrive only where there are people, because they are a low rosette-growing plant. If we're not tromping down all the other stuff, they get overshadowed and die out. The plantains need us. We're part of their preferred ecology. Going into a store and buying the world's highest-quality herbal preparation misses this construct. This goes beyond plant spirit medicine into plant fantasy medicine. One, it's no longer the plant, and two, assuming that it's medicine, this is really coarse biochemistry. Standardized extracts have a little bit of extra just to say the constituent is there. It's like shooting mosquitoes with a shotgun—you're bound to hit something. All the rest of the biological ritual of interdependence has not been attended to in this wishful thinking. Our hope lies in having a living relationship with the plants used for medicine.

*Our rootedness with community seems to be broken as well.*

Living in the same place, eating from the same soil, seeing the same people for twenty-five years meant I knew their ups and downs, their successes and failures. I saw how they generated their own pathologies as a consequence of their way of life. When they came to me as the free community herbalist, I already knew hours worth of intake about them. This just eludes me when I'm in clinical practice in a large urban area, where I see fifty people a week that I've never seen before in my life, and may not see more than half of them again on a follow-up. That's mystery work. Familiarity with individuals in your community makes for more precise medicine. I'd often have some idea of what's going on. And if not that, the plants would come to me in no rational way—just be in my head—these are the plants that would work. I would trust that completely, and if it didn't work, then I'd try something else. But almost always they did. I just used the plants that were around me; I don't need to import wild and crazy, powerful plants like chaparral from the desert. Unless someone came from that place, or had been visiting that place and brought a developing pathology with them. Then my local medicine many times would be ineffective against a distant obtained pathology. I would ask, especially if something seemed opaque or resistant to therapeutic resolution, if people had been traveling, doing something different, or introducing something new and exotic to their diet. That was one of the beauties of living within a very proscribed five-square-mile area for twenty-five years.

---

A fascinating list of constituents has been recognized in plants. Their juices and volatile oils, starches and acids, gums and fatty oils contain the chemical basis that we find in an herb's medicinal effect. As herbalists, we learn about these physical attributes through our five senses. Chewing on a leaf and subsequently discovering a sensation of "cotton mouth" (where one's saliva seems to dry up totally) typically indicates the presence of tannic acid. This quite prevalent plant constituent produces an astringent action, drawing together or constricting tissue. Tannins act on proteins to form a protective layer on mucous membranes, and thus are used to bind the tissue of the gut to reduce diarrhea or internal bleeding. Tannins act much the same on the skin, where astringent herbs are used in the treatment of burns, for sealing wounds, and to reduce inflammation. By recognizing the presence of this constituent in a plant, we're on our way to knowing how a particular herb may be of use to us as a medicine.

This direct experience of plants through tasting, smelling, and observing medicinal effects ultimately teaches us more than any field guide can. The first people learned to recognize certain constituent tastes and characteristic smells, just as we can. So often in an herb class we take exacting notes on uses for each plant, somehow forgetting that the teaching herbalist knows about these things from experience. One tries different remedies when one is feeling ill—call it a good guess, call it the ability to divine medicine power—and only then passes along what worked for that situation. So often in herbalism we encounter various recommendations for the same herbs. Personal medicine based on relationship does not always follow strict guidelines of cause and effect.

"We were always taught that the stronger valerian smells then the more powerful it is, which is actually inaccurate because the more the constituents break down, the stronger the smells," says California herbalist Jane Bothwell. She never felt much of an affinity to valerian because of this strong aroma (sometimes described as dirty socks) and she wasn't attracted to using this herb. Jane admired its beauty, yet didn't consider valerian to be among her personal medicine plants. "One time we were on an herb school trip and I had menstrual cramps that I didn't usually ever get," continues Jane. "We stopped for an herb walk but I just felt crampy and contracting. I looked over and there was a valerian plant that seemed to be blowing in the wind, when there didn't seem to be any wind. This has happened to me a lot since, when a plant seems to be moving but it really is not. Anyway, it happened to me with this plant and the energy caught my attention. I looked and saw that a bit of the root was showing. I went over and took a piece of root and tasted it. I marveled at how almost sweet it smelled and tasted. I ate a small piece, about an inch of the root, and thanked the plant for it. I was happy for such a positive experience with valerian. I walked on and very soon, ten to fifteen minutes later, I realized I didn't have any more cramps. It was a really wonderful experience of meeting a plant in a different way."

Society places the healing herbs on a pedestal, a medicine that belongs in the hands of trained experts. Meeting the plants—herbalism—is far more. It is about all species being friends and neighbors. The long evolutionary path that connects everything on this planet back to the first bacterium suggests connection. Animals have numerous biochemical ties to plant life. All living beings on Earth partake of infinite spirit. If we don't set humanity apart from Nature, suddenly those "why" questions behind the gifts offered by medicinal plants seem answered.

## PLANT ALLIES

Certain plants resonate with our hearts at different points throughout our lives. Finding that very first plant friend brings a recognition of what every plant can offer just as readily thereafter.

Herbalists use the term *plant ally* quite literally. A plant can be a partner in many ways, supporting us on the physical, emotional, or spiritual level. We form a bond with that plant: Perhaps we have healed ourselves of a chronic condition with the aid of a specific herb; perhaps we have meditated side-by-side in the garden during a time when we really needed guidance. The plants do have messages for those who listen receptively. Our essence mingles with that herb, and, as the friendship grows, so usually does an inherent understanding of healing possibility. We relate to the plant in a way completely different from that made possible by the purchase of any commercially prepared herbal extract. A resonance comes from deep within, knowing that another being has helped us.

Finding plant allies might seem like a fairy tale to some. To others it might be as easy as making a new human or animal friend. Mind-set determines individual reality. Believing that Earth and her various aspects are full of intelligence and wisdom—and that we as humans can learn from this guidance—is a huge step in the right direction. One doesn't have to be a full-fledged shaman to hear these messages of shared spirit. Quite frankly, we all hear them on some level all the time. Subliminal feelings draw many of us to green kinship in the garden. Hunters eventually recognize a similar sense of kinship when the acts of walking through the woods and sitting for long hours in a tree become as important as taking their prey. We absorb the healing energies of Nature on many levels. A rejuvenating walk outside can leave us feeling fulfilled and might help us find resolution on some pressing matter. Our wholeness of being gets restored in the presence of plants.

We can all learn to intuit messages from plant friends, be it practical information about planting and cultivating or more encompassing lessons about healing and love. This admittedly comes easier for some people than for others. Once in a while these messages come to people with actual images of the plant spirits and audible voices, but more often, the messages come as an inner knowing, a feeling, a new insight. The message may be as simple as sensing that a potted geranium is in dire need of water, or that the mint is unhappy, crowded in its container, and asking to be divided. That bloodroot wants to be moved out of the sun and into a completely shaded area. The catnip, glowing with vitality, shouts out as we walk by, "Pick me! I'm in my prime today." Certainly these first perceptions are linked with the physical aspects of the plant, but when we pause and consider each situation, we perceive how these plants are actually feeling, and thus what they are telling us.

Let's take this relationship deeper. Plants provide direction in our daily lives through metaphors and by example. A bountiful garden can be admired to no end . . . yet if we don't graciously gather those vegetables and fruits, the gift goes to naught. Unruly seedling volunteers need to be thinned so the remaining plants grow complete, just as tough love with an unruly child may be needed to nurture integrity and honor. We determinedly battled burdock—that harbinger of prickly seed burrs—when we first moved to our farm, yet in her persistence burdock clearly said, "I am what you need. Tincture my seeds, eat of my root." That unspoken desire for a liver tonic now finds concord in a far less pervasive weed that we may actually start cultivating more intensively.

Some plant teachings come to us in directed meditation. Seeking an unfamiliar plant with which to communicate over the course of a three-day workshop, Nancy found herself repeatedly drawn to the common dandelion. Knowing that she already knew much about this plant did not deter the messenger. "Why you?" asked Nancy. "People are digging and mowing me down all the time," said dandelion. "Yet I am tenacious. I persevere and remain strong. I continue to give freely even when mistreated. This is the medicine you need now." Energy flashed bright yellow in kindred recognition.

Michael's bond with apple trees brings explicit teachings that only mutual friends can explore. The loss of leased orchard ground and a water-powered cider mill weighed heavily on his mind when he came to the same workshop on sacred plant medicine. When asked to seek a plant companion Michael sat beneath an apple tree he had pruned earlier that spring. The message came: "You too are pruned in order to be stronger," and the apple grower knew this cut would not only heal but allow room for a bolder vision to bear fruit someday. Such an ongoing relationship with tree friends bespeaks the intimate nature of every plant ally.

All this begins only when we truly understand the sacredness of all matter at all times. Creation endows everything with spirit. Stephen Buhner, who guides a fascinating plant medicine workshop, teaches four basic attributes in broaching sacred relationship with plant spirit. Integrity is absolutely essential: We must keep our word and never, ever break it. Certain things can only be revealed to the extent that we are morally developed. Second, we must transcend our regard for human beings as the central element of the universe. This type of anthropocentric thinking is particularly prevalent in Western culture. Interpreting reality exclusively in terms of human values and perception limits our experience of the plants as kindred spirits. Third, we need a commitment to travel to ever deeper levels of meaning. The door to the soul has been unlocked; we need to keep it open. Last is our willingness to engage in self-examination. We can see clearly only if we're willing to do the same with our selves.

People gifted with green consciousness seem to need little or no practice at making this two-way relationship with plants work. The rest of us get better at listening to the plants the more time we spend with them and by actively cultivating our communication skills. The following exercises will help you become more tuned in to the plants.

Connect with a plant by sitting next to it, observing it, and listening for its voice. Go out and sit with a plant. Relax and let the right plant choose you. Start by sketching the plant, observing the minute details of its existence. Botany can come later; for now you are truly looking to see. Write down everything you see. Write down whatever impressions and intuitions seem to come. Later you can look up the botanical facts and explore its healing knowledge. Go back to the plant, preferably every week

and in every season. Ask it questions. Answers will come.

Nancy calls the next exercise her Blindfolded Tree Activity when teaching classes aimed at connecting students to Nature. (No snickering . . . no one is about to blindfold a tree!)

## THE MAGIC OF FINDHORN

An intentional community in Scotland voiced connection to the Nature kingdom when *The Findhorn Garden* was published in 1975. Our talk of plant allies and plant spirit medicine would not be complete without sharing some of the magic of that book. The term *deva* is a Sanskrit word meaning "shining one," and was chosen by community member Dorothy Maclean to avoid the stereotyped images suggested by "angel." The herb devas were found to be especially amenable to contact with people.

> We are part of human consciousness. You have discovered much about us and we can easily dance into your awareness. But remember, this is a new contact on a new level and not one from which you can compile dictionaries of long words about our abilities. I do not mean that we will not give you information about our use, but the contact comes when you rise to a level of joy and purity. You must respect us and love us as part of God's life before we can trust you with more secrets about ourselves. Plants are not here just for man's use, but when you learn that man's chief end is to glorify God and enjoy Him forever, then we can be part of that enjoyment and glorification, each in our own way, in your consciousness.

#### ❧ ❧ ❧

Forces work through us in the soil, and extra strength is given them through your consciousness of them. Everything belongs to one world, but if each thing or life lives to itself, it cuts itself, it cuts itself off from the one great teeming force field. If each opens out to the all, then currents flow through unhindered. So realize that your recognition of us opens up strength to us and to you, because it lets the forces flow naturally.

*Remember all things are of the spirit. Everything is sacred. There is never spirit without matter and never matter without spirit. Keep this in mind as you get to know the plants. Approach the plants with respect for their sacredness and they will share their medicine with you.*

SHAROL TILGNER, *Herbal Medicine from the Heart of the Earth*

Team up with a partner. Take turns blindfolding each other and then navigating the blindfolded person to a tree within a given area. While blindfolded, feel the bark, hug the trunk, smell the wood, and ease yourself into the essence of being a tree. Then you are led back to where you started, untie the blindfold, and try to find your tree. Amazingly, without fail, both children and adults can do this. Paying attention in all ways initiates the connection.

In this last exercise, beginning students can contrast "store herbalism" to direct experience.

Have students go to the store and buy peppermint tea bags. Then have them gather, preserve, and prepare their own peppermint tea. Next have students discuss which peppermint experience enriched their lives more. Connection begins whenever we have students make an herbal preparation, starting outside in the garden or field, with the plant that offers so freely of itself. Offering a prayer of gratitude to this living being stirs something in people they may have yet to touch. Doing then becomes a lesson not only in preparing medicine but in preparing the spirit to awaken.

Doug Elliott is a naturalist-herbalist as well as a downright captivating storyteller from Painter Gap, North Carolina. He spends much of his time observing the natural world. Doug has this to say about our connection to both the plant and animal worlds: "The true lessons we can derive from an animal, or any being of nature with which we identify, do not come from our own narrow-minded projections. They come from a true relationship, which is based on paying attention to the being, spending time with it, observing its way of living, and feeling its spirit."[1] The plant beings speak for themselves, offering lessons and insights that go beyond any attempts on our part to create this communication. Some call this inner knowing intuitive, but it's more. Spirit wraps around us and tucks us into her fold. We listen and then we understand.

Plant allies often seek us out and tell us how to use them. All plants will communicate in a general sense, but the ones that seem to volunteer themselves in a personal way become our allies. One of the first plants Matthew Wood came to understand was agrimony, which he now touts as an excellent remedy for tension, either physical or psychological. "Agrimony is so effective it will change the things around you in your life, especially pertaining to work situations," notes Matthew. "If somebody is having trouble at work I have them wear or take agrimony, or its cousin cinquefoil, or put it on top of work-related papers. It will change the situation for the better. After ten years, agrimony said to me one day, 'You can tell I'm a wolf medicine because of the leaflet on the end—it's the leader of the pack.' Then I knew I had a plant ally in agrimony. And I knew I could use the plant to change things in a magical way."

One story about a plant ally caught our attention for its earthy humor and focus on that ever volatile love between sisters and brothers. Rosita Arvigo grew up in Chicago, going on to apprentice with the late Don Elijo Panti, a Mayan bush doctor who lived to be 102 years old. Rosita continues to live in Central America, where she offers her healing skills as an herbalist in Belize. She shared this story about her girlhood days:

> There was a patch of mint in our backyard garden. I'd go there for sustenance when I was sad, often making mint medicine for my dolls. One day I stole my brothers' bicycle to ride to Lincoln Park. Riding down the steps, the chain on the bicycle broke. My brothers tended to be very rough in dealing with an unruly little sister—I was hauled three stories up in a swing, my hair starched and sticking out in all directions. Then my brothers charged five cents a kid to show me to the neighborhood! I immediately started to plan my revenge. The perfect day to get even came. It was hot. Frankie and Jimmy were sitting on the porch. I went inside and peed in a big bucket, poured that into glasses, and added sliced lemons and sprigs of my beloved mint. Out I came with an offer of cold lemonade. They knew on the very first swallow, but by then I was already running down the street. That mint was my very first plant ally.

The first time Bob Liebert was directed to a plant for others was when a woman came to his home to escape an abusive episode. She developed a very alarming fever and had pains that wouldn't let up. Bob went out to pray for guidance and was shown a plant that was totally vibrant and in flower when everything else in late summer had withered. "It was glowing," recalls this Ozark herbalist. "I made a tea and gave it to her, and all symptoms went away. She had a spiritual healing as well. It was not a plant that any book would say was good for much." Such can often be the case when we open ourselves to healing messages that come direct.

Plant allies continue to reveal great gifts over time as we deepen our link with Nature. We add new dimensions to our healing when we come to know these living beings as our friends. Putting up medicines and cooking meals with a green ally throughout the seasons builds the giving relationship.[2] Plant wisdom—its essence, spirit, and generosity—become a part of our own being.

*Text continues on page 84.*

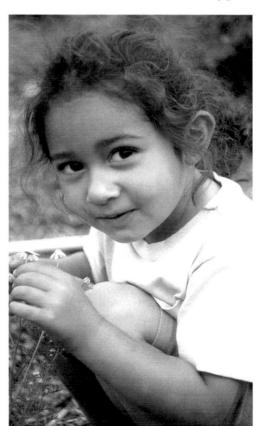

*Our very own chamomile girl*

# TEN HERBS FOR FAMILY HEALTH

*by Herbalist Nancy Phillips*

GROWING AND wildcrafting my own medicinal herbs and making herbal preparations with them is one of my greatest joys. I've become empowered to take charge of my health, to nurture my family's well-being, and to find myself deeply connected to Earth in the process.

Choosing ten herbs to get to know and befriend is a great way to begin on the herbal path. Research and experiment with them. Use these herbs for minor family illnesses and to promote overall health and well-being. Practice making herbal preparations such as teas, tinctures, salves, syrups, and body care products. Choosing plants you can grow or wildcraft yourself deepens this relationship considerably. The real insights of herbalism come when you spend time with living plants. A year spent cultivating and harvesting your medicinal plants provides a far better understanding than just reading about an herbal remedy purchased elsewhere.

We grow well over a hundred medicinal herbs on our farm, so narrowing the list to ten family favorites is always difficult. How do you decide which good friends *not* to invite to a party? Nevertheless, the following are ten plants I wouldn't want to live without here in New England.

1. **Echinacea** was the first herb I used to make a tincture. Tinctures are highly concentrated extracts of herbs. (Making them versus buying them is a little stepping-stone in an herbalist's life.) Echinacea is a beautiful perennial that grows about three to four feet tall. There are at least nine species of echinacea, three of which are commonly grown for medicine: *angustifolia, pallida,* and *purpurea. Echinacea angustifolia,* native to the midwestern United States, is relatively difficult to grow in the Northeast. We have been growing *Echinacea purpurea* successfully for years, as

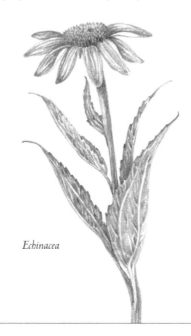

*Echinacea*

it's very easy to grow and highly effective as a medicinal. We start it inside from seed, but it also readily self-seeds. The first year we don't harvest anything from the plant, but we speak sweetly to it when passing by or cultivating. The second year plants are lightly harvested for leaves, flowers, and seeds to dry for tea and use in tincture form. We wait until plants are at least three years old to harvest the roots.

Echinacea is known as the king of the blood purifiers. It is used to help the liver function better and is widely respected as a natural immune enhancer. Native Americans used it for treating venomous bites and stings and other poisonous conditions. Modern research has shown that echinacea increases white blood cell growth, thus helping to fight infections and viral conditions. We do not use echinacea every day in our family, but rather to "jump-start" our systems at the first onset of an itchy throat or a sniffle. This herb always helps when it is combined with other good health practices and enough of it is used. One-half to one full teaspoon of tincture given every couple of hours is usually an effective dose for an acute situation. This varies depending on an individual's weight, physical stamina, the quality of the tincture, and the affliction.

2. *Garlic* stands tall as one of our family's most called-upon herbs. It has been used for food and medicine in many cultures for centuries. Often it is recommended to help control high blood pressure and arteriosclerosis. We feature this antibiotic herb regularly in miso soup whenever any of us shows signs of flu symptoms. I occasionally suck on a whole clove to rid myself of a sore throat. A few other brave souls in the family now use this sure cure as well. One coworker responded to this suggestion with, "Yuck! I would rather be sick" . . . and I guess she would. Olive oil can be infused with garlic alone or a mix of garlic and mullein flowers for ear infections (but not if the ear is perforated). I also formulate these potent cloves with other herbs to make a strong immunity tincture. Plant garlic cloves in the fall, a few

*Garlic*

inches deep, and come the next summer you'll have gourmet medicine aplenty.

3. *Valerian* can grow as high as six feet. This beautiful perennial herb is grown easily from seed and also self-seeds regularly. We harvest the roots in the fall after a hard frost to use in tinctures or tea. Valerian is probably the most commonly recommended herb for insomnia. This natural sedative can also be used in smaller doses as a general nerve tonic.

Although valerian is relaxing and sedating for most people, 4 to 7 percent of the general population have the opposite reaction to it: They become stimulated. So try out your valerian at an opportune time, rather than waiting until you are tossing and turning and need a good night's rest.

4. *Comfrey* is another favorite. I can't imagine having a medicinal herb garden without a comfrey plant to grace it. The trick with comfrey is to pick the spot you want it to be in forever when you first plant it. The roots can grow to be ten feet long, and a new

*Valerian*

plant can grow from a one-inch piece of the broken root. Comfrey has been used internally and externally for hundreds of years, though currently a controversy centers on its safety for internal use. You'll need to research the subject to make your own decision. A poultice of the leaf helps heal fractures, sores, and cuts.

My favorite healing salve features this herb. I also find comfrey to be a beneficial ingredient in formulas for respiratory tinctures and teas because of its soothing, mucilaginous, and expectorant qualities.

5. *Catnip* deserves a place in your garden or herb pantry, cats or no cats. This stimulant for kitty is a very gentle, relaxing herb for the rest of us. A nursing mother can drink its tea to help a colicky baby, or she can give the baby

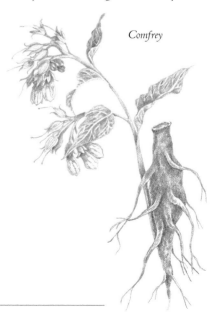

*Comfrey*

small amounts of an infusion in a bottle or by spoon. Catnip tea helps a stomachache or indigestion caused by gas. Combined with elder, peppermint, and yarrow, catnip aids in bringing down a fever. This plant readily self-seeds, so once you get a plant started, it will continue to sprout somewhere in your garden each year. Harvest the upper third of the plant when it is just beginning to flower or when it looks vibrant enough to call out: "Hey, look at me. I'm ready to share my healing spirit!"

6. *Stinging nettles* planted in the garden may seem like the act of a madwoman, but if you don't have easy access to a great wild patch, then find a secluded spot in your garden for it. Nettles can be started easily from seed, cuttings, or root divisions. This plant demands our attention—you'll get stung if you're not mindful— reminding us to tune in and listen to our green teachers. All parts of the nettle can be used medicinally. I use the leaves almost daily as tea, but we also steam them to eat plain or in any recipe that might

*Catnip*

call for spinach. We dry plenty of nettle for winter use. This herb helps the liver to purify the blood, as it is loaded with vitamins, iron, and life-giving chlorophyll. The formic acid in the little hairs on the stems and leaves causes the sting. Some people use the sting itself to help in their treatment of arthritis. The sting goes away when the herb is dried or cooked.

7. *Peppermint,* my dear peppermint, I wouldn't want to be without her! When most of America wakes up in the morning and longs for that first cup of coffee, some of us can't wait for our gently stimulating cup of peppermint. This herb nourishes the nervous system and keeps the emotions on an even keel. Peppermint does have the habit of want-

*Stinging Nettle*

ing to run all over the garden, spreading by its root runners. This plant needs a contained area or a strong disciplinarian to chop it out when it sneaks beyond its assigned spot. You can keep it happier in its contained area by taking chunks out each spring and composting the rest.

*Peppermint*

True peppermint should be started by root division or cuttings, not from seed, as the seed does not always produce the same strain of mint as the mother plant. My absolute favorite variety is the black peppermint *(Mentha × piperita)* grown for commercial production because of its strong flavor. Peppermint is invaluable for adding to other formulas to help improve the taste and palatability of the remedy.

8. *Chamomile* is gentle enough to give to a baby, but a tea of it is strong enough to help ease tension headaches and painful menstrual cramps. This antispasmodic herb also helps as a digestive aide. The annual German chamomile *(Matricaria recutita)* is our favorite. We started it by seed directly in a

prepared garden bed twelve years ago, and it has faithfully self-seeded somewhere in the garden every year since. Picking these dainty little flowers in early summer can be meditative and healing in and of itself.

*Chamomile*

9. **St. John's wort** has gotten a lot of media attention for being a natural antidepressant. It is used to treat anxiety and depression without many of the negative side effects that synthetic drugs such as Prozac induce. This wild herb commonly grows in fields and along roadsides, but if you want to harvest a lot, plant an abundant patch in your own garden. Harvest the beautiful yellow flowers right before the buds open to make infused oils and salves. We clip the top three inches of leaves and buds to dry for tea and tinctures. You don't have to be severely depressed to benefit from a little St. John's wort—a gentle nervine tea can be made with equal parts of lemon balm, chamomile, milky oats, and St. John's wort. Someone who is severely depressed should

work with a knowledgeable health care provider in determining the proper dosage and other therapies.

10. *Goldenseal* is not easily grown in every garden. I mention this valuable medicinal here to encourage you to try cultivating your own. This somewhat delicate woodland plant grows best in 75 percent shade in deciduous forests. A moist, rich, woodland area is its preferred habitat, but the shade beneath a hedge has been known to serve as well. Because it is scarce due to loss of natural habitat and overharvesting, only cultivated goldenseal should be used. The powdered root is quite expensive to buy, running about $100 a pound. Goldenseal roots

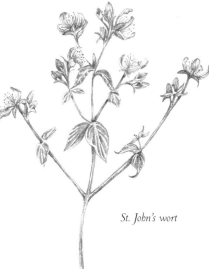

St. John's wort

are small, and the plant does not reproduce readily. Harvest occurs from the fourth year on. This natural antibiotic and infection-fighting herb should not be used for extended periods, because it can irritate the body.

You can get started with my

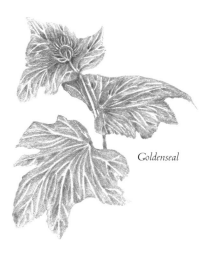

*Goldenseal*

ten suggested herbs or choose from many other valuable plants, but start to use herbs for family health. Pass on your newfound knowledge to your children. Gracie loves to take people on a stroll through our gardens, grazing on edibles and explaining the virtues of peppermint, echinacea, and her favorite heartsease pansies, the Johnny-jump-ups. No one goes away without the offer to eat "a jumper." It warms my heart knowing the chain of herbal knowledge will continue with my daughter.

## THE HERBAL LIBRARY

Well-written books enhance our botanical knowledge of plants and form our materia medica of how to utilize their healing properties. We will discuss our favorites and guide novice herbalists in their use, and open doors to further study. A passionate embrace of the art of healing will never be satisfied by a single point of view. Learning from books empowers and enhances the lessons taught both by the plants themselves and by the people we assist with holistic assessment and herbal recommendations.

It's fitting to begin this discussion of an herbal library with the words of Harvey Wickes Felter in *The Eclectic Materia Medica, Pharmacology, and Therapeutics,* written in 1922.

> Were we to start a working library for a young practitioner, or an old one for that matter, first among the books chosen would be, not one book but several on the practice of medicine and materia medica and therapeutics. Many practitioners begin and end with one book . . . failing to recognize that while there are many works touching on these topics in a general way, no one as fully presents them as a collection of books, each devoted to some particular phase of the subject. He who purchases only a pure materia medica, searches in vain for some fact concerning a medicine, and is disappointed that the writer has failed to include that fact—perhaps therapeutic—or some other he is seeking. The doctor who so frequently asks, "What is the best work on medicines?" does not realize that what he desires must be looked for in one or the other of five classes of books. . . . materia medicas, pharmacopoeias, dispensatories, formularies, and works upon therapeutics alone.

The Eclectics often combined two or more such classes into broader reference books. A *materia medica* is a work describing the characteristics of selected plant or chemical drugs. Preparations and dosages are given along with specific indications (ailments for which the drug has shown an effect) and known physiological actions. Brief toxicological notes may be included as well. Herbal materia medicas will include botanical specifics about each plant's habitat, the parts used, and its identified constituents.

*Therapeutics* is the art of applying drugs and other measures to alleviate or to cure a disease. Eclectic works often included within the materia medica a therapy section that offered the "wisdom of the ages"—the experience of the author with each medicine. Herbalists should never regard the known use of plant medicines as a closed book. Personal discovery with previously unlisted indications and herbal therapies adds our own experience to the materia medica. David Hoffmann sagely advises each of us to disagree freely when our insights vary from the recorded experience of someone else.

A *dispensatory* expands considerably beyond any one materia medica by including every known medicinal or pharmaceutical drug in use. The actions of each—physiological, toxic, and curative—are given fully and briefly. Formulas are given for compounding preparations. Official and common names of each plant are given, along with marks of identity (including microscopic appearances) and a discussion of possible adulterants. The conciseness achieved in a good dispensatory attests to encyclopedic thoroughness. A *formulary* can be little more than a collection of prescriptions, but to pharmacists it expands into a standardized reference that lists the working formulas for the preparation of medicines. A *pharmacopoeia* is the official manual of standards for the identification of drugs in a given country, usually revised every ten years by delegates from the medical and pharmaceutical institutions. It lists the standards for quality, uniformity, purity, and integrity of each drug deemed applicable for medical use. *The United States Pharmacopoeia* of today differs considerably from turn-of-the-century editions when plant medicines where in the forefront of accepted treatments.

Our eclectic collection of herb books starts with the old doctors themselves, whose detailed works fall within the categories described above. Today's herbal medicine books tend toward a more conversant style, with a materia medica included as a separate section. We've grouped the books below according to emphasis, and have highlighted several choices in each category. The challenge has been to pare down many favorites to a few.

We like the advice often given to herbal students: Look for books on herbal medicine written by experienced herbalists who really know and honor the plants.

## The Old Herbals

Botanical treasures from a century ago await herbalists who peruse early published works on herbal medicine. Doctors then did not necessarily limit themselves to an allopathic mind-set. Some practitioners worked diligently to determine the medicinal efficacy of plant remedies, and their exacting knowledge about dosage and positive therapeutics were duly recorded. Folkloric wisdom with its rich oral tradition could have

been lost in the succeeding generations, but thankfully we still have these empirical references to bring us up to speed.

*King's American Dispensatory*, first published during the latter part of the nineteenth century, tops many herbalists' wish lists. Its two volumes consolidate the known uses of hundreds of North American herbs at the time. Harvey Wickes Felter compiled the eighteenth edition with the help of pharmacist John Uri Lloyd. *American Materia Medica Therapeutics and Pharmacognosy* by Finley Ellingwood came out about the same time (1898), and dealt with the therapeutic application of plant remedies. John William Fyfe delved into the practice of herbal medicine with an update of John Scudder's similarly named classic work a generation earlier. The 1909 edition of *Specific Diagnosis and Specific Medication* details a singular approach to choosing herbs based on identified disease. *The Eclectic Materia Medica, Pharmacology and Therapeutics*, edited as well by Felter, sums up this branch of botanical wisdom as of 1922. Medicine makers will want to keep an eye out for any pre–World War II editions of *Remington's Practice of Pharmacy*. Plant medicines were unquestionably in vogue with our great-grandparents.

Many classics have been reprinted by Eclectic Medical Publications, so don't despair about finding these books. People with Internet access will appreciate finding a number of Eclectic volumes freely available on the Web sites listed in our appendices. One site lists the most useful tidbits in *King's American Dispensatory* along with the unabridged details of more than seven hundred herbs. Michael Moore currently posts dozens of such works for free perusal, including Benjamin Colby's *A Guide to Health* (1848) on Thomsonian Medicine. David

Winston offers scarce titles for sale through Herbalist & Alchemist Books. Any book lover will be sated by a visit to the Lloyd Library in Cincinnati, Ohio, where every conceivable old text on plant medicine is available Monday through Friday.

### General Herbals

Most of us get started in herbalism with one or two favorite reference books that provide a broad overview of working with the plants, making remedies, and staying on a healthy track. Those first herbals click with something inside us, prompting further exploration of this fledgling relationship with the plants. They not only encourage us to try our hand at medicine making, but also provide basic instruction to help us get started. A clear presentation guides us to understand the connections between body systems and how we feel. We learn the theory of herbs and the delight of herbs by beginning with a good basic herbal.

David Hoffmann's *The Complete Illustrated Holistic Herbal* wonderfully weaves together the science and spirit of all aspects of herbalism and holistic health. David explains how to use herbs in the right way to support the body's innate balance. This authoritative herbal, with more than three hundred color photographs, is a visual gem as well. *The Way of Herbs* by Michael Tierra offers up an equally comprehensive view of herbal possibility from a planetary perspective. A sound understanding of how plant medicine works is coupled with many practical applications of both Western and Chinese herbs. Christopher Hobbs took on a cultural trend in writing *Herbal Remedies for Dummies*. Despite the format, it's one of the best guides available for layperson.

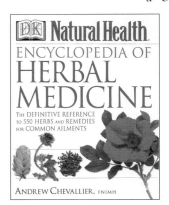

*Andrew Chevallier profiles more than 550 plants in the* Natural Health Encyclopedia of Herbal Medicine. *The color photographs and constituent details help considerably in making each plant medicne better understood.*

We really enjoy the thorough integration of Native American medicine, homeopathy, Traditional Chinese Medicine, and Western herbalism brought together by Matthew Wood in *The Book of Herbal Wisdom*. This book goes deep into the nature of more than forty plants. In the end you understand how each tradition views that plant and how you might apply this generously shared wisdom. An initial section on signatures, elements, and constitutions makes the vitalist connection between different traditions clear.

*A Modern Herbal* by Maude Grieve can never be overlooked. This twentieth-century version of a medieval herbal contains information on the lore, growing, cooking, medicinal uses, chemical constituents, and preparation of more than eight hundred herbs. Mrs. Grieve kept a fine herb garden in Buckinghamshire, England. During the First World War when imported plant medicines were in short supply, her understanding of local plants for local medicine proved to be of sterling value.

A delightful book intended for home herbalists deserves mention here. Joyce Wardwell shares generations of herbal common sense in *The Herbal Home Remedy Book*. Her sound advice on gathering and using twenty-five basic herbs for family medicine keeps this ancient healing art from becoming overwhelming. And, quite frankly, the plants never intended anything different.

### Herbals for Pregnancy and Children's Health

Naturally we want to start right in all regards with our dear ones. Herbal medicine for children needs to be understood by all parents, and these are the books that impart that knowledge gently and thoroughly.

Susun Weed shows how herbs can support the natural functions of pregnancy and childbirth in her easy-to-understand *Wise Woman Herbal for the Childbearing Year*. Aviva Romm, who is a midwife, nurtures women in *The Natural Pregnancy Book* by addressing all those concerns that come with the blessing of new life. Natural health care is the bedrock of continuing wellness, and knowing about nutrition and other holistic choices empowers the precious journey of motherhood.

Aviva shares her practical experience as a mother of four in *Natural Healing for Babies and Children*. This savvy herbalist advocates for home care whenever possible, and clearly explains the medical implications behind how our children feel. The classic *Nature's Children* by Juliette de Baïracli Levy dances with poetic spirit. This wise elder goes beyond offering remedies for common ailments (which are here in plenty) to looking at the wonderful choices we can make in life. Ultimately we are all children, here to savor a generous and meant-to-be-happy world.

Linda White and Sunny Mavor bring together the best of medical and herbal thinking in *Kids, Herbs and Health*. A holistic doctor and the founder of Herbs for Kids combine their views in a language that resonates readily for today's parents. Conventional treatments are explained alongside herbal remedies in a sensitive way that guides mothers and fathers to choose what's best for their children. Assurance takes the form of easy-to-read sidebars that indicate when calling the doctor should be considered.

## Women's Herbals

Women have always used herbs to cope with a wide variety of health problems and conditions. In *Herbal Healing for Women* Rosemary Gladstar describes how to create remedies for common disorders that arise in different cycles of a woman's life. This book rates high as a preeminent introduction to herbal medicine as well as a comprehensive look at girlhood, the childbearing years, and menopause. The wisdom intended to be transferred from mother to daughter, generation after generation, can be found here.

Deb Soule writes from personal experience in both the garden and the apothecary in *A Woman's Book of Herbs: The Roots of Healing*. Her book covers the process of creating a botanical medicine chest for a variety of female health concerns. Deb trusts strongly in Earth's healing abilities and in the ancient power within every woman to call on the sacred connection with plants. That same strength emanates in the Wise Women Way books by Susun Weed. *Menopausal Years* and *Breast Cancer? Breast Health!* encourage women to ask the important questions emanating from inner wisdom. The energies of touch, pleasure, love, whole food, and green healing plants provide the nurturing answers.

The respected traditional herbalists Christopher Hobbs and Kathi Keville teamed up to write *Women's Herbs, Women's Health*. They explain how herbs can be part of a healthy lifestyle that includes a good diet, quality sleep, healthy habits, and an active social life. The authors provide clear information about many common female disorders and offer a variety of approaches to treat them. We also recommend the *Women's Encyclopedia of Natural Medicine* by Tori Hudson. She is a naturopathic doctor with twenty years of experience in clinical practice. Christiane Northrup's *Women's Bodies, Women's Wisdom*, is not an herbal per se, but it is invaluable for its penetrating exploration of female health issues and women's spiritual well-being.

### Men's Herbals

Which brings us to the Wise Guy Way, right, men?

Menfolk have a tough act to follow, but the gifts of the plants and a nurturing manner serve us equally well. James Green assembled *The Male Herbal* to help move men beyond their oblivious attitude toward health care. Building self-reliance is something men can understand as particularly suited to the male psyche. Herbal medicine offers one venue for rediscovering our relationship with the natural world. This book offers a holistic understanding of male issues such as prostate trouble, hypertension, virility, heart health, and hair loss.

The notion that the only herbs for men are those with a reputation for increasing sexual performance reveals the usual gender bias. When you come right down to it, with the exception of reproduction, the bounds of the human condition are neither strictly male nor strictly female. Male spiritual and emotional health matters just as much as how men treat their bodies. Rosemary Gladstar makes that message clear in *Herbal Remedies for Men's Health*. She shares formulas that are effective, invigorating, and flavorful. She includes recipes for potency soup, Damiana chocolate love liqueur, and aphrodisiac balls, as well as long life elixir, male toner tea, bath salts for relaxation.

### Green Medicine

How *we* prepare plant medicines deserves our utmost attention. The scientific component of an herbal pharmacy offers useful lessons in extracting the whole of a medicine. Regardless of our view on isolated constituents, knowledge gained from Eclectic observation and in today's laboratory reveals technique and nuance that matter. Choice of solvents and concentrations for each herb affects medicinal quality, a subject we will explore in chapter 7. Books written expressly with the medicine maker's art in mind provide details needed in every herbal apothecary.

James Green's *The Herbal Medicine Maker's Handbook* provides a basic overview. Its down-home style makes medicine-making accessible to everyone. Debra St. Claire wrote *The Herbal Medicine Cabinet* with home herbalists in mind. Making basic herbal preparations gets the ball rolling, and then one can try a hand at less common products such as solid extracts, wines, and elixirs. A thorough resource section launches dreams of a home business venture.

Gilian Painter, an herbalist from New Zealand, provides a clinical perspective in her *Herbalist's Medicine-Making Workbook*.[3] The advantages and disadvantages of various preparation methods are discussed from both safety and efficacy points of view. Sections on posology (determining proper dosage for an individual), setting up a dispensary, and herb incompatibility are especially useful to practitioners.

*Making Plant Medicine* reflects Richo Cech's experience of more than a decade working for Herb Pharm in Oregon. Richo pays attention to solubility factors and shows how to figure tincturing recipes for both fresh and dry herbs. He tackles those mathematical aspects some folkloric herbalists avoid. Richo includes a gardener's herbal formulary, in which he discusses the best medicinal preparations to make with plants readily cultivated in any temperate-zone garden. He explains those invaluable nuances that make for good medicine. You can purchase this book (along with all the seeds) directly from Horizon Herbs.

Sharol Tilgner of Wise Woman Herbals, a tincture company in Oregon, couples her pharmacy experience with her training as a naturopathic doctor in *Herbal Medicine from the Heart of the Earth*. She provides herbal formulas galore (arranged according to body system) with the clear rationale behind each tincture formulation. A dose-and-duration chart shows how many days each prescription can be expected to last. An impressive solvency range chart lists more than 120 herbs . . . but be aware that the best strengths given here for some plants tend to have equal parts of solvent to herb.

# BOOKS FOR THE HERBAL CHILD IN US ALL

*Wise Child*, 1987
*Juniper*, 1990
Monica Furlong
Although these books were written for children, any herbalist will enjoy these journeys back in time to Wales and Scotland. "Good witches" work with apprentices to heal and counter the influence of evil magicians attempting to usurp the kingdom.

*The Herbalist of Yarrow*
Shatoiya de la Tour, 1994
Not many Daddys get to be the fearful Duke of Allopathy for

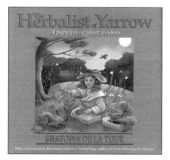

*What fun we have with Shatoiya! The Herbalist of Yarrow definitely heads our list of delightful children's books.*

weeks on end. But Michael did after we read and reread our friend Shatoiya's delightful herbal adventure to our Gracie. Wee herbalists win out in the end, with the Duke destined to embrace complementary medicine or face banishment from the land of Yarrow.

*The Midwife's Apprentice*
Karen Cushman, 1996
Back in medieval England, Jane the midwife needs a helper. A homeless girl comes to understand the deep-rooted satisfaction of helping others with herbs. The audio version of this book, narrated by Charlotte Coleman, is smashing.

*The Root Children*
Sibylle von Olfers, 1906, 1990 (English translation)
Nature spirits awaken each spring under the care of wise Mother Earth to lead a grand procession of greenery and flowers. This imagery of the earth coming alive guides our stewardship of the precious soil here on our farm.

*Song of the Seven Herbs*
Walking Night Bear and Stan Padilla, 1987
Each herb has been gifted to us as powerful medicine helpers. The tales behind these gifts make healing insights come alive for kids and adults alike.

*The Education of Little Tree*
Forrest Carter, 1990
A young boy raised in the mountains by his Cherokee grandparents learns firsthand about living in the natural world. The clash to come with white culture over proper schooling and the like determines the better path for Little Tree.

*The Shaman's Apprentice*
Lynne Cherry and Mark Plotkin, 1998
The story of an Amazon tribe that learned the importance of their own knowledge about the healing properties of the rain forest.

## Clinical Herbals

*Principles and Practice of Phytotherapy*, written by the highly respected clinical herbalists, Simon Mills and Kerry Bone, has been called "the guiding therapeutic manual of herbal medicine." This book offers the most coherent approach to melding the vitalist understanding of tradition with a thinking person's use of herbs in the scientific age. Assessing the synergy and complexity of herbs in light of medical physiology gives herbal practitioners sound footing to march past allopathic convention. The materia medica of forty herbs is backed by scientific research and clinical relevance. Herbal approaches to system dysfunction correlate specific herbal actions to biological fact. Clinical herbalists and doctors will be able to move ahead on common ground by referring to this advanced text.

The German doctor Rudolph Weiss initiated this journey between the two camps with the publication of *Herbal Medicine* in 1960. The English translation of the sixth edition became available in 1988.[4] Dr. Weiss examines an impressive body of plant medicines, arranged on the basis of clinical diagnoses to particular systems. Our appreciation of specific constituents began with this book, precisely because whole plant remedies are still regarded as the guiding principle behind any prescription recommendation.

A book that speaks clearly to our hearts comes from the compassionate experience of Donald Yance's work with cancer patients. *Herbal Medicine, Healing and Cancer* goes deep into proper diet, vitamins and other micronutrients, and herbs that can help create the right conditions for maximum healing. Yet Donald reaches further (again, as he should) into the spirit that animates that full possibility for healing. Bringing together body and spirit, humanity and nature, lies at the core of this good man's work.

## The Botanical Perspective

Botany gives us a shared working vocabulary for identifying plants. The knowledge to grow and wildcraft herbs successfully comes with experience and a good growing guide. Many works that focus on the ways and the needs of plants are recommended throughout this book. We list specific field guides for herbalists in chapter 6 that help to identify plant species and list their healing virtues.

All herbalists include some of the following books in their herbal library: *Botany in a Day* by Tom Elpel shines at making plant classification simple. Michael Moore's guides to medicinal plants of the Mountain and Desert West continue to set the standard for this genre. *Wild Roots* by rambling Doug Elliot artistically profiles the roots, rhizomes, corms, and tubers to be found below ground across North America. Works such as the *Manual of Vascular Plants of the Northeastern United States* by Gleason and Conquist (published by the New York Botanical Garden in 1991) provide complete botanical detail. Similar books are available for every region and most every family of plants.

The commercial growing advice proffered by Tim Blakley in *Medicinal Herbs in the Garden, Field and Marketplace* gives prospective herb farmers a leg up on the reality of a medicinal harvest. We like Tammi Hartung's *Growing 101 Herbs That Heal* for home herbalists. This pictorial guide delves into gardening techniques and ways to use many different plants as medicines. *Planting the Future* speaks expressly to our wild hearts. This collective work put together by United Plant Savers addresses the critical issues facing native healing herbs. The precious gifts of the plants goes far deeper than notions of sustainable harvesting. This book celebrates right relationship as told by individual herbalists who share their insights into more than thirty plant species.

You can keep abreast of the many herb books these days by tapping in to the opinions of Montana herbalist Robyn Klein. You'll find feisty reviews on her *Robyn's Recommended Reading* Web site (see appendix) which provides a look at literature relating to herbal medicine. The perspective of an herbalist attuned to the plants and appreciative of medical factuality (a tenacious clarity junkie, as she puts it) makes Robyn's comments worth noting. The content listings from numerous phytotherapy journals help the rest of us keep aware of the cutting edge driving herbal discovery today.

A thorough catalog of herb books is available from the American Botanical Council. Many classics on specific herbs and ethnobotany can be found there, as well as many of the books we've mentioned. Several publishers are quite keen on herbal subjects—Storey Books, Healing Arts Press, Crossing Press, Interweave Press, and Keats come to mind. Request their catalogs to find out what each house has available. Many authors of herb books who speak at conferences and gatherings will sell their books directly. These herbalists are always happy to take a moment to inscribe your book, so don't be shy. Just think what a treat it would be to have a copy of a turn-of-the-century work such as *King's American Dispensatory* signed by John Uri Lloyd and Harvey Wickes Felter!

## CHOOSING A MENTOR

Every herbalist follows a unique path in his or her training. Either by chance or through astute inquiry, we discover teachers with whom our heart resonates. The oral tradition of herbalism suggests the one-on-one learning opportunity promised in a mentorship. A knowing herbalist can take us under their wing and can draw out those vital lessons waiting within each of us. Reading about herbs in home study courses and books can't compare to direct encouragement, getting our hands in the earth, and truly knowing the plants. A mentor's inspiration sends us soaring to our fullest capabilities.

The evolving nature of an apprenticeship suits these fast-paced times. The old model of a wise counselor accepting an apprentice for years on end is rare. Some herbalists have undertaken such journeys with shamans and traditional healers in indigenous societies, but in North America the dynamics of this learning period have taken a turn toward apprenticeship programs or volunteer summers on the farm. These are wonderful experiences for serious herb students who desire an initiation into wild foods and plant medicines, making remedies and personal care products, gardening skills, and a holistic understanding of health. Developing an ongoing relationship with a chosen teacher is more likely in a smaller group. Bonding with supportive friends definitely happens among the group itself regardless of its size.

These apprentice programs are set up in many different fashions. Susun Weed has live-in students for six weeks at a time. Eagle Song and Sally King offer a similar approach at Raven Croft in Washington, set up as three-week sessions exclusively for women. Many, many herbalists schedule intensive weekends, one weekend a month, over the course of seven months or so. People often tent or bunk in small cabins, share meals provided as part of the course package, and basically absorb herbal teachings from dawn till dusk. Herb walks, saunas, ceremony, and playtime throughout the day keep these sessions balanced. Nonresidence programs can be organized over longer periods of time with an express goal of moving beyond beginning herbalism into intermediate and advanced studies. The new notion of apprenticeship still applies, as the teaching is done primarily by the chosen mentor.

Tammi Hartung has set up such a program at her Colorado herb farm for groups of ten apprentices at a time. Each of the first three sessions includes forty-eight hours of formal study over a period of three months. This includes topical classes shared with the public, apprentice round-table sessions, six private sessions spent one-on-one with Tammi, and a research class chosen by the group. Students progress from a well-grounded base of herbal knowledge to a very deep perspective on the interaction between plants and people. The final two sessions include fifty-two classes—each two hours long and spread over six-month periods— again including that invaluable one-on-one sharing time. Tammi gives homework as well, with an expectation that very few classes will be missed and all work will be finished before moving on to the next session and the eventual completion of the course. The ongoing commitment to this type of local program results in herbalists who are ready to embrace community work where they already live. An option to pay part of the program fee through work exchange helps students both financially and in experiencing the plants on an honest-to-goodness working herb farm. Often these less-structured opportunities to

work with or near one's mentor are delightfully instructive.

Nancy has many herbal heroes and heroines. Her own path to choose a particular mentor from among so many good herbalists was inspired first by a book, then by a correspondence course, and then came the opportunity to take Rosemary Gladstar's apprenticeship program at nearby Sage Mountain. Nancy had to sign up for this seven-month course a year in advance to reserve a place. Her first day on the mountain started with drumming and the opening circle in a woodland yurt. She was a bit taken aback by the size of the group—more than twenty-five apprentices—because she was dreaming of an intimate relationship with this wonderful herbalist. That disappointment lasted about three minutes. Her time at Sage Mountain was transformative, filled with deep connections to plants and people.

This personal mentorship in truth began after Nancy graduated from the apprentice course. Offered the opportunity to join the teaching staff and assist Rosemary with her programs at Sage Mountain, she leaped at the chance. Finding an experienced herbalist whom you admire and to whom you can be of service opens some doors. Many teachings and untold blessings have come our way ever since, thanks to our generous, loving herbal sister.

The chance to offer helping hands and a commitment in exchange for working alongside a good teacher is more like the traditional apprenticeship arrangement. Busy community herbalists can use help, partly to make their own living, partly to serve the people they help with herbal advice and care. If the time is right, the personalities match, and the desire to learn is sincere—and we absolutely trust our inner guidance—anything is possible.

"My pursuit of Native American ways from age five on has led me to a number of wonderful teachers who have taught me the spiritual basis of herb use," says Bob Liebert. "None have any desire to be known by the public at large, as they don't lead workshops and work mostly in their own communities." This Missouri herbalist learned from many wise people along the way by simply asking to share their paths for a while. The amazing diversity of plants in his chosen home called him to learn more about them and their uses for food and medicine. Some of the last old-timers shared Ozark herbal lore with him, thus continuing that vital link between generations.

*Text continues on page 98.*

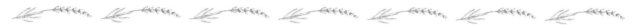

# UNEXPECTED MENTORS

Life lessons come in many forms. Matthew Wood generously shares his path of herbal destiny with us.

### Mentor number one: The kindly old gent

I was about ten. We went to the Northern Yearly Meeting of Friends [Quakers] in Wisconsin. The first-day schoolteacher was Francis Hole, a soil science professor from Madison. He was so animated; he jumped around telling us fascinating little tidbits of natural lore. We went up on Rib Mountain, the geological core of Wisconsin—an old weathered chunk of black crystal and basalt. This feeling just emanated out of Francis: "Nature is alive, Nature is alive." It sank into me, like an initiation. After that, Nature was always alive for me.

### Mentor number two: Bizarre, otherworldly, and incomprehensible

About twenty years later. One exceedingly cold day—it was about thiry-two degrees below zero—I drove up to Cloquet, Minnesota, with an Indian friend to teach a class on herbs at the home of an Anishinabe woman up there. The second I walked into the kitchen, in a burst of steam and relief from the cold, I felt like there were years of relationship with this person and it wasn't all good. Several of us visited for an hour and I went in the other room. When I came out Kathleen was pale. She said, "I was just showing everybody pictures of my grandfather. You remind me of him so much, it was like he was here." His picture was posed in a photography studio in the 1930s. He was dressed in an eagle-feather headdress and beaded leather clothing. This was in the days when nobody wanted to be an Indian, but he hammed up the part. I could see and feel a mantle of authority and responsibility on his shoulders. This was a man who took care of the young and the old, the women and children, the sick and the vulnerable: Charles W. Brunelle, 1883–1959. Later that night I felt the mantle on my shoulders and merged with it. A few days later I felt a feeling coming down my arms from the shoulders, to my hands. A feeling popped into my hands. "Oh, the healing hands," I realized. Then Mother Nature came and presented me with a diploma that said I was recognized by Her as a true doctor.

### Mentor number three: If you see the Buddha on the road, kill him

My third teacher was a younger Indian man. A genius and an egomaniac. I learned a lot from him, but in the end, he wanted to own me (his exact words, as a matter of fact), and I had to break my connection with him or die.

# Herbal Visionaries

G OOD HERBALISTS pass along
Earth awareness and plant
wisdom to each generation.
Many of us today are indebted
in one way or another to certain
influential teachers whose
insights have helped enliven these
times. For these profiles we have
chosen people who have founded
schools, written invaluable
books, or worked actively as
practitioners at one time or
another. Their diverse perspectives have created a strong warp
in the herbalist tapestry. These
good folks truly are among the
integral voices of today's herbal
renaissance.

## Christopher Hobbs

Few herbalists serve as a bridge
between the scientific community and earth-centered herbalism as well as Christopher
Hobbs does. This highly sought-
after teacher and practitioner is
known to his friends as something of an absent-minded professor, with his nose constantly
in a book or a few inches from
the ground observing a plant.
His many excellent books on
herbal medicine include are
listed in the bibliography.
Christopher's clarity and compassion shines in them all.

A fourth-generation herbalist
and botanist—his grandmother

and great-grandmother were
herbalists, and his father and
great-uncle were professors of
botany—he has more than
thirty years of experience with
herbs. Christopher
has been a
licensed acupunc-
turist since 1995.
He helped con-
ceptualize the
American Herbal-
ists Guild and
continues to be a
senior member of
the admissions
committee. He
cofounded the
American School
of Herbalism in Santa Cruz,
California, in 1989, and now
directs the Christopher Hobbs
Clinic of Phytotherapy.

Some very well-known
herbalists consider this man to
be their "family doctor" when it
comes time to seek another
opinion. Christopher considers
himself more like a health coach.
"The best qualities of a practitioner are active listening, keeping an open mind, compassion
and caring, and nonattachment,"
says Christopher. "My Western
mind was very skeptical in the
beginning about some of the
concepts of Chinese medicine,
like pulse and tongue diagnosis,

yet when I started practicing, I
saw so many dramatic things on
the tongue—hepatitis C patients
or other patients with advanced
cirrhosis all had deep cracks on
the sides of their tongues—I
became a true believer." He went
to China to study more. His
advice: "Learn one system well

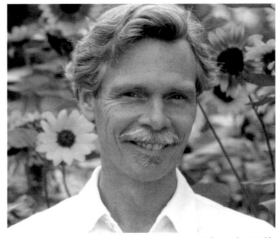

*Christopher Hobbs*

and then you can wander off
from it and let your intuition
and creative energy work their
magic. We see health and disease
more clearly when we see from
different angles."

## David Hoffmann

David Hoffmann trained at the
National Institute of Medical
Herbalists in Britain, where he
has been a member since 1979.
He started his herbal practice in
Wales, then he moved to the
Findhorn community in Scot-
land. He has been practicing in
California since. The inaugural
president of the American

Herbalists Guild, David has written numerous highly regarded books, including *The Holistic Herbal, An Elder's Herbal,* and *The Herbal Handbook.*

Highly trained and steeped in a medical approach to phytotherapy, David is also one of the heralds of Earth-centered herbalism. He integrates detailed scientific information and much empirical knowledge into his teaching, yet he stands out particularly for emphasizing our relationship with Gaia, the living Earth. "The use of herbs touches us in an experience of the green," writes David. "The medieval herbalist and mystic Hildegard von Bingen talks of *viriditas,* the greening power. The healing offered so abundantly and freely by the plant kingdom is indeed a greening of the human condition, pointing to the reality of a new springtime. The health

*David Hoffmann*

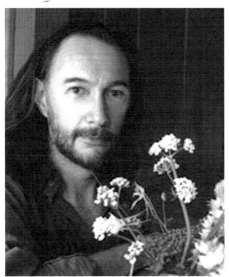

of Earth and our relationship to her is directly connected to our own lives and health."

This affable Welshman knows quite clearly where the valuable lessons are to be found in herbal medicine: "The most important herbal information you'll ever get is your own experience."

## Rosemary Gladstar

The tradition of the healing herbs was handed down to Rosemary Gladstar from her Armenian grandmother. Rosemary is a woman deeply connected to Earth. Her great love of people and plants and her skillful and magical way of bringing the two together, propels American herbalism today.

Our lady of the herbs founded the California School of Herbal Studies in 1977, teaching and inspiring many students over a ten-year period. *The Science and Art of Herbology* (her home study course) seems to be a starting point for many of us on the herbal path. We cannot imagine an herbal library without her book *Herbal Healing for Women.* She continues to teach at her home at Sage Mountain in Vermont, offering both apprentice courses and advanced programs that honor the wisdom of our ancestors while blending in holistic insight.

Rosemary has set the standard for all present-day conferences. From the first herbal gathering in 1974 that evolved into Breiten-

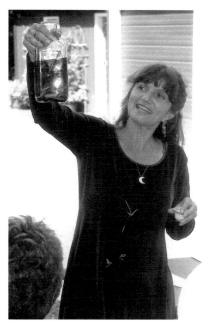

*Rosemary Gladstar*

bush, to the annual Women's Herb Conference in New England and the International Herb Symposium, this woman has brought us together. One place or another, you'll soon be embracing her incredible spirit.

Rosemary became concerned about the potential demise of the medicinal wild plant populations in North America. She realized she and her peers were partly responsible for the resurgence of the use of herbs. She took action and founded an organization that focuses on the long-term conservation of medicinal plants. Under her direction, United Plant Savers (see page 307) is currently making a positive impact on the herbal community as well as on the herb industry. "We've made tremendous inroads these past thirty years," says Rosemary. "Thousands of people are working in quiet ways

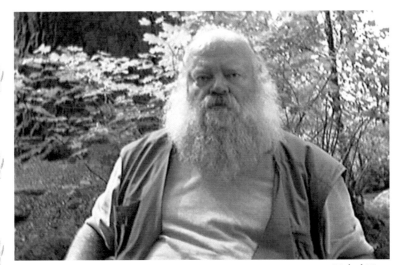

*Michael Moore*

for their families and communities. All this now depends on our learning to preserve our precious plant resources."

## Michael Moore

The grandfather of the contemporary herbal movement, Michael Moore has been an herbalist since 1968, plying his trade as merchant, picker, therapist, teacher, and writer. His universally respected books include *Medicinal Plants of the Mountain West, Medicinal Plants of the Desert and Canyon West,* and *Medicinal Plants of the Pacific West.* A depth of information flows from this marvelously eccentric character—spiraling out in a vortex of spontaneity in a lecture, or illuminating his point his point in a practical, down-to-earth manner on the written page. Michael founded and has directed the Southwest School of Botanical Medicine for more

than twenty years. He now offers a five-month residency in Bisbee, Arizona. This rigorous training program for herbalists fills rapidly each year. The focus is on the plants, and includes four weeks of field trips into widely varying ecosystems.

The school catalog reads: "Using whole plants (herbology) or constituents (phytopharmacy/pharmacognosy) has always been a primary or secondary part of medicine. If you start with the clinical observations of the older Eclectic, Physio-Medicalist, and Homeopathic physicians, mix them with the uses to be found among traditional peoples, integrate those with current knowledge about human physiology, and toss in the accepted medical uses of plants in Europe and Asia, as well as current Naturopathy and British Medical Herbalism, you can end up with a solid body of

knowledge. The pharmacology and therapeutic implications of herb use are well understood, and the methods for their preparation and extraction has long been a part of standard pharmacy. All you need is a way to learn these things."

Generosity bespeaks good in any person. You'll strike gold checking out Michael Moore's Web site at http://chili.rt66/hrbmoore/homepage to access all sorts of herbal information, including all his teaching manuals, classic works in botanical medicine from the Eclectic literature, more than 1,700 photographs of medicinal plants, and all sorts of research abstracts. This old bear sets the Internet standard for what individuals can accomplish for everyone's collective benefit.

## Susun Weed

Susun Weed speaks for the Wise Woman tradition: "We don't treat diseases. We don't have herbs that counter diseases. We have herbs that nourish the wholeness and flexibility of each unique being."

Susun has been living the simple life for more than thirty years as an herbalist, goat keeper, homesteader, and feminist. She has influenced millions of women to attain better health and empower themselves. Her four books—*Healing Wise; Menopausal Years the Wise Woman*

*Way; Breast Cancer? Breast Health! The Wise Woman Way;* and *Wise Woman Herbal for the Childbearing Year*—are a must for anyone interested in herbs, health, and healing. Her "Six Steps to Healing" is an invaluable framework for making wise choices on the path toward wellness.

Expect to get your cage rattled when Susun Weed presents her intriguing point of view! Susun teaches internationally. Her day-long and weekend workshops at the Wise Woman Center in Wood-stock, New York, launch people into new ways of being. She also offers on- and off-campus apprenticeships and correspondence courses. Training in the shamanic arts with this self-proclaimed green witch encompasses hands-on herbal medicines, moon lodges, trances, magical plants, ceremonies, Goddess archetypes, and

other avenues for developing Earth-based personal power and ceremony.

"Herbal medicine belongs to everyone. No licenses are needed or wanted. I am excited to see M.D.s becoming comfortable with herbs, but what really thrills me are three-year-olds putting plantain on their boo-boos. That," says Susun, "is the revolution."

## Michael Tierra

One of our most dog-eared reference books is *The Way of Herbs,* written by Michael Tierra. Its pocket size makes it just right for travel. Michael integrates herbal wisdom from many traditions.

Michael has traveled through India and China and has lived with Native Americans to learn the secrets of herbology. He has further advanced his own medical wisdom by obtaining degrees in naturopathy and acupuncture and has more than twenty-five years of clinical experience. His books and teachings have helped to infuse present-day Western herbalism with Traditional Chinese Medicine techniques and philosophies. Some of his other internationally acclaimed books include *The Way of Chinese Herbs* and *Planetary Herbology. Chinese Traditional Herbal Medicine,* coauthored with his wife Lesley, covers diagnosis, the Chinese materia medica, and specific treatment of diseases. Through East-West Herbology he offers correspondence courses for both the

home herbalist and the professional consultant. A yearly spring seminar at the Tierra's clinic in Santa Cruz, California, gives students a week of hands-on herbal practice with them and guest teachers.

A founding member of the American Herbalists Guild, Michael continues to be a strong

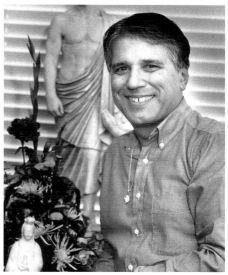
*Michael Tierra*

advocate for establishing professional standards. This is his advice for someone just entering the field of herbalism: "Don't enter it for the money! Herbalism is a sacred art that goes far beyond knowing constituents, pathology, and contraindications. Embarking on the path of an herbalist for me—and for the best herbalists and students who I know—is a calling rather than a profession. If one focuses on one's life passion and purpose, money and all good will come as a result." ✆

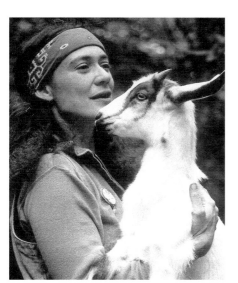
*Susun Weed*

Not all mentors necessarily teach us the lessons we may expect initially. Joyce Wardwell had a wonderful teacher, one of those who teaches by doing a horrid job. "She took on the role of being everyone's expert, everyone's guru, so to speak," remembers Joyce. "Instead of learning to empower ourselves, we were expected to go back to this very well-respected herbalist for each step. Most students would do this unquestioning. If there was a problem or a complication when they were taking the herbs, like feeling bloated, they would just continue on, figuring she knows what is best." That message—"she knows, I don't"—obviously struck a chord in Joyce, who now actively encourages self-reliance in others.

Naava Koenigsberg, who works at Bear Creek Herbs in Silver City, New Mexico, is a shining example of a community herbalist. "When I was searching for the right teacher, I thought some of the herbalists with big reputations were a bit intimidating. I was looking for someone I could relate to. Someone that wasn't larger than life. I wanted to study with someone I could look at and think, *I could be that person, I could learn to do what they do*. Naava ended up studying with Pam Montgomery, whom she loved dearly. "The focus of my apprenticeship with Pam was on each herb and getting to know them in depth."

Choosing a mentor basically comes down to the law of attraction in most instances. We attract to ourselves that which is like ourselves. How we really feel deep inside determines what kind of experience we are likely to attract to ourselves. Each and every day, energy is in the air to make of that what we will.

## HERB SCHOOL

The rich experience of being a full-time student can be embraced at any point in life.

Herb schools attract students of all ages who are eager to learn about plant medicine. Young idealists on an Earth path meet up with seniors who have discovered only recently their gypsy passion for plant ways. Others raise their kids, patiently awaiting that year when finally some directed time for their own education fits the family agenda. Practicing herbalists and medical professionals have been known to take an educational sabbatical when in-depth studies will lift them to a fuller perspective. The choice of good herb schools somewhat parallels this wide-ranging student body. The experience you want to find exists, but plan to put some serious effort into evaluating the numerous choices.

Start by asking yourself, "What do I want to do with this education?" There are a number of paths to become a community herbalist. An introductory course in herbalism may be all one needs to work in a health food store and give people broad advice. Growers and medicine makers don't necessarily require full training in therapeutics but they absolutely do need to know the plants. Consulting herbalists must understand the nature of all sorts of disease and constitutional protocols. For those who envision interacting in an integrative medical clinic, an actual degree of some sort may be needed to establish professional acceptance.

Most people equate an investment in schooling with a degree. Our culture tends to make such blunt distinctions, as if the college degree has more relevant value than the education itself. North American herbalism, with its roots in folklore and a growing desire to find approval within today's medical constructs, has only recently been able to offer an accredited graduate degree program for herbalists. The Tai Sophia Institute in Maryland offers a

Masters of Arts in Botanical Healing that requires approximately twenty-seven months to complete. Herbal students who want an accredited degree have three other options: (1) going abroad either to the College of Phytotherapy in East Sussex (where many noteworthy British medical herbalists received their licensed training) or to the International College of Herbal Medicine in New Zealand; (2) self-designing a degree program under the auspices of a progressive university that will recognize the validity of certified study by correspondence or through a more traditional herb school; and (3) pursuing an adjunct degree in herbalism from a naturopathic university such as Bastyr in Seattle. Accredited programs either require that basic college course work be completed before entrance, or they offer English, biology, and chemistry courses in conjunction with herbal studies.

There is a notion that letters following one's name presumably assists people looking for an herbalist who they can trust to be qualified. We appreciate both sides of the ongoing debate (see page 23) in the herbal community. Professional membership in the American Herbalists Guild serves just as well as a college degree for numerous herbalists who see lettered distinction as helpful to their clients and their employment prospects. Acceptance into the Guild means you have met certain standards and thus the AHG designation can follow your name. Quite frankly, such peer recognition may well hold more meaning than the achievement of a university degree in herbalism, as both clinical experience and a living relationship with the plants mark this accomplishment. Each herbalist must decide for him- or herself which kind of accreditation to pursue. The Guild suggests that students acquire 1,200 hours of education apportioned among the

basic sciences (200), materia medica/therapeutic herbalism (400), herbal pharmacy (80), plant identification and botany (60), Western herbalism (40), career preparation (20), and clinical skills (400). An additional 400 of clinical experience is recommended. The serious study represented in those 1,600 hours is a worthy goal for any aspiring herbalist.

What counts in education is embracing a wide range of knowledge and making it our own. Spirit and intuition and all the other traditional approaches to holistic healing should be explored as well. Critics of the Guild's certification requirements are right: hourly totals are beside the point. Not every herbalist needs to put a scientific emphasis on his or her experience. The underlying goal for any health care practitioner is the same: helping people feel better. Those allegorical 360 paths that lead to the center of the circle are an apt metaphor for our schooling as well. Respecting all truths allows an open mind that seeks to understand the bigger picture. So, shall we add 400 hours in "plant communication" to the above list?

An herbal education can be undertaken at home through correspondence courses. Clayton College refers to this as a "distance learning alternative," which costs less than a campus-based experience. Motivation and discipline are integral to any self-study. A student at home deserves the same dedicated time and space to pursue an education as someone who attends a school with established schedules and semesters. Teacher interaction is limited to comments on homework via telephone and e-mail, so don't expect hands-on guidance in making medicine and identifying plants. It goes without saying that diagnostic skills are best learned directly from an experienced practitioner. Some correspondence programs do include week-long practicums where home study is reinforced with direct lectures and hands-on application.

Rosemary Gladstar offers a wonderful home study course in herbalism. "The Science and Art of Herbology" insightfully guides students to listen to the plants, to make medicines, and to draw out their inner wisdom. The homework assignments that are submitted with each lesson are returned promptly with encouraging commentary.

The EastWest School of Herbology with Michael and Leslie Tierra integrates both Traditional Chinese Medicine and a Western perspective into their basic course. Students have the option of continuing with the professional herbalist course, which features an extensive global materia medica and clinical therapeutics for specific diseases.

More than fifty hours of videotapes feature Tieraona Low Dog in her course "Foundations in Herbal Medicine." This comprehensive study program incorporates an element of tradition along with Tieraona's fifteen years of clinical practice as a biochemist, midwife, and M.D.

The School of Natural Healing, originally founded by John Christopher, has established twenty-two levels of progressive home study that culminate in a six-day advanced seminar in Utah and a final exam.

Herbalists in Canada have both Wild Rose College and Dominion Herbal College in British Columbia to consider. Of course, anyone can go to Canada for either of these two great options. Former Wild Rose students have expressed high regard for Terry Willard who teaches there. Credits toward an herbalist diploma here can be earned through a combination of correspondence work and class-room courses. The college's correspondence course in phytopharmacy for health care profession-

als who are already familiar with basic human anatomy, physiology, and pharmacology provides a thorough grounding in Earth medicines.

Dominion Herbal College was founded in 1926 when Dr. Herbert Nowell brought his knowledge of botanical medicine back to the people. The basic course reflects the use of herbal medicine as practiced by natives, Thompsonians, and Eclectics. A four-year tutorial in clinical herbal therapy from Dominion combines this excellent home study program with an annual summer seminar and 500 hours of supervised clinical training in either Vancouver or Toronto.

Some of us thirst for the chance to break away for a bit to study intensively. College students take such focused time for granted (remember those wild days?), often without realizing how precious it is to be free to learn about a deep passion. But then, heeding an inner call is entirely different from training for a profession. The California Herb School offers a campus setting and a devoted staff of herbalist-teachers. Guest faculty here includes internationally known herbalists as well.

Those who want lectures in the field will enjoy five intense months with Michael Moore at the Southwest School of Botanical Medicine. The botanical and constitutional emphasis here is second to none.

At his Northeast School of Botanical Medicine, 7Song offers a similar focus. Time with the plants should be a given in any good herb school.

The educational experience you are looking for exists. The American Herbalists Guild has assembled a comprehensive *Directory of Herbal Education,* which is well worth checking out. Search the listing of herb schools at the Herbal Hall Web site, and you'll immediately be struck by how varied the options are. How about aromatherapy summer school in Provence, France, during the height of the lavender flowering season, just as harvesting begins? The Australasian College of Herbal Studies offers this opportunity. Whether you undertake learning from a distance, can only get away for the occasional weekend, or really want to dedicate months at a time to clinical learning and botany field trips, the right teachers and schools await you.

## GATHERING OF THE CLANS

Conferences are an excellent way to enjoy an extended weekend learning about all aspects of herbal medicine. Many respected herbalists teach at these gatherings, often presenting two or three workshops apiece. Topics range from home herbalist basics and plant identification walks to advanced clinical application of herbs and therapeutic intensives . . . the hardest part of these events always comes down to choosing which classes to attend! Gatherings recharge us with all the good energy you'd expect to find when folks smitten with the green world come together to celebrate herbal wisdom.

We have numerous choices of herb conferences throughout the year. More events seem to be announced each year, reflecting the burgeoning interest in natural health and Earth connection. The better-known gatherings draw five hundred to a thousand incredibly focused attendees intent on furthering their herbal knowledge. Such learning opportunities have their roots at the Rainbow End Ranch in Sonoma County, California, where fifty or so people gathered in the mid-1970s to hear from four teachers who had each discovered their own herbal way. The cost of that weekend was

$25 and included food, lodging, and all classes. These were "happening" times and the gathering grew quickly, eventually moving to Breitenbush Hot Springs in Oregon's Cascade Mountains in 1984. Herbalists continue to meet at Breitenbush today, soaking in the hot mineral springs and enjoying thousands of acres of wilderness at what can easily be called the most relaxing herbal mecca around.

Gatherings become known for particular focal points. Medicines from the Earth, sponsored by Gaia Herbs, is held each spring in the mountains outside of Asheville, North Carolina. It tends to be clinically focused, and an equal number of naturopathic doctors and herbalists teach at this event. In late summer the Women's Herbal Conference calls women forth to share the wisdom of the plants and natural healing methods at a retreat center in southern New Hampshire. Green Nations comes together in the Catskill Mountains of New York each September to embrace connection with plant spirit and the teachings of tradition. The growing conference sponsored by the Richter Herb folks in Toronto, Ontario, provides farmers with a strong medicinal focus while the earth rests beneath the snow. Herbs from the desert bioregion come to the fore at the Southwest Conference on Botanical Medicine in Tempe, Arizona, where continuing education credits are approved for nurses, acupuncturists, and pharmacists.

The chance to study with well-known teachers (albeit briefly) certainly plays a big part in bringing herbalists to gatherings. Here we can touch on their wisdom, sense their healing energy, and perhaps consider the possibility of further study with a mentor-now-revealed. Not every worthy teacher is available for public speaking, but

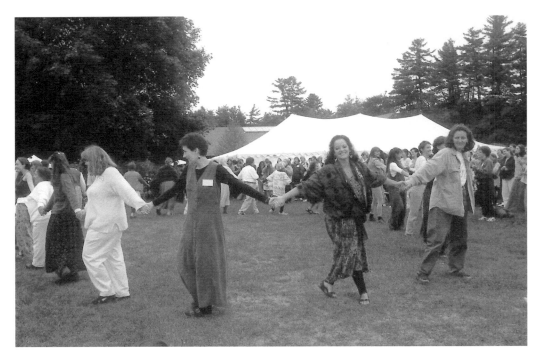

*Herbal gatherings such as the Women's Conference held each year in southern New Hampshire celebrate those precious relationships we share with the plants and each other.*

many are. Some travel from coast to coast on the herbal circuit; others choose to favor home ground. Traveling farther afield to attend a conference introduces us to a wider array of inspiring individuals. Northwest Herb Fest in Oregon regularly hosts many excellent teachers who don't usually leave their bioregion for East Coast events. Similarly, the International Herb Symposium (held every few years on the campus of Wheaton College in Norton, Massachusetts) gives herbalists from other cultures a chance to share their knowledge with aspiring American herbalists.

The largest gathering of all brings teachers from both coasts to the cornfields of Iowa. HerbFest draws families from throughout the Midwest to the home farm of Frontier Herbs each August. The boisterous enthusiasm of this gathering reflects an eagerness to learn what the healing plants of the prairie have to offer. HerbFest focuses equally well on celebration—from the powwow dance around a big bonfire to the

pulsating rhythms of reggae and nighttime volleyball. If it sounds incongruous but absolutely delightful, you'll understand why some refer to this festival as HerbStock. Frontier Herbs delights in bringing its customers in for three days of fun combined with in-depth learning. The research farm features a 22-acre tall-grass prairie habitat where native species grow in amazing diversity, as well as cultivated plantings of more than three hundred species of medicinal herbs. Frontier also hosts educational field days for potential commercial growers at other times of the year.

Regional gatherings tend to be more intimate and offer the best opportunity to meet herbal peers from nearby communities. Montana, Cape Cod, and Maine are now several years into their respective events. Panel discussions allow local herbalists to interact with nationally known teachers who hail from that same bioregion. What an opportunity to focus on local plants and regional health concerns! Medicine makers and herb growers get good exposure to their primary market by offering their products and crops at these assemblies. Get-togethers of regional herb groups offer similar educational and marketing opportunities. "No one is in teaching mode [at NEHA's annual meeting] so everyone is equal," says Mary Pat Palmer of the Northeast Herb Association, "which one doesn't always feel at the big conferences."

United Plant Savers hosts a variety of inspiring conferences throughout the country in collaboration with regional groups. The theme at these plant-focused sessions is vitally important: The cultivation and preservation of native medicinal plants involves us all. The teachers at these confer-

ences generously donate their time, and all proceeds from these events go directly to support the work of United Plant Savers. The Appalachian Herb Gathering in southeastern Ohio, for example, offers seminar tracks on farm development and management, sustainable forestry, tours of both the UpS Botanical Sanctuary and the neighboring National Center for the Preservation of Medicinal Herbs, herb growing, and using herbs in an Earth-connected way.

### THE LEARNING NEVER STOPS

Experience will always be our ultimate teacher. Reaching greater depths in herbal knowledge involves seeking out further education, openness to lessons the plants

# CONTACTS FOR HERB GATHERINGS

**American Herbalists Guild Symposium**
1931 Gaddis Road
Canton, GA 30115
770-751-6021
www.americanherbalistsguild.com

**Breitenbush Hot Springs Herbal Conference**
c/o Tracy Bosnian
503-236-0473
www.trilliumeducation.org

**Green Nations Gathering**
c/o Pam Montgomery
1525 Danby Mountain Road
Danby, VT 05739
www.greennations.org

**Herb Fest**
Frontier Natural Products Co-op
P.O. Box 299
Norway, IA 52318
800-669-3275
www.frontiercoop.com/about/herbfest/herbfest.html

**International Herb Symposium**
and **Women's Herbal Conference**
c/o Sage Mountain
P.O. Box 420
E. Barre, VT 05649
802-479-9825

**Northwest Herb Fest**
c/o Wise Woman Herbals
P.O. Box 279
Creswell, OR 97426
800-476-6518

**Southwest Conference on Botanical Medicine** (Arizona) and **Medicines from the Earth** (North Carolina)
Herbal Educational Services
P.O. Box 3427
Ashland, OR 97520
800-252-0688
www.botanicalmedicine.org

**United Plant Savers Conferences**
UpS
P.O. Box 400
E. Barre, VT 05649
www.unitedplantsavers.org

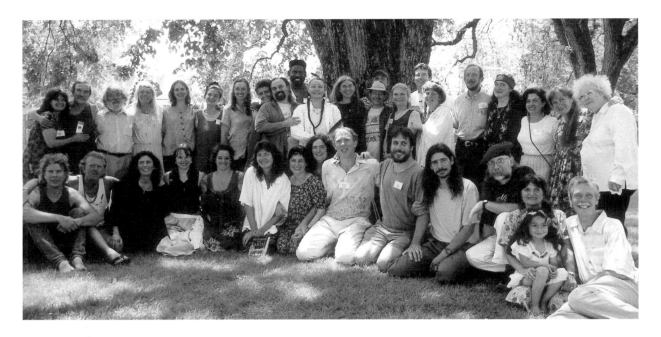

The teachers at the 2000 International Herb Symposium represent a broad cross-section of herbal wisdom, even if Matthew Wood showed up too late to be included in this picture.

and your clients offer, and maintaining a humble heart filled with universal awe.

We add to our herbal repertoire by getting to know each plant in our personal pharmacopoeia well. Really well. "The woman I studied with for twelve years told me to try to learn one plant a year and no more," points out Ryan Drum. "Otherwise you tend to just get confused." Learning everything we can about one plant at a time from both a scientific viewpoint and an experiential viewpoint—especially the experiential viewpoint—is refreshing. It does not need to be directed intellectually. The right plant seems to jump into our herbal laps saying "Here I am" when the time comes.

"This is the year of the thistle," says Ryan, who is well known for exploring the nuance of each herb he gathers. "We've been introduced before and had a few dances, but haven't been intimate. I'm going to have a committed relationship to the bull thistle, the biennial thistle. It's such a nasty plant superficially, but underneath it's tender and scrumptious, therapeutic, nutritive,

and giving. It knows it has to be tough for it only has two years alive. The seeds are eaten by the goldfinches: This spiny plant essentially turns into these beautiful black and gold birds. Seeing these birds is heartening, just like the bull thistle is particularly good for the heart. I expect spirit will provide even more therapeutic opportunity. I'm getting the message that it's the live plant whole that's important, which means peeling off the spines very carefully and eating it as a fresh green. And juicing it in a wheatgrass juicer and drinking that juice to feel its vibrancy."

An herbalist just starting out should not be too quick to give up the idea of a traditional apprenticeship. School settings can be both intensive and extensive, but they don't necessarily cater to an individual pace. Developing a personal relationship with a mentor happens over a longer period of time. The everyday becomes the classroom where reality doesn't get any more real. Taking time for long-term learning may not be as difficult as the financial vagaries of modern-day life seem to insist. Ultimately, what we have and what we pursue are choices we make. A determined will can always find a way to let the heart lead.

A Traditional Chinese Medicine education follows four to six years of schooling with two to eight years of clinical tutelage with a senior practitioner. The older doctor diagnoses patients and composes a traditional prescription while the doctor-in-training watches and writes down the prescription. Medical school attempts to do the same with a residency program for physician graduates to learn their profession under the watchful eyes of an experienced doctor. Naturopaths refer to this period as a *preceptorship*. Herbalists often lack this critical exposure to clinical practice. This weak link in our educational paths, thankfully, is becoming easier to put right.

Real learning in medicine and healing comes by doing. We have lacked experts to train us as herbal clinicians for the last generation or two simply because botanical healing has not been promoted in our culture since the turn of the twentieth century. Watching clinical herbalists at work—conducting patient interviews, performing physical examinations, explaining differential analysis of symptoms and signs, formulating/prescribing/dispensing herbal medicines, and following up cases—teaches us far more than reading books and attending lectures. Taking a turn under the guidance of experience allows students to stretch their herbal wings while getting vital feedback on the spot. Assessing disease in people and determining a therapeutic course of action from a holistic perspective is a skill best learned under direct supervision.

The highly respected clinical herbalists, Donald Yance and Chanchal Cabrera, have teamed up to offer a week-long advanced practicum to provide students with exactly this opportunity. Each patient is scheduled for a two-hour appointment, allowing plenty of time for discussion and detailed consideration. Students take turns conducting the client interview while the others observe. After discussion and agreement on the optimal treatment protocol, the patient returns to the consulting room to hear about the conclusions, options, and expectations. On some occasions, Donald or Chanchal will conduct the patient interview to demonstrate intake techniques and style. Other herbalists have also begun to offer similar clinical guidance in their programs, a few of which we point out in chapter 8.

Wouldn't it be absolutely smashing if such extraordinary opportunities became ordinary? The integrative medicine being promoted today suggests that holistic-minded doctors can and should work with clinical herbalists, naturopaths, midwives, acupuncturists, and so forth. People then choose the kind of health care that best suits them as personally responsible individuals. Extending this open-mindedness back to the practitioners themselves creates an integrative opportunity for clinical training. New practitioners and community herbalists alike could participate in any local medical center to learn about interacting with patients *and* an array of health care providers. Community-wide healing can happen when we stop being rigid about professions, competitive advantage, and pocketbooks.

We must remember one thing—

Project Projimo fosters the use of indigenous healing methods in poor villages in Mexico, where no modern doctors practice. One healer in Ajoya, a man named Martín, sums up his training: "I learned [folk medicine] here and there, but mostly by treating people every day, and every day you learn something. It's a lie, whoever says, 'I know how to do it.' There's always something else to learn. Every day one has to learn by trying different methods of how to cure the people more actively. You can learn things in hospitals, schools, everywhere, but the best school is practice."[5]

## NOTES

1. Doug Elliot, *Wildwoods Wisdom: Encounters with the Natural World* (New York: Paragon House, 1992).

2. One of Susun Weed's correspondence courses is based on intimately getting to know one plant throughout a full year.

3. This author distributes her work directly at a price of $25 plus $9 for shipping (U.S. postal money order, please). Contact Gilian Painter, 651 West Coast Road, Oratia, Auckland, New Zealand.

4. Dr. Weiss's book was revised in September 2000 by V. Fintelmann, M.D., the former chairman of the German Commission E. The reworking of a classic text in order to promote a pharmaceutical agenda is wrong. *Herbal Medicine* is worth reading only if you can find the original edition.

5. Robert and Michèle Root-Bernstein, *Honey, Mud, Maggots, and Other Medical Marvels:* (Boston: Houghton Mifflin, 1997), 43.

# CHAPTER FOUR
# *Considering Your Niche*

ELDERBERRY
*Sambucus* spp.

My friend Lynn, a former student and a blossoming young herbalist, just called to share her joy with me. She has signed papers to buy some land. She's happy about being able to sink her roots into a beautiful, isolated, woodland spot and become a homesteader herbalist. Excited as she may be, she's also in a big dither and more than a bit overwhelmed. "I have resolved that I can't put in a garden this year," says Lynn. "There just won't be time. I have to keep my teaching job and my waitressing job to be able to afford to build my house. I want to pay as I go and not go into more debt. I have been trying to teach herbal classes in my area, but sometimes nobody shows up, or I get about three people. I should be designing and printing new labels for my products and writing up a new brochure, but I just can't keep up with everything. I need to spend more time with the plants getting to know them, and also I need to meditate more. I am hoping to take some more classes this year and go to some good conferences. Which ones do you think are really the best? I can't afford all the ones I'd like to go to. I just don't know about charging people for herbal rec-ommendations or even for my tinctures. I usually just give them away. But I really want to be an herbalist." ℘ We all have our dilemmas. We can't do it all: grow our own herbs and market them, too; teach classes; make and sell medicines; do consultations; continue our education; keep harmony in our personal relationships; and stay connected to the plant and spirit world. Each of us needs to find our special gifts and focus on those. Trying to do too many things doesn't work. The goal is to find out what we really love and are good at—and then to pursue honorable and effective ways to do these to make a right livelihood—N.P. ℘

MAKING A LIVING depends on a complexity of choices. Each of us has particular talents that animate our inner being. Recognizing one's skills and desires, and matching these to a viable herbal livelihood, is the way to find one's niche. We will find plenty of people who can benefit from what we have to share about plant medicine.

We promote our niche by how we identify ourselves to our community. A wide-ranging array of words defines herbal practice. Anyone who honors the plants and has an innate desire to understand and share their healing properties is an herbalist. A tradition rooted in centuries of human experience certainly includes everyone who cares about this Earth-based approach to health. Using the term *herbalist* does not, however, indicate an individual's abilities as a healer. Herbalists who call themselves master herbalists or clinical herbalists or certified herbalists or medical herbalists understandably are seeking to do just that. Discerning the nuances of the clarifiers (as we tried to do in chapter I) may allow the herbal community to reach consensus as to what these terms can reliably mean. Still, as we each seek to proclaim our herbal niche, we must do so with an honest assessment of our abilities. Some of the best herbalists choose no adjectives at all. Other healers that these distinctions are both important personally and useful to the communities they serve. Good intent comes with either point of view.

## HEAL THYSELF

Naturally enough, people expect that herbalists are going to be hale and hearty, bright-eyed and cheerful. They must have a strong sense of inner knowledge and peace, right? We are the folks who commune with plant spirits, after all, with every remedy at hand for each possible idiosyncrasy of our own dis-ease. The advice we offer again and again centers on being attuned to mind, body, and spirit. We know how to find balance. Most certainly we eat right, exercise regularly, and earnestly tend to our relationships. Right? We do have stellar immune systems, don't we?

Meeting our own expectations can be a struggle. Breaking a lifetime of patterns can be hard even when we know better. Living each day with healthy resolve takes effort. The holistic pathway begins with a personal encounter with ourselves. *Physician, heal thyself* doesn't necessarily mean we achieve every good intention; it means that we go through the very same processes as every human being on the path toward wholeness. Compassion flows from having been sick ourselves. Strength can be shared when we have weathered our own storms. We face personal frustration, embarrassment, and pettiness, knowing damn well that healing is about moving beyond our shortcomings. If we can't forgive, how can we ask others to forgive? Life humbles us so we can offer the spark of love deep within our hearts without fear. The mark of a healer goes beyond his or her knowledge of herbal facts. The journey begins with accepting oneself.

Many of us start out intending to help our families, but the first recipient of this help is always oneself. As herb students, we learn to make tea, to taste tinctures, and to apply a soothing poultice. As we come to understand what a good diet is, we can incorporate changes in our own eating habits. We listen to wise teachers who share their holistic insights while our inner dialogue digests each lesson in a personal way. The plants always welcome us home regardless of how far away we've been. A passion is kindled deep in our souls like a sapling that begins to reach for the sun. Growing strong heartwood now assures that someday the tree will shelter family, friends, and community.

The process of self-care—relaxation, meditation, nutrition, and exercise—is a sacrament. We enable our innate abilities to heal by honoring our bodies, minds, and spirits. The gift of being able to help someone else become empowered proceeds from our own ability to do the same for ourselves. Walking in balance ensures that we will have the enormous energy and attentiveness to share with others who seek plant wisdom and personal guidance. There are times to heal and times to be healed, just as there are times to love and times to be loved.

Eventually we will come to see our own illnesses and down times as opportunities. Symptoms are messages from our bodies that perhaps the whole is not as we perceive—or insist—it to be. We need to listen and take such messages to heart. "Healing thyself" also means giving ourselves a break when the good work of helping others becomes a burden. We need to slow down. Breathe deep. Understand. Be. This is the place where healing starts.

## WALKING IN BALANCE

These days of the new millennium readily fill with commitments and urgency. Herbalists with a pulse on the rhythms of Mother Earth would seemingly have a handle on joyful balance. Yet the call for help is vast, and we can lose that vital sense of self by becoming overwhelmed. Here are some dependable tips shared by practitioners who have learned how to lessen that inevitable risk of burning out.

"The number one, most important thing for me in keeping balanced is to

*Those who dwell . . . among the beauties and mysteries of life are never alone or weary of life. Those who contemplate the beauty of earth find reserves of strength that will endure as long as life lasts.*

—Rachel Carson, *The Sense of Wonder,* 1965

have alone time," says Rosemary Gladstar. "Deep, alone time. Time alone in Nature where I can shut the chatter off. I don't need long periods, like months or years. Though that probably was the most influential time in my life in becoming who I am, when I had those long months by myself in the woods. Being alone restores me more than anything. More than good food, more than spiritual teachings." Rosemary recounts how she had been doing a vision quest every year. Spending four days and four nights alone on a mountain, without food or water, can open doors to the essence of oneself. "I never had big visions. I never saw bear spirit come or eagle spirit come. Vision quests," says our herbal mentor, "are mostly about restoration for me, for being quiet."

Many of us get a continuous lease on life doing what we do. Healing work can fill as well as empty us. "Reaching out to another to help her heal and connect with her spirituality also helps me heal and connect with mine," says Dr. Christiane Northrup in her extraordinary book, *Women's Bodies, Women's Wisdom.*[1] The truth is that the advice we proffer might apply on the home front as well. Sometimes what we need the most is exactly what we advise for others.

Spending time with the plants—growing, harvesting, or meditating—takes us to our source. Time with Mother Earth is healing. Working in the garden can be as restorative as a walk in the woods. Nancy's

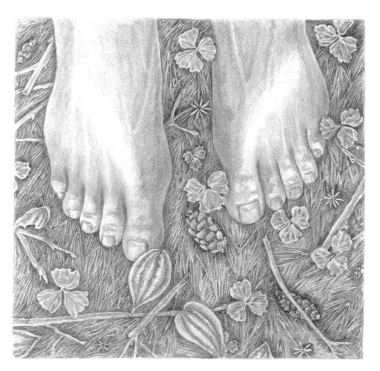

*Connecting with the Earth Mother means simply being and giving thanks for the life that surrounds us.*

ideal morning starts with a dawn walk through our fields and along the brook to her special place. "The Sisters" are an encircling grove of fir, spruce, and pine trees that offer their peaceful embrace in any season of the year. A luxurious layer of needles and mosses covers the forest floor. Staring up through the branches into a blue sky and lets the spirit soar. We love going on family canoe trips for that very reason. Out beneath the blue sky, paddling on a lake or lazily drifting with the current, we again come to feel a part of the real world.

The spirit of the plants shines provided that we get out to visit them now and then. "You miss that nourishment if you are not out walking with the plants," says Phyllis Light in Alabama. "Last year I let myself get too busy seeing people and teaching, but this year I am getting out more. Even if it's just going out behind the house and lying on the ground to feel the Earth energy. Or getting out with the kids and letting them

run in the woods while I lag behind. The plants sing to me, and I, in turn, find a much deeper connection for myself."

We can bring a sense of the sacred into everyday life. "My tendency over the years," says Pam Montgomery of the Partner Earth Education Center in Vermont, "has been to do simpler ceremonies on a more daily basis. Every morning I take my cup out to the spring by our stream to drink its sweet water and give thanks for the day. I include ritual in my daily life the same way I include wild foods. It has become a part of who I am instead of a special occasion. Wanting to be in that conscious place has become a part of my daily walk."

"I do ceremony regularly as a Cherokee medicine priest. Evoking the spirit certainly gives me a sense of renewal," says David Winston. The sweat lodge has long been revered by Native Americans as the womb of Mother Earth. The sacred fire, the sacred stones, the sacred dark all give of themselves in birthing us anew. Creating ceremony around the turning of the seasons keeps us in touch with Earth rhythms and strengthens us for change. Coming together in spirit creates magic no matter what our religious path.

Practical solutions to going about busy days help keep balance, too. Bartering our skills in exchange for work help gets more things done than if we attended to every detail ourselves. "I have people clean my house, help me with the gardens, set up for classes, and put out posters and flyers," says Jane Bothwell. "I pay $7 an hour for work trading. They might work in the garden for three hours, so that is $21 toward whatever class they are interested in. I am pretty selective, but I really appreciate what people are doing to help me," says Jane. "And they really appreciate it too, because they are able to take a class. It works best if you have a regular time, like Mondays from nine o'clock to noon, instead of just whenever they have time to drop in."

Being a parent is a high calling in itself. Time to be together as a family can get waylaid easily by herbal doings unless we carefully tend to making it a priority. "I learned to say to people, you can stop by at these times, which works better than saying stop by anytime. This is when I'm available. It is a challenge to balance your practice with being a mom," says Kate Gilday. "You ask yourself, 'Am I abandoning my kids?' The times we are together have become more meaningful because another part of me is also being fed."

Rest is essential for all of us. The centered-within time of winter is part of

*Text continues on page 114.*

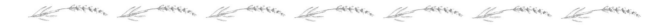

# FLOWER ESSENCES

Herbalists around the world are incorporating flower essences into their health care practices. Though sometimes confused with herbal tinctures, they are not the same thing. Flower essences are highly diluted with springwater, and a small percentage of brandy is used as a preservative. Yet many people have had tremendous impacts on their lives using them.

The essences work in an energetic way to effect emotional and spiritual well-being. They are completely mild and can complement many other healing modalities. You can buy prepared essences, or you can make your own. The one most commonly used is Rescue Remedy. It is a combination of five essences developed by Dr. Edward Bach in the 1930s to treat trauma and extreme stress.

Making the essences is relatively easy. Here are abbreviated instructions:

Fill a clean glass bowl with fresh springwater. Go out on a beautiful sunny day. Either choose a flower in bloom or let it choose you. Sit with the flower and meditate. Ask permission. Listen. Then, using scissors or two stems from the flowering plant, pick enough blossoms to nearly cover the bowl. Leave the flowers uncovered in the sun to infuse, using your inner guidance to determine how long. Use a twig or leaf from the plant to remove the flowers from the water. Offer your words of thanks and return some of the infused water to the plant. Use a tinted, sterilized glass jar. Fill the jar wth equal amounts of brandy and the infusion. This Mother Essence is then diluted to make a stock bottle, and the stock bottles are diluted again to make dosage bottles.

"I have found while preparing flower essences over the years that this connection with plant spirit brings me grace, balance, and joy in all that I do," says our friend Aurora, the founder of Green Angel Flower Essences. "Flower essences have helped revitalize my creative spirit. Old patterns of limiting thoughts have been shed and replaced with more healthful choices."

To learn more detailed information, we recommend the following books:

*The Healing Herbs of Edward Bach* by Julian and Martine Barnard
*The Flower Essence Repertory* by Richard Katz and Patricia Kaminski
*Flower Power* by Anne McIntyre

# Phyllis Light

My Granny and Granddaddy Light were herb walkers, and so was my cousin, Calvin, on the same side of the family," says Phyllis Light, an herbalist from Alabama. "People still come to him for herbs and he is in his seventies. People got around with mules and wagons when my grandparents were growing up. It was a long trip to the doctor, maybe several hours away, so people learned to take care of themselves. You just didn't go to the doctor unless it was very desperate, almost a life-or-death situation. . . . Everyone was very self-sufficient."

As a girl, Phyllis went along into the woods with her grandparents. The Light family gathered herbs in the spring and again in the fall. "Of course I hated it. You know how little kids are. I loved being in the woods, but I just thought it was work. My grandparents and other family got cash money wildcrafting the plants. Seng [ginseng] was the first plant I learned to gather and use. Pink root was another big one, as well as bloodroot and yellowroot. These were sold to fur trappers, who then sold them to jobbers, who then sold them to pharmaceutical companies and exporters."

The plants first sang to this herbalist-to-be in that subtle, glorious way all Earth-connected people know. Phyllis was about nineteen, out in the woods with her father, when he announced it was time she learned this craft. "We went way out where I had never been before, about four or five miles from our house, a place called Moon Holler. We walked and walked and walked. Then Daddy stopped, took his paperback Western novel out of his pants pocket, and nestled his butt up against the tree roots. He said, 'Between this rock here and that tree over there and that creek, there are six ginseng plants,' and then he started reading. I don't know if you ever looked for seng, but it's not always that easy to find. The berries weren't showing, so I didn't have that signal," remembers Phyllis. This mission was more about sensing the plant than seeing its green leaves among the equally green groundcover of summer. Gathering time would come in fall, when the red berries flag this venerable root. She walked the perimeter of the area, then back and forth, and two hours later still hadn't found any ginseng. "Daddy looked at me and said, 'You better find them so we can get home and eat dinner.' I stood there in the middle of the greenery, took a deep breath, closed my eyes, and felt the frustrated tension leave my body. I found myself disconnected to the world and just connected in to the plants. I could clearly see the seng outlined from all the other

> *I could clearly see the seng outlined from all the other plants, like in an ethereal light.*
>
> —Phyllis Light

plants, like in an ethereal light. That was really my first heart connection with a plant. It would be several years before I noticed that there were other plants in the woods and started listening to their songs just as vividly."

Phyllis had begun on that long, winding herbal path that leads many of us to our true calling. She learned about anatomy and physiology, and became certified to teach physical education. Her uncle introduced her to yellowroot. Other plants started to move into her consciousness as well. She worked in a mental health center and saw firsthand the devastating effects of psychoactive drugs. A decision to go back to college full-time at the age of thirty to study psychology—while working three part-time jobs and being a mother—set Phyllis up for a classic crash. "I totally wrecked myself. My adrenal system was exhausted. My immune system was gone. Then I was expecting another child and realized that this poor baby was hitching a ride in on a broken vehicle. I had reached a healing crisis for myself," she admits candidly .

"Spirit brought my knowledge of plants, physiology, and psychol-

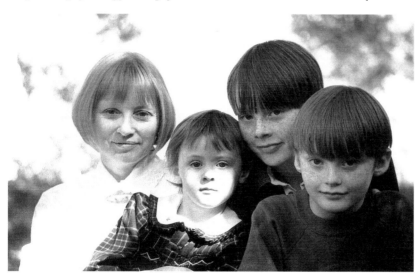

ogy together. Everything started to gel and I started to heal. I learned about dandelion and Queen Anne's lace. I started to find nettles and plantain, even though they are not easy to find in my area. Sumac is wonderful. I began talking to my cousin more and learning about the native plants. I met Tommie Bass [a well-known Appalachian herbalist] for the first time. He was

just a character and knew so many niches for each plant. I began to move past my ginseng—although I still consider it an ally—and to look past the yellowroot, even though there are a 101 uses for yellowroot. I didn't have a good library at this time. I was getting an old education and a plant education. I was working with my own health. Other people would just drive up to the house and say, 'Are you the herb lady and do you have time to talk to me?' I had the plant information and the dietary information to help them. It seemed like it was all wonderfully coordinated," smiles Phyllis. "I was making brews for all these fine people."

A brew can be made with either a single herb or a combination of herbs. This southern extraction process involves cooking the herbs until the brew is thick, not quite a soup, but thicker than a beverage. It can be sweet-

ened with honey or sugar, but now Phyllis uses licorice or violet leaf to "cut" her brews. People receive a quart jar of the brew to sip, taking a quarter cup a couple times a day, depending on their problem. Phyllis's grandmother canned her brews for a long time, until a freezer made all that canning work unnecessary.

"Now I package the herbs in muslin bags and give people directions on how to brew their own." says Phyllis. She is well aware that convenience figures into client compliance today. "People here in the Bible Belt are very hesitant to use tinctures. Putting alcohol in your body is thought to not be a good thing, even if it is medicine." She doesn't make tinctures, but will occasionally recommend them for a plant remedy not found locally. Burdock, for instance, works well for gout and ovarian cysts (combined with other herbs) and helps with the thyroid.

"I still live in the same town where I was born. People come by the house on weekends or after work, or chat with me in the grocery store or in the park about remedies. I consult two days a week in a health food store in Huntsville—people have to get on a waiting list to see me—and have an actual office in Birmingham one day a week. I also have a working relationship with a physician in a medical clinic. This takes me away from that down-home feeling, almost to where I feel I need to put on a white jacket," says Phyllis. "One day I can be doing the real folksy stuff and the next I'm using the proper medical terminology. I appreciate both, and both have their place.

"Some people need a more earthy approach and others need the more medical approach. What's important is that they listen and hear what I have to say in the way that works for them. The vocabulary changes to meet the needs of the person. Just like everybody doesn't need the same plant, why should everybody need the same vocabulary? We come from different cultural backgrounds and orientations. I have gotten comfortable with meeting some of those other needs as an herbalist and not feeling that it is diminishing something in me."

Phyllis currently directs the herbal studies program at the Clayton College of Natural Health. "Both Lloyd and Nancy Clayton, as well as the whole staff, are very dedicated to educating folks on how to take care of themselves and their families with natural remedies," says Phyllis. "But also important for me is that they honor the plants and the Earth and work hard in the environmental arena. The honoring brings it all together." ✌

---

the Creator's plan for seasonal renewal. Honoring a sabbath each week is a gift to ourselves as well as a time to nurture that precious connection with spirit. Set aside a portion of that day—a single, uninterrupted hour at least—to have no plans. Serendipity makes an excellent companion for nurturing the child within, forgetting ourselves, and letting the world meander by. Such a sabbath becomes a highlight of the week, a time to look forward to and savor amid the busyness of commitments and schedules. Being content in the moment at hand, simply being attentive to where we are, is a pleasure not to be missed.

A good night's sleep fills us with the vigor and vim to start every new day. And don't forget the gentle art of taking a nap. Adults seem to assume they've lost the right to give themselves a few moments of complete relaxation in the middle of a busy day. The herbalist Svevo Brooks offers sound advice on this score: "As children, each of us knew how to relax, and we took time to relax. We could lie down in the middle of a roomful of noisy people and go instantly to sleep. . . . Relaxation is the empty space before and after 'doing.' It is the nothingness that defines and makes possible what we do."[2] Setting a pace for yourself that embraces naptime as good time is but one of many insights Svevo shares in *The Art of Good Living*. Walking in balance involves the simple steps we can take to regain our health and our joy in life.

Certainly we need to be realistic. As herbalism becomes more popular, it's easy to think, *Gee, I'm an herbalist, I'm somebody*. Yes indeed, but so is everyone else doing the things they do. Staying in touch with our families hones that sense of reality. "They don't let you get away with much," laughs Rosemary Gladstar. "Anytime you feel you've begun to get your life together, spend time with your grown kids or go to your parents' house and spend two weeks there. Then you start to realize how much stuff you still have to work on.

"A sense of serious humor is absolutely important or else one starts thinking one is an expert at something, a problem that does occur occasionally in our herbal community, especially as we grow older," observes Rosemary. "Jeannine Parvati is always quick to point out that an 'ex' is something past, and a 'spurt' is nothing more than a dribble."

That ability to laugh and shine in the moment at hand seems to be universal among herbalists. If we are going to help others with our herbal knowledge and healing gifts, we need to have fun along the way—to dance, to drum, to sing. We are doing well when we find our work as enjoyable as our play.

## BEING OF SERVICE

Albert Schweitzer once said, "One thing I know: The only ones among you who are really happy are those who will have sought and found how to serve." Healing each other and our precious planet will always be about loving one another as we love ourselves.

Some of us feel the call to serve by being a healer. We might have a "healing gift" that we feel compelled to offer. In some traditional societies a young child was chosen as a medicine person because of certain physical characteristics or position of birth (the seventh son, for instance). These children were given special opportunities from an early age to build character and gain knowledge. In other traditions a person would find his or her calling during a vision quest in adolescence. These individuals would then work as apprentices for most of their adult lives. Some would not work independently until the elder or master died.

Our paths today are more far-flung. Sometimes those vision quests don't come until we reach a midlife crisis. For some, our learning is gradual, and rarely is it under the steady guidance of a master herbalist for an appreciable amount of time. Plant medicine somehow piques our interest and as we learn, opportunities to help others seem to come. We build our knowledge base plant by plant through personal experience. A lifetime will pass in learning all we need to meet our call. And yet, from that very first moment, we can begin to help others. The healing plants, once revealed to us, insist on being shared.

"If all you know is dandelion, but you know that you know it, then that's what you gather and tell people how to use. You can only work with what you know," says Joyce Wardwell. "When I first started, if somebody came to me and said, 'I have a fatal kidney disease, I am taking this and that,' I'd tell them, 'it sounds like you are more experienced with this than I am.' I will be very honest. I do tell people I am more than happy to research a particular disease for them and provide leads for their own research."

Making time to be there for others is one of the critical components of being a community herbalist. Amid the bustle of family and commitments to other work comes this growing reputation of being someone knowledgeable in natural ways of healing. The opportunity to serve has arrived at our door. These first encounters will not necessarily bring a financial reward. Getting to practice our skills and share treasured medicines is as much a learning venture for the new herbalist as it is for the people seeking holistic remedies. We can relish the healing relationship entirely as one of service. Such profound satisfaction should be remembered when earning a livelihood from healing work may seem to counter this precious dynamic. First and foremost, our call is to help out just because we can.

Our culture expects this of its healers. However, making ourselves available twenty-four hours a day to help anyone in distress is one sure way to burn out. "I urge anyone getting into herbalism to kill that myth," says Susun Weed emphatically. "It is very important to set your limits. That does not mean that you cannot on rare occasion extend beyond those limits. But I know dozens of people that have gone out to be the village herbalist who fall for every sob story in the book, don't charge people, and then wind up having to work some hideous job forty hours a week to support themselves. Just so they can continue to give to people who, let's face it, don't appreciate them too much.

"One of my earliest teachers said to me, 'Susun, you may give your fruit, you may give your seeds, you may give your flowers, you may give your leaves, you may give your stalk right down to the ground level, but you may never give anyone your root.'"

We need to take this apt metaphor to heart. The seeming dilemma between serving others and our personal needs should not be a stumbling block. We're each responsible for acknowledging our limits—all the more so when others don't take heed. There is no guilt in arranging for an appropriate energy exchange. Grateful thanks may be all that's needed in the beginning. But later, as we become more knowledgeable and thus able to help more people, we devote considerable chunks out of the week to healing work. That fine line of having *time enough to make a living* is likely to be crossed. Feeding the soul doesn't always put food on the table.

Building community is a process. Offering yourself to the community in ways that go beyond individual consultations is another form of service. Free herb walks introduce people to plant medicines nearby. An afternoon volunteering in the local natural foods store advising people about health options can help make your presence in the community known. An introductory course in home herbalism offered at the town library may be just the nudge needed to stir interest in more specific courses. Taking miso soup to a sick friend and pitching in to help with the chores is just plain neighborly. Kindness is an essential human act.

"I set aside a day each summer, four to six hours, for an extended herb walk with a picnic lunch of wild edibles for the community. Anyone can come for free," says Ryan Drum. "I also teach in the school at least once a year on marine biology or medicinal wild plants. The kids learn what greens would make a wild salad, what herbs to use for wasp stings and minor cuts and bruises. This is empowering, not just more esoteric information. The way to teach kids is about things that fit into their daily lives." The next generation will honor Mother Earth to the extent we teach them about her marvels. Each of us is charged with inspiring children to learn about what the plants do for our species and what we, in turn, can do for the plants.

Empowering people to effect their own cure often turns out to be the greatest service we offer. Remedies and good advice take on fuller meaning when people realize their innate capabilities to heal. "Your ultimate goal as a practitioner," says Joyce Wardwell, "is getting people to a position where they don't need you." She carries the notion of a people's medicine back to our own laps: "I would rather teach people to grow their own herbs. They don't need to rely on me. I am looking at moving away from marketing products altogether to focus on teaching, writing, and maybe some belligerent bumper stickers. We now have to explain why organic or wildcrafted herbs are better than what you can get at Wal-Mart. If I am not selling an herbal product (and thereby not pocketing the sale) the message goes home a lot faster."

There's a basic human need to feel that we are serving and making a contribution to the world in some way. As our society becomes more complex, many are losing that sense of connection. The personal touch of giving and receiving can get lost in the isolation of technology and the need to work merely to pay the bills. Conventional health care has sadly become a study in efficiency. Doctors and nurses alike have trouble finding their Hippocratic ideals in the shuffle to keep up with paperwork and the constant turnover of personnel. Making a living needs to be about fulfilling spiritual and emotional needs as well as physical ones. Satisfaction with our work comes from being able to help when someone else depends on us. Being paid is another discussion entirely.

## MAKING A LIVING

Everyone wants a good home and a pleasant life. *Trusting to the Universe* generally requires initiative on our part to bring herbal intentions to fruitful reality. Sometimes the humble need to blow their own horn.

People show appreciation for their healers in various ways. A valued member of any community should expect to be upheld and supported in that community. Indigenous societies made this far more apparent before money arrived to cloud the relationships among people. Value was based on practical worth. A sack of heirloom beans or a pair of finely stitched moccasins equaled the time spent conducting a healing sweat. A man treated by a healer's remedy might be expected, after recovering, to thatch the healer's roof in exchange. The village midwife needed help in her garden and chicken coop when birthings kept her away from home. The purpose of a healthy economy is to assure everyone's living within a commu-

*To serve is to make whole in some way. Service . . . it's more of a grace. It's very close to love, but a very pure kind of love. A befriending of the life in others, unconditionally.*

—Rachel Naomi Remen

nity. *Making a living* does not have to mean *making big bucks.* Cash is only one form of exchange.

Some contemporary herbalists think they'd like to paddle down the medical mainstream—let's shoot for the moon and claim both scientific respectability and a piece of the insurance pie—but in truth, ours is a fringe culture in North America. Holistic healing and Earth wisdom have little to do with six-figure salaries and investment futures. This is a very good thing. We have a chance to engage in some serious economic healing precisely because we do struggle to make a steady dollar. Understanding barter and in-kind payments as legitimate earnings can make a difference. Every person's work has value. Recognizing that value means being able to embrace those who lack the same dollars that we often lack. Regardless of whether an herbal consultation brings in a monetary fee or a weekly loaf of whole-grain bread, a fair transaction occurs. We can apportion value for different talents, with a sense of equal exchange. Hard labor gets granted its due from skilled finesse. Time dedicated to another has relevance. Experience should be rewarded. But all within sight of each other. Parity needs to be instilled as a guiding principle in the project of implementing a people's medicine.

"There does need to be an energy exchange, but not in a harsh way," says Ryan

Drum in a discussion about the value of an herbalist's skill and time. "Anybody needs enough to survive. If you're important enough to your community, that will happen. For a few years I didn't charge. When I reached a low point in personal economics, not having worked for a living for a long time, then I charged. I charged then the same thing I charge now, which is a dollar a minute of contact time. I don't charge for investigation time or forty-five years of serious preparation. I do charge for contact time when people are basically consuming my consciousness."

Ryan came to understand payment-in-kind on his island home off the coast of Washington. If there were things that he couldn't do, such as repairing the motor on his boat, or that needed doing, such as cutting firewood, he traded for herbal care in exchange. "People put an equal amount of energy into supporting each other this way," observes Ryan. "I would get a salmon for dinner from the island derelict who had time to sit all day at the wharf and jake for fish, whether he caught them or not. These payments-in-kind seemed to just flow."

Material reality hinges on paying the piper, of course. Herbalists need hard cash as much as anyone. Blending context with trust—and a prevailing sense of frugality—seems to work for most of us. We become more established over time. Confidence builds while the transition from a full-time job elsewhere becomes a home-based herbal livelihood. We graciously welcome those patrons of the herbal arts who can afford to pay in full for our knowledge and care. But we also welcome all comers who respond to that inner spark to heal. Good things happen when you take steps toward your vision.

There is no piece of paper on Kate Gilday's wall that says, *I am this so I can charge that.*

*The sign at the end of the driveway tells neighbors where to find you.*

This community herbalist started by charging just for her medicines. Some people offered a donation toward consultations, but she didn't feel ready to put an hourly rate on her time. Spending a couple days a week doing this work left more of the financial burden for four children and a house on her husband. Kate began trading to provide herbal care. People worked in the garden; someone built her a beautiful bench. Yet these things weren't what her family really needed. "I began charging $15 an hour, and asking people to pay for their medicines as well. Now, ten years later, I have a sliding scale fee ranging from $25 to $45 an hour," says Kate. "I do a lot of pro bono work with people that don't have any money; I have lots of people that just pay me as they can. If I lived in New York City or Boston, I would charge more. Money is a big issue for people, especially when insur-

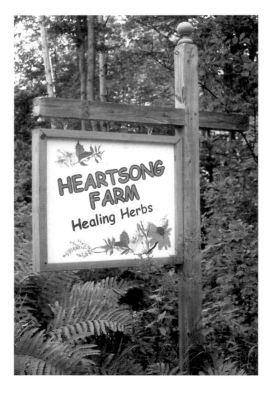

ance won't cover it. You have to look at the community where you live and decide what is affordable to the people that live there."

"I often get people who have cancer, say, who want an herbal program but have only $20 to spare. This has actually been valuable in forcing me to bring things down to a bare-bones approach," says Bob Liebert. This herbalist chooses not to charge for consultation time, relying instead on the sale of Teeter Creek Herbs to make a living for his family. "I've discovered that as much can be done with one or two herbs or a simple formula as by practitioners who prescribe hundreds of dollars worth of supplements. I tend to use simple, time-honored healing herbs over the latest craze herbs. So much is in the intent, the prayerful gathering of herbs, the potency of the herb, and the receptivity of the person to healing from the Earth."

Placing a value on our experience and herbal education can be intimidating. "The concept of selling my knowledge—or even of selling the herbs that the Earth gave to me—was very foreign," says Mary Pat Palmer. "That was my hurdle [in the beginning] and at times still is." A holistic psychotherapist practicing in the Boston area, Mary Pat charges on a sliding scale for time spent with clients in therapy for depression, anxiety, mood swings, or a history of abuse. She makes tinctures for her clients with herbs from her gardens, but does not charge additionally for the medicines. "I put up so many tinctures as an act of love," explains this urban herbalist, "that I would run out of space in my house if I didn't give them away! I make my living in spiritual terms as a grower."

That question of setting a value on our time deserves some pondering. Most practitioners working out of the home do not

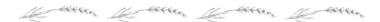

## AND NOW A WORD FROM THE DALAI LAMA

THE DALAI LAMA has shared a simple practice that will increase loving and compassion in the world:

1. Spend five minutes at the beginning of each day remembering we all want the same things (to be happy and be loved), and we are all connected to one another.
2. Spend five minutes breathing in—cherishing yourself— and breathing out— cherishing others. If you think about people you have difficulty cherishing, extend your cherishing to them anyway.
3. During the day extend that attitude to everyone you meet. Practice cherishing the "simplest" person (clerks, attendants, and so on), as well as the "important" people in your life. Cherish the people you love and the people you dislike.
4. Continue this practice, no matter what happens or what anyone does to you. These thoughts are very simple, inspiring, and helpful. The practice of cherishing can be taken very deeply if done wordlessly, allowing yourself to feel the love and appreciation that already exists in your heart.

employ help or rent office space, so overhead costs can be basically nil.[3] Our gentle advertising campaigns tend to be limited to neighborhood flyers, a well-designed business card, and word-of-mouth recommendations. An hourly consultation fee can sometimes amount to several hours of time devoted to one client: spending two hours in the initial consultation, researching a particular condition, perhaps asking fellow practitioners their opinions, customizing herbal remedies, following up with the person by phone to see how it's going. Let's say one wishes to earn a modest $600 a week

*Text continues on page 122.*

# Joyce Wardwell

THE MEDICINE of the people flows most assuredly on a self-reliant herbal path. Joyce Wardwell lives in northern Michigan and has not purchased herbs for more than a decade. She grows and wildcrafts all the healing plants she needs for her immediate family and community. She admits to buying kelp from Oregon—"It's pretty hard to grow seaweed in the Mid-

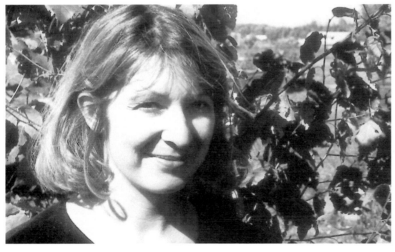

west!" Selenium or iodine are lacking in the foods grown in the soils of the Great Lakes region. Joyce and her husband are true homesteaders, living close to the land in a 10 × 20-foot cabin with their four children. Their kitchen is more outside than in; an outhouse is out back. Raised-bed vegetable gardens are kept neatly and appreciated voraciously. Nettles, comfrey,

and other medicinal plantings are scattered here, there, and everywhere. The Jordan Valley Wilderness Area, with 5,000 acres of woods, lies 200 feet from their door.

"Some people are taken aback when they first come and see how humble our place is," says Joyce. "We started from scratch, borrowing $10 from everyone we knew for a down payment on the land and a mailbox." The family lived in a wigwam until their homestead cabin was ready. Ten years have gone by working on a new home, with hopes to move in soon. "We've hauled in the rocks for the foundation, cut trees, and I don't even want to think about how many logs we've peeled. We've learned to make do with what we have, growing much of

our own food and using the herbs that are around us."

Joyce began her herbal journey when she was a child. "I started on this path back in about 1970 when I was around thirteen. There weren't any teachers to be found then, and if there were, I probably couldn't have paid them anyway." She gained a wealth of knowledge by listening to the stories of elders in her community, and by directing the stories back to herbs, folkloric wisdom began to take hold. *Use what you've got on hand* was a particularly apt tenet. "Another one of my teachers was a Native American, and, again, you have the atti-

> *The mere act of getting out to gather and grow is healing.*
>
> —JOYCE WARDWELL

tude of use what you have. The mere act of getting out to gather and grow is considered healing. To deny yourself of that relationship is to deny yourself of healing. When I purchase an herb from someone, I forgo that relationship. This is a part of my training and this is what I teach. Pretty much everything I could use is here, or, if it isn't, I try to grow it. And if that doesn't work, I can try to makeshift it."

Encounters with these Native American healers gave Joyce stories that taught her the essence of herbalism. "Gathering with respect so that the plants will always be there for you and also for your great-great-grandchildren is part and parcel of the whole thing. I can tell you how to gather your herbs with a reverent heart, or I can tell you the story of 'How Rose Got Her Thorns.' "This medicine story is included in her delightful book, *The Herbal Home Remedy Book.* Stories teach us how to approach the plants wisely and instill deeper meaning into everyday life. Good teaching resonates in traditional tales, weaving Joyce's readers gently into the practical ways of herbal wisdom.

Back on the home front, herbal wisdom for Joyce takes the form of keeping a somewhat low community profile. "My business is mostly word of mouth. I work as an educator, teaching classes at the local university, middle school, and at our home. I also give a lot of classes for local garden clubs. I do some consultations, usually seeing people out in the garden whenever possible."

One positive change Joyce has noticed recently is that people are seeking herbal alternatives. People get a diagnosis and a prescription from a doctor, but wonder about its side effects. They want to know if there is else something to take. "It wasn't like that before. I usually got the people who had terminal cancer and already had ten rounds of chemotherapy. The doctor had given them three months to live. Then they come to the herbalist and ask, 'What can I do now?' My work is to help them find the research to answer their own questions, so they may empower their own path of healing, whether it be herbal or otherwise. It is wonderful that this change has occurred.

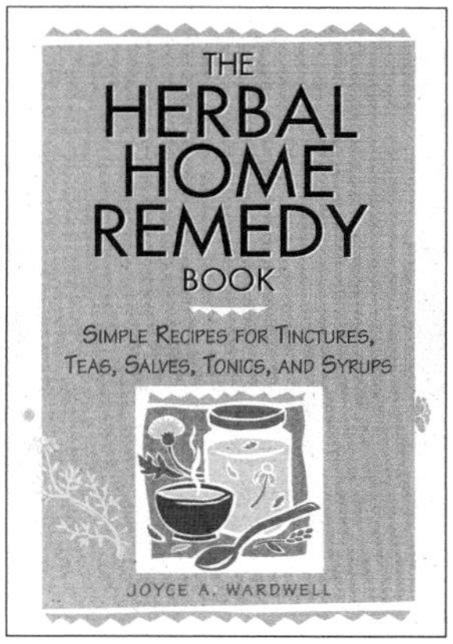


*Joyce's* Herbal Home Remedy Book *is a "must have" book for any home herbalist.*

"I have a great dichotomy of clients here. I see blue-collar workers and people that have second homes near the water, where, if you make a couple of million dollars a year, you are in the poor end. My clients are pooled from those two extremes." Joyce estimates that half of people's problems are job related. "They work sixteen hours a day trying to keep up with the image they think they need to maintain, with expensive cars and hundred-thousand-dollar homes. Pursuit of this image leaves a person very little time to take care of themselves." The Wardwell homestead, meanwhile, is anything but posh. "We do have running water now, having put in an artesian well, but still carry it inside to our original cabin. We have a combination of solar panels and line electricity. It works wonderfully, but sometimes it takes people aback when they come here for a consultation. They see that you don't have to have all the material items to be happy."

Simple treasures can be profound. "I have always been drawn to the plants first. It brings me joy to stick my nose in a flower and get my nose full of pollen and just smell the fragrance. That's the kind of thing that keeps me going. That's what pulled me in. I'm in awe when the snow melts that there are violets and Johnny-jump-ups awaiting under the snow. I get into the magic powers of leaves and the vitality of the roots. But the flowers! I look at their intricacy and marvel at the beauty and the pink-and-white universe that lies within each bloom." A good journey starts for each of us caught up in such admiration of the green world. Herbalism begins with self-reliance—going out in a wild place or the garden to gather herbs. "We go on from there to learn the plant's chemistry, the plant's abilities, the plant's spirituality, so that we can apply it to the next plant that we use," says Joyce. She is always building her herbal knowledge base.

(before taxes) from a community practice. Herb sales might provide a third of that amount after expenses. Payment from teaching opportunities are an added bonus. Perhaps three or four people are seen each day over the course of four days, leaving time for the gardens, medicine making, community building, and all the other things one does. Of these, ten to twelve people can afford to pay in full. A consultation fee ranging from $35 to $45 would achieve the income desired. Now apply this reckoning to your own circumstances and your community to see what's affordable. Some herbalists can charge more, some less, but at least personal finances can be considered alongside the ideal of serving humanity.

A $30,000 annual income (on which we based that theoretical $600 a week) works for us on our farm in part because of lifestyle choices we've made. Our combined herbal efforts amount to about half of that, with the bulk of the money coming from the sale of dried herbs we grow and wildcraft. Nancy teaches far more than she consults. A community practice evolves over time, of course, so this might change. You never know by which path people might come seeking herbal guidance. Twelve people a week asking for an appointment seems like a lot of folks to us right now. Figuring a consultation fee gets a lot more complicated the more you introduce reality into the equation.

Splitting responsibility for family income with a partner or an outside job certainly gives a community herbalist helpful flexibility when it comes to reckoning someone's ability to pay. Just as we ask our friends and neighbors to trust in us as healers, we in turn need to trust that they want the healing exchange to be fair. Posting a *barter sheet* that lists things we need helps reduce the awkwardness anyone short on cash might feel. People can respond to such a clear statement of needs—splitting firewood, grading a gravel driveway, tending animals, patching clothes, whatever it is— knowing we honor in-kind contributions as much as they honor our healing abilities. Negotiating a fair trade follows from there. A holistic economy won't always insist on money.

Being empowered to ask for what we need is okay. People have become accustomed to paying for bad health without a second thought. Cheap food and insurance premiums don't add up in the long run. Most folks can grasp good health as a far better deal without too much prompting. And yet convincing them (and sometimes ourselves) to pay more for organic food, to take time to prepare whole meals, and to step out of the material mainstream can be a real struggle. Patterns may be hard to change, but, by golly, that's a huge part of what this collective journey toward planetary healing is about.

Herbalists reap other benefits in addition to an eventual modest income. We don't have a collective retirement plan going, but we do have basic insurance coverage of a different sort: we are healthy from the get-go, and are able to take care of ourselves and our families in most situations. (Obtaining a policy for catastrophic coverage for accidental injury will have to come out of pocket, however.) Our pace of life reflects our values. "What I'm really getting," says Monica Rude from her New Mexico herb farm, "is being able to live in this beautiful place, eating fresh organic produce, drinking clean water out of the tap, having the kind of lifestyle I want. It's quiet and peaceful here. We can see the stars at night. I feel very rich."

## RESTORING OUR COMMUNITIES

A local living is tied intimately to those of our neighbors. The mythical dollar at one time recirculated seven times within the loop of community. The corporate world now grabs that dollar bill before it has a chance to turn around twice. Envision a sustainable society and you quickly realize local jobs depend on the renewable use of local resources. The goods we need—real food, a decent shelter, practical clothing—can be found locally. The services that matter—medical care, education, and foot-stomping music—can be provided locally. The culture at large, however, seems to be fixated on shopping elsewhere for the lowest price. Community health has lost much ground in the broken hoop known as the global economy.

Herbalists play an integral role in any local economy. The need for care and plant medicines will always be with us. Our livelihoods in turn depend on a fair exchange of goods and services with our neighbors. This direct relationship holds promise if all involved can see the need for mutual support. Not being privy to insurance reimbursement means two things. First, herbalists need to provide care at a cost people can afford. And second, the people coming to see us need to recognize the value of an early investment in their health, long before chronic conditions develop.

Opportunity lies like a pearl in the jaws of any challenge. Perhaps in our struggle to work the edges of a health care system that's just beginning to accept clinical herbalism in an integrative setting, community herbalists will be the ones to reintroduce self-reliance to the public at large. People who assume personal responsibility for their own health are the ones most likely to realize the ethics behind manifesting community and planetary health.

That holistic message to honor ourselves naturally includes this holy Earth. Our culture tends to pay lip service to environmentalism because no one wants to reduce their take of material goods: *Yeah, yeah, save the whales, save the rain forest, save the Quebec watersheds. But don't affect my pile!* How much wiser we will be when we view Creation as a sacrament. Chief Seattle advised that what we do to ourselves we do to Earth. Maybe the message for us today should be: What we do to Earth we do to ourselves.

A sustainable society ultimately needs to address population, the distribution of wealth, and destructive human habits (such as gas guzzling and lawn care) as a whole. Asking farmers to provide us with a "sustainable agriculture" without committing ourselves in all other regards falls short of the mark. We nurture local agriculture by getting involved in the growing of our food and by supporting small farmers in our communities who have the gumption to work with Nature, not against her. Eating the products of the corporate farm makes you sick. As the food activist Sally Fallon put it, "Those of you not eating healthy food are going to die out. The corporations will then need a contingency plan to maintain their markets. I look upon this as a natural selection of the wise. People who become wise about foods and supporting local farms are the people who are going to survive."[4]

That same kind of discerning wisdom applies to our relationship with the plants. Eco-herbalism involves knowing where our medicines come from and the proper way to nurture that source. A respect for diversity is the key. When we realize that human diversity is part of the deal, we tie community health to our vision and work as herbalists. Holistic considerations matter as much collectively as individually. The answers to our seemingly earth-shattering problems lie in bringing our attentions back home. Every dollar spent can amount to an economic vote for a worse world. Or, as we optimistically prefer to think, a far better local world. Consciousness will always be a big part of the journey.

"Everyone has the potential for greatness," says David Winston, "great good and great evil. It is our choice. Life is about becoming a human being. The Cherokees don't believe that you are born a human being. We believe that you are born a two-legged animal. A two-legged animal is only driven by instinct: If you are hungry you eat, if you are sexually aroused you do that, if you have to go to the bathroom you do that. You are working off your instincts, your fears, and your passions. A human being is somebody who strives for greatness, who reaches for their potential, who makes mistakes and learns from them and grows. Someone who lives a caring, giving life and who grows their spirit."[5]

We have both a prescription and a prognosis to offer humanity. The first is to become that human being David describes so eloquently. We can choose to nurture and honor this incredible Creation. We can choose to love one another. And if we do indeed succeed in leaving this temple we call Earth in better shape than we found it, there will be many generations to come.

## NOTES

1. Christiane Northrup, M.D., *Women's Bodies, Women's Wisdom* (New York: Bantam, 1998), 614.

2. Svevo Brooks, *The Art of Good Living* (Boston: Houghton Mifflin, 1990), 21–25.

3. Which isn't to say business expense for use of one's home doesn't enter into income tax considerations.

4. Sally Fallon speaking at the MidWest Small Farm Conference in Indiana in November 1999.

5. David Winston speaking at the Fourth International Herb Symposium at Wheaton College in Norton, Massachusetts, in June 1998.

# CHAPTER FIVE
# The Offering of Herbal Medicine

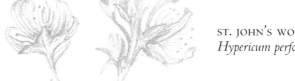

ST. JOHN'S WORT
*Hypericum perforatum*

*W*hen do we really know enough to start seeing clients? ❧ A few years ago I was sitting in my first dream-comes-true Advanced Herbal Training Program class at Sage Mountain. I had been growing and using herbs for a long time already, for myself and my family. I had completed an in-depth home study course as well as a seven-month herbal apprenticeship program. My confidence about starting a formal herbal practice was on the rise. I was quite excited and started to feel like a real herbalist. ❧ Our first guest teacher was Chanchal Cabrera, a respected clinician and founder of Gaia Garden Herbal Dispensary. She opened the class by talking about her feelings and experiences at the beginning of her herbal career. After four years at the College of Phytotherapy in England, four more years of supervised clinical practice, and then eight years of private practice, she finally felt competent. Not good, but competent to be let out on the streets. Well, that burst my bubble! ❧ Later that year we heard more encouraging advice from Kathleen Maier, the founder of the Dreamtime Center of Herbal Studies. "Don't ever believe that you can't help [with herbs] anyone who comes to your door," she said. These two wonderful teachers seemed to be offering conflicting advice. Their statements, however, actually represent two sides of the same coin: Encouragement to share what you know comes with a proper admonition not to go beyond your limits. ❧ The desire to help people experience healing plants permeates my being. I finally know with all my heart and soul "what I want to be when

*I grow up." I want to be a wise woman, a healer, an herbalist. I want to be old and wise and inwardly powerful, knowledgeable and resourceful.* ❧ *I am a practicing herbalist and always will be one. When people come to me with health concerns, I practice my healing skills and techniques with them. Sure, it sounds scary, practicing on people as they come to you for help. But we are always practicing, always learning. Most important, we must be honest with ourselves. A good community herbalist knows what can be done to help people and knows when to refer them to other health care practitioners, including doctors, naturopaths, psychotherapists, energy workers, body workers, acupuncturists, and so forth. Herbs can complement other healing modalities.* ❧ *Being in close contact with other herbalists helps to speed up one's learning. We can share with each other when something works well. We can ask advice when we just aren't sure. Reviewing case studies together (keeping the personal information private) adds to our experience.* ❧ *Experience brings knowledge and wisdom followed by confidence and trust in one's abilities. Each experience makes me stronger, more solid, more deeply connected to life. With my roots deep in the Earth Mother, and my branches reaching out and open to the guidance of the Creator, my foundation is strong, my spirit is willing. Every day I am able increasingly to be of service to others.* —N.P. ❧

UNDERSTANDING the difference between healing and curing is essential. Healing goes deeper than a curative fix. The latter emphasizes technology, analysis, and fixing broken parts *from without,* usually by chemical or surgical means. Physicians shoulder the responsibility for a cure—this is their training, the mantra of a patriarchal system. A holistic healer does not take on this burden. Healing comes *from within.* Healers help people to look at the whole of their lives. Together we find ways to set right the underlying imbalances behind the symptoms to be cured. The internal mechanisms of mind and body are equipped to repair virtually any type of trauma or disease. The innate ability to heal endures in every human body.

"Our job is to not always come in and try to fix everything or cure the person," says Candis Canton, a community herbalist in Placerville, California. "That journey is theirs and they are responsible. Maybe we help them to stop sinking in the river by helping them learn to swim . . . though it may not be our job to pull them out. Some situations may not even call for herbs. A person may just need prayer or touch."

Recognizing our role as that of a healing partner is liberating. The ability to help a partner begins with doing no harm. We can offer the herbs we know from firsthand experience and share holistic approaches to wellness. Any early self-doubts can be eased somewhat by allowing one's nurturing nature to assist in the healing process.

Think of the role of a consulting herbalist as that of a *health coach*. A coach is a guide with expertise, but he or she is not ultimately responsible for building muscles, stamina, and skills. A coach works hard figuring out strategies for the team as a whole. A coach inspires each player to do better and ultimately to realize his or her full potential. The players must decide what they want to accomplish. The coach encourages but never does the actual work.

The French philosopher Voltaire put it this way: "The efficient physician is the man who successfully amuses his patients while Nature effects a cure."

Understanding the strengths of one's medicine makes it clear when herbs are particularly appropriate. Herbal medicine can treat many chronic illnesses by bringing the body back into balance. The long-term overall building of health is an herbalist's forte. Evoking the body's healing response differs from masking or attacking symptoms. *Time enough to heal* distinguishes this work with the healing plants. We aim for the lowest level of intervention whenever possible to allow the body to respond. A crisis situation or severe pain, however, is often best addressed by allopathic medicine. Most of us want to have a skilled doctor on hand in an urgent, life-threatening situation.

Chronic illnesses involve a weakened or debilitated system. Often many organs of the body are affected. The illness is ongoing, perhaps having developed over many years, and can become quite serious and even life-threatening. Asthma, osteoporosis, diabetes, allergies, and arthritis are typical examples of chronic conditions. A person with an acute problem, in contrast, is oftentimes healthy but currently ill or traumatized. Headaches, constipation, and colds are usually acute. Should such problems become frequent, however, a chronic imbalance is likely to be indicated.

We start off as herbalists working more with acute situations. Successes such as calming an upset stomach with peppermint tea or fending off the flu with echinacea give us confidence in herbal wisdom. Eventually we encounter a wider array of chronic diseases and learn to work with long-term therapies. Each herbalist determines his or her own level of competence. The golden rule to honor throughout is honesty: Always clearly state your experience and knowledge to the people with whom you work. By trusting what we do know and being clear about what we don't, we bring integrity—as important as any license—into the healing relationship.

"If somebody says to you, 'I have this condition, have you ever treated that?' say no if you haven't," advises Aviva Romm. "You can tell them you are happy to hear their story and that you can share resources and learn about this together. I don't think there has to be any difference between a community herbalist and a clinical herbalist. They are different levels of the same thing. The more you see, the more you know, and the more you'll have experience to help people. But just be honest with people."

## LAWFUL SEMANTICS

Herbalists have found ways of maintaining legal decorum in order to practice. While some pursue legitimating herbal medicine in the eyes of the law, others carefully fulfill their heart's desire to help others. A clear sense of what we're about—empowering people to feel better—marks out a gray area that medical bureaucracies prefer to leave alone. If we truly support the notion that each person is his or her own healer, then herbalists will never deviate from emphasizing their role as a supporting partner in the healing process. Recognizing that healing choices are both the right and responsibility of every individual places a protective moral context around our work.

The rub comes when we apply the core definition of medicine to herbal parlance. "The science of diagnosing, treating, or preventing disease and other damage to the body or mind"[1] is physician-ordained territory. Medical doctors are currently granted a fairly exclusive license to practice medicine in this country.[2] Each state drafts its own legislation for the establishment and enforcement of laws regarding the practice of medicine, but, in effect, the implications from state to state are one and the same. Take away that word *medicine,* as one surgeon friend told Michael in casual conversation, and doctors as a rule have no problem with people helping other people feel better.

Herbalists can give care as long as they don't diagnose a particular illness or prescribe particular herbs to cure a patient's condition. Avoiding catch words such as *diagnose, prescribe, cure,* and *patient* does seem a bit ridiculous when much of what we do in an herbal practice at first blush seems so similar to the basic medical conventions. Nor does changing one's language ultimately insulate herbalists from a shift in medical enforcement policy. On the other hand, the notion of holistic partnership suggests friendlier terms anyway. We speak instead of *assessing* one's *whole health* in order to *recommend* particular herb(s) for our *client's consideration.* An intention to allow the body to regain its natural balance and self-healing process is not considered to be "medical" by state licensing boards. Herbalists have ways to safeguard the sharing of specific herbal advice: "Traditionally this has been used for _____; you can read about _____ here." Passing along historical documentation and scientific validation from clinical trials is information sharing, not the practice of medicine. A typical brochure for a consulting herbalist reads "Offering herbal treatments for those that wish to incorporate them into their diet." Use of the word medicine is sidestepped entirely. Diet and nutrition are not directly claimed by authorities as a relevant area of medical concern.

Maintaining the appearance of "not diagnosing" by herbalists is most important. Doctors take a special pride in their ability to analyze the state of the body and precisely identify physical cause and effect revealed by acute symptoms. Chronic conditions tend to be more subjective. Skilled insight comes with a problematic shortcoming of its own. The whole situation of body/mind/spirit underlying symptomatic cause and effect is often not revealed (let alone considered!) in a typical medical diagnosis. Many herbalists appreciate the diagnostic clues provided by physicians through laboratory analysis. Medical training in physiology and anatomy often does pay off in understanding the working mechanics of the human body. However, limiting our assessment of a matter to anything less than the whole does a considerable disservice to the people seeking assistance. Medical diagnosis can often be enhanced. A health assessment could be construed as constituting diagnosis if undertaken solely by a consulting herbalist. However, taken in conjunction with a physician's opinion, the ramifications belong most truthfully to the patient/client/human being who wants to feel better.

"If an herbalist is not diagnosing and is not claiming that the herbal products will 'cure' the client," advises attorney Ken Collins, "there is little danger of being attacked for the unauthorized practice of medicine." Ken (who also happens to be the husband of herbalist Jane Bothwell) points out that a regular pattern of conduct in the course of pursuing an herb business fans the flames of desire on the part of authorities to prosecute. In other words, several complaints received are viewed as far more serious than one. The occasional advice we give to family and friends, based as it may be on a singular assessment of their illness, will not trigger trouble. The *chicken soup exception* allows that people do indeed have time-tested advice for each other to gain relief from the common cold. Even medical zealots have to be practical.

The desire to not call attention to a very desirable healing collaboration determines how we go about helping others. As David Hoffmann puts it, herbalists can get a license for a gun but not one to practice herbal medicine. The reality of the day needs to be acknowledged. Yet the regulatory radar is choosing more blazing targets such as health fraud, cancer cure exploitation, and medical incompetence when enforcing licensing codes.[3] Rooting out herbalists as medical heretics is not viewed as either politically or economically expedient at this time. Abiding by the unspoken rules of fringe practice works for herbalists willing to accept humbler rewards. No one is fooled here. Herbalists have been preparing and dispensing herbal remedies for many thousands of years regardless of legalities. We should consider the source and nature of any law that fosters anything less than the freedom to choose our medical care. The philosopher Thomas Aquinas determined three levels of lawful hierarchy: laws of spirit, laws of nature, and laws of man. Natural law had to obey spiritual law, and humankind's law had to obey both natural and spiritual law. Furthermore, people have a duty to challenge any law not in accord with higher law.

"Everyone is a healer," says Ryan Drum. "We all have healing opportunity every second of our lives to do something therapeutically positive for ourselves, our families, and others. To feel it's the special privilege of a few to thwart native ability when it's needed at the moment is wrong. . . . The way it is now, unless you have license to touch somebody or give medical advice, you're facing potential fines and imprisonment for practicing medicine without a license." Ryan quietly adds, "I do it at every opportunity. Anywhere. Strangers, friends, family, community. I insist on my right to be helpful no matter what."

Minnesota recently passed a bill called the Complementary and Alternative Health Care Freedom of Access Act, which gives people the freedom to attend to their health problems as they wish. In essence, this law recognizes the nonlicensed right to help people feel better. Matthew Wood was one of the herbalists who worked hard to see this commonsense legislation enacted. "I was tormented the first five years I practiced, because it meant I was outside the law," says Matthew. "I was mildly tormented the next five years. The next five years I didn't care. The past two years I worked to change the law."

Many herbalists establish *health care agreements* with their clients. These specify the roles and duties for both the herbalist and the individual seeking health care advice. People are asked to acknowledge their personal responsibility in forging a healing path; the herbalist honors the essential right of each client to choose the preferred services. Unrealistic assumptions are revealed when you openly discuss the process up front. After all, the nature of any herbal practice is to provide information. Clients assume responsibility for ingesting any supplements discussed and agree to report any unexpected side effects. In the case of adverse reaction, people need to seek medical attention and fully inform their medical practitioner of all supplements taken. Having clients affirm their integral role in committing to a healthy lifestyle is a nice way to start the healing relationship.

The American Herbalists Guild believes one of the most effective means for avoiding legal trouble is through the use of such an Informed Consent/Full Disclosure form. This form discloses your professional training and standards of practice, and informs a client of what is to be expected from both parties. Informed consent will not protect a practitioner from legal action so much as minimize the chance for client dissatisfaction that might lead to subsequent legal action. Most complaints against health professionals are based on miscommunication. Clearly spelling out expectations and money matters in black and white at the initial interview is much easier than waiting until after the consultation.

"Some practitioners have each of their clients sign an informed consent form. I just tell people the information I am sharing with them has helped other people in the past. I am not a doctor. I tell them what my training and experience has been. Maybe it's just me being the eternal optimist," says Kate Gilday, "but by not giving them this piece of paper to sign, a bond of trust is formed in the very beginning that follows through our relationship."

## ASSESSMENT SKILLS

Examine the tongue, feel for distinct types of pulse, peer deep into the eyes of the soul . . . healing traditions offer a wide array of paths for tuning in to the body. Discerning the whole of a client's health enables us to recommend potential plant medicines specific for that person. The two abilities go hand in hand. *Differential diagnosis* seeks out the individuality of each situation, while *differential therapeutics* senses which herbs are appropriate for this person now and, as changes occur, over time. Experience and knowledge merge with art and intuition at the core of herbal practice. The assortment of assessment tools will be unique for each herbalist, for in truth the paths of discernment are many. The more tools we have to enhance a physician's diagnosis, the more ability we have to reveal constitutional patterns and system imbalance. The one thing that does seem applicable across the board is that holistic discernment is learned only by doing. Again and again and again.

Working on one assessment skill at a time, ideally under the tutelage of an experienced herbalist, is how we learn. Reading that someone having a yellow complexion around the mouth and nose indicates stagnant digestion isn't going to mean a thing until you meet that person and work with herbs to help that person. Observing different body postures and constitutions, and then actually experiencing the vitality and typical ailments of all sorts of people, teaches us about the outward clues to health. Don't be surprised when you next head off to a concert or ball game if you soon spend more time observing facial indications as you scan individuals in the crowd.

Taking blood pressure provides yet another window to look through. Pulse and tongue diagnosis are intricate and sensitive arts to be learned only by taking pulses and looking at the tongues of many, many people.

"The tongue is like a map," says Christopher Hobbs. "Once you learn to use this skill, it is really an ally. It takes time—you must observe thousands of tongues. Just because a person has certain signs on the tongue does not mean that they will be symptomatic. They may be predisposed to an imbalance or moving toward it. Pulse

# INTEGRATING GLOBAL TRADITIONS

WESTERN HERBALISM blends the generational knowledge of Europeans about flowers, leaves, and seeds for medicinal use with the traditional Native American wisdom about root and bark remedies. The understanding of the body itself—whether expressed as the Galenic humors, the empirical insight of the Eclectics, or seemingly simplistic folklore—reflects a strong emphasis on physical cause and effect. People in other cultures have contributed equally vital perspectives on energy flow in the human body and the use of plants to harmonize our dynamic nature.

The word *Ayurveda* literally means "the knowledge of life." This centuries-old tradition from India focuses on connecting mind, body, and consciousness. Disease or illness results when the primary metabolic forces in the body, known as *doshas,* are out of balance. Stress, accordingly, is understood to be a causative factor in the disease process, responsible for lodging toxins deep within the tissues of the body. A *rasayana* (herbal

preparation) is designed to remedy stress and its effects. It can be a combination of many herbs and minerals put through an extensive preparation process designed to enhance potency, or a single herb such as ashwagandha, sometimes referred to as "Indian ginseng" for its rejuvenative and tonic actions. Ayurvedic herbs are considered to be effective only when our behavior is uplifting and our lifestyle is in harmony with Nature—when we are rooted in universal consciousness. A concise guide to this holistic approach to health can be found in *Ayurvedic Healing* by Candis Canton.

Practitioners of Traditional Chinese Medicine (TCM) view the body in terms of energetic flows and polarity. Blockages or disruptions in the *chi,* or life force, are seen as damp or dry, hot or cold conditions. The balanced polarities of yin and yang—where yin refers to the tissues of the body organs, yang to the activity of the organs—cannot work independently of one another. If a yin deficiency occurs, the body

is likely to lack proper nutrients or adequate physical structure to perform its functions. A yang deficiency indicates the body cannot react to metabolic stimuli. Chinese herbs are used to maintain proper energetic flows and polarity in the body. *Between Heaven and Earth* by Harriet Beinfield and Efrem Korngold offers a lucid and penetrating introduction to Chinese medicine.

The oldest method of acquiring herbal wisdom is shamanic journeying. Aspirants who seek knowledge go out alone to fast, pray, and cry for a vision. Sometimes the spirits of the plant and animal worlds come unsolicited. The properties of the plants are explained to the shaman by a spirit guide, who often appears in the form of an animal or person. These teachings become integrated into native herbal medicine through stories that establish clearly this link to spirit power. Shamans continue to journey today, bringing back both new cultural messages and undiscovered plant uses.

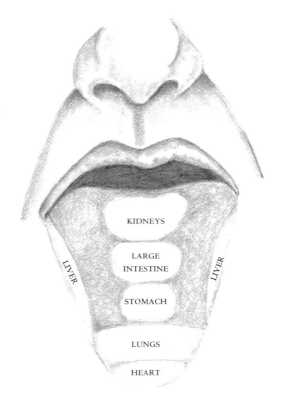

*Knowing which organs correspond to specific locations on the tongue only initiates the subtle art of tongue diagnosis.*

KIDNEYS

LARGE INTESTINE

LIVER

LIVER

STOMACH

LUNGS

HEART

instance, are indicative of hemorrhoids, cystitis, and urethritis. A yellow mucous coating around the edge of the tongue suggests looking at liver and gallbladder function.

Pulse indications, on the other hand, are not so obvious. We are considering more than how many beats per minute can be counted. Three positions on each wrist reveal internal possibility to practitioners attuned to the pulsating feel of the blood. The positions correlate to the upper (thoracic), middle (abdominal), and lower (pelvic) areas of the body: lungs, stomach/ spleen, and kidney/intestines/adrenals are sensed in the right arm; heart, liver/gallbladder, and kidney/intestines/bladder are sensed in the left arm. A deep low pulse, for instance, may indicate a deep-seated chronic ailment in the organ indicated by position. Still, you can't begin to differentiate *low* from *hollow* or *empty*—let alone *bounding* or *scattered* or *resistant*—until a master identifies pulse possibility with you.

The traditional approach to determining the nature of someone's health emphasizes observing physical characteristics. Assessment can also be aided by muscle testing (where tension response of the arm when holding a prospective herb affirms receptivity) and other intuitive techniques. Folklore has relevance too. Phyllis Light watches to see if ants take interest in a urine sample poured on a flat rock in the warm sun. A person with insulin-dependent diabetes has large amounts of sugar in the urine . . . so if the ants come to get the sugar, confirming the presence of diabetes mellitus is merited. Modern urinalysis, using chemical reactions and automated techniques, quantifies what the physician's tongue, eye, and nose have been doing for thousands of years.

diagnosis is much harder to learn. Pulses change so easily, while the tongue takes days to change. Some aspects of pulse diagnosis are very subtle. I have been practicing for ten years and am always learning."

We look at a good-sized piece of the digestive tract and mucosa when we observe the human tongue. The Chinese divided the regions of the tongue into compartments that corresponded to different organs in the body. Tongue observations work to a great extent, but always need to be checked against other indications. The color and condition of the tongue provides this opportunity to perceive what is going on with the soft internal organs (viscera) of the body. Raised red papillae on the back third of the tongue, for

Tuning in to the body by many different routes strengthens our judgment. "We need a variety of tools and techniques to practice well," explains Michael Tierra. "A clinical differential diagnostic model should include a variety of diagnostic parameters, and even then the diagnosis is only hypothetical until the treatment that would follow shows results." Asking meaningful and incisive questions helps reveal the complexity surrounding the essence of each individual. We try not to ask leading questions but rather get the person to confirm what we suspect may actually be going on with them. We look for salient clues revealed on the intake form (see "Individual Health Profiles," page 141), and by asking about all aspects of their complaint and health history. A doctor's input is important—hopefully we see the results of all blood work and hear a detailed report of the physician's diagnosis from the client. An amazing amount of information from test results is often overlooked in conventional medicine.

"I not only look at values," says Phyllis Light, "but also where within the range the value is located. I look for trends over time as well." The herbalist's job then becomes one of tying all these indications together in terms of body, mind, and spirit.

Western herbalists use three basic points of view to contemplate the whole of a person. We move from the general to the specific. *Constitutional considerations* help us recognize where people belong in terms of broad patterns. These point in turn to certain innate tendencies toward both health and disease for each constitutional type. The three doshas of Ayurveda, the four qualities of Greek medicine, the five elements of traditional Chinese medicine, the Native American medicine wheel, the four psychological functions—whatever most resonates with your ken—can be used as a basis for considering someone's constitutional nature.

*Text continues on page 136.*

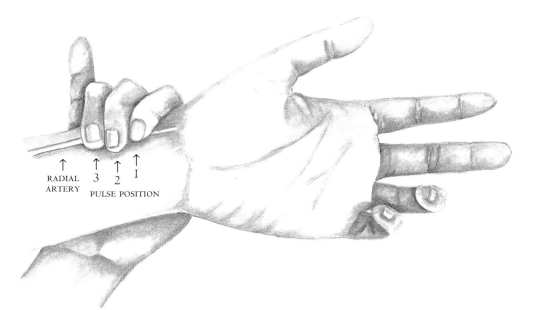

RADIAL ARTERY    3  2  1
PULSE POSITION

*The three pulse positions on each wrist correlate to the thoracic, abdominal, and pelvic regions. The lungs, stomach/ spleen, and kidney/ intestines/adrenals are sensed in the right arm; the heart, liver/gallbladder, and kidney/ intestines/bladder are sensed in the left arm.*

# Margi Flint

A THRIVING HERBAL practice befits the Old World flavor of Marblehead, Massachusetts. Sailboats abound in this beautiful seacoast town, where people of all ages and coping with all manners of dis-ease come to Margi Flint's home for herbal consultation. "I practice as I learn each issue, each herb, each constitution, each spiritual effect," explains Margi. "That's where my term 'practicing herbalist' comes from." She prefers seeing one new client in the morning, one new client in the afternoon, with follow-up visits scheduled around these longer intake sessions. The rest of her day is spent formulating, preparing tinctures and salves, brewing teas for the office, organizing classes, unloading herb orders, or answering the never-ending phone calls.

"I do receive many referrals from doctors. Most don't know the answers to the questions their patients are asking them about herbs." Margi notes that in many countries a license to practice medicine is not given without a degree in phytotherapy and that herbs are often prescribed prior to pharmaceuticals. "I for one am delighted that America is waking up."

Margi honors the choices people make concerning their health care. "One of my clients said, 'I come to you because you are a real person. Neither too radical nor extremely rigid. I can tell you I've taken an antibiotic or an aspirin and know you won't judge me for it.' I certainly hate to judge anyone, because I don't want to be judged myself. I work closely with doctors, and I try to learn as much as I can about the pharmaceuticals so I don't hurt my clients. You need to know what the action of the pharmaceutical is so the actions of the herbs don't make it work too strongly or offset its use or completely go in the opposite direction. Once I know how a drug works in the body, I know what to avoid. If someone is taking Coumadin, then don't give them turmeric."

The long and winding path of Margi's herbalist training began at the first Gaia Herb Conference. She met David Winston, who agreed to return to Massachusetts on occasion and teach additional classes that Margi organized so she could learn more herself. She eagerly joined the first apprenticeship Rosemary Gladstar offered in Vermont. "I began my path with those two teachers," says Margi, "and local seminars on herbal medicine. Then it took over my life completely. Closet by closet, hour by hour, began to fill with herbs. My approach was to gradually take in information. I would fluctuate from feeling that I was getting a grip on herbal knowledge and then go to another class and feel that I didn't know anything." This slow progression of confidence serves as a safety measure for most herbal novices. One apprenticeship does not establish lifetime

*We need to teach people to go into their backyards, that real healing is all around us.*

—MARGI FLINT

credentials for any of us. "Making medicinal products and using them was all romantic to me. I was being courted by the herbs. People began showing up at my door and saying they needed this or that, yet I wasn't ready." Margi humbly offered what she knew. And practiced. And practiced. And now that practicing has led to a busy herbal practice in its own right.

The application to become a professional member of the American Herbalists Guild asks, "Why do you want to join the Guild?" Margi wrote that she wanted to bridge the gap between herbal and allopathic medicines. The next day a person called asking her to give a lecture on herbs at Tufts University School of Medicine in Boston. "Sure," she responded. "Then they asked if I would teach a ten-week course, for free, at the medical school. I taught two years, two ten-week blocks, once a week. When the students' eyes began to glaze over with the overload of information that dominates med school, I would jump into preparation of

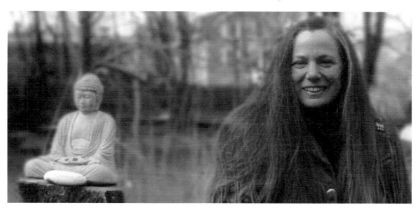

products and play. We made tonics, teas, salves, lip balms, massage oils. The third and fourth year I got smart and asked to be fully reimbursed for travel and supplies." Margi treasured the opportunity, but eventually found that teaching at Tufts took more time than she could afford. "I miss my students. I was making a big impact on how they think about health and our connection to the planet."

At first Margi was quite scared of facing the medical modality in such a core place. "How could I possibly go and teach a class about herbal medicine at a bona fide medical school and not use the big

taboo words *medicine, cure,* and *remedy*? I decided that I would just teach honestly, that as long as I told the truth, I couldn't get into trouble.

"I also think I helped my students survive medical school. I would give them an overview of respiratory care and herbs, and later in class we would do aromatherapy. I brought plants in for them to experience the actual source of our remedies, and so remind them to connect to Earth. I taught them how to feel energy and how to meditate." Fourth-year medical students were offered a four-week clinical rotation in herbal medicine with Margi as an accredited portion of their medical degree. "Those four weeks were truly amazing. We covered the entire beginning-level apprentice program, saw clients daily, and had seven visiting herbalists in to teach. We taught about flower essences, aromatherapy, herbal preparations, formulation, and diagnosis. We ran an herbal clinic at the hospital to serve the com-

munity. We had sacred drum and prayer circle weekly. The exchange of information from this blend of spirits was fantastic for all.

"We've been in a huge tidal wave of energy these last several years with herbal medicine, but now I think there has been a shift. I think this change has affected the spirit of the herbs. The night that *20/20* [the television show] spotlighted St. John's wort, all the St. John's wort in my backyard died. Much of the St. John's wort in this area diminished. The areas that had huge stands of St. John's wort were no longer there. It was so strange. Our collective mind had tuned in to this wonderful plant, all of a sudden thinking that St. John's wort is a panacea for everything in the universe. I think when a message like that goes out that affects so many hundreds of thousands of people, the spirits of the plants pull back. They withdraw, because there is something inappropriate about it. No one herb is the cure for everything."

"We need to teach people to go into their backyards, that real healing is all around us. I get very annoyed when people say, 'Oh, you healed me.' I didn't heal anyone; the herbs did. I don't want people to detach from the Earth Mother and think a pill in a bottle healed them. Keep in mind that plants live in the earth. We need to take care of the earth so that the plants are taken care of, so they can take care of us. Life is truly a big circle." ℘

Next we look at the organ system that's off. This approach of the old physiomedicalists has been adapted by medical herbalists in Britain. The basic functions in the body are correlated to five observable states of tissue: hot/irritated, constricted/tense, damp/relaxed, dry/atrophic, and cold/depressed. The goal here is to visualize the *physiological dysfunction* behind the symptoms being revealed locally. Intuition and imagination help us sense the energetic connection between body systems and spirit. Thoughtfully observing the body's state of being allows us to "see" what is going on in the hidden interior of the body.

Nobody gets as precise as conventional medicine, of course, in detailing the specific disease revealed by symptoms. Technology unveils biological facts that can indicate clearly which illness is at hand. Identified drug therapies follow from there. And yet the specific diagnosis techniques outlined by Dr. John Scudder, a leading figure of the Eclectic movement in the nineteenth century, get down to therapeutic nitty-gritty quite well. Our clients want a ready answer—*I have this problem, I don't necessarily need to know what's going on in the big sense, please just tell me what will help now*—which we provide by directing them to specific herbs known to work well for a particular condition. Herbalists begin with a sound footing in empirical medicine and return many times to this same trustworthy knowledge base. We gain confidence and become effective healers by first relying on specifics. Only later do we fit constitutional and physiological considerations into the incredibly intriguing assessment puzzle. Empirical recommendations become that much more precise as we learn to make differential diagnoses of our own.

People often come to us wanting help for a specific problem. They expect us to treat what's bothersome. As herbalists, we want to help relieve these symptoms as soon as possible, but we should not stop there. True healing comes in addressing the underlying reality. *Treat the branch, then the root* aptly describes how we should work with our clients. A person with heartburn (the branch) can be treated for digestive upset, and the likely liver imbalance (the root) behind this distress can be addressed as well. We may suggest demulcent, antispasmodic, and carminative herbs as a tea blend to help with the branch condition. Second, a custom formula derived to moisten and cool the liver keeps rooted balance in mind. Keeping herbal medicine doable for folks often means not overwhelming them with tiers of concurrent remedies chosen to deal with every possible aspect of their situation. A tea and one formulated tincture are not so daunting.

The entry complaint might not be the right thing to treat immediately when a more poignant factor gets revealed in *peeling off the layers* during the interview or physical examination of a client. Or perhaps the herbs in our repertory would better address another branch of a complex situation first. A good explanation will make any shift in focus workable for most people. Keeping immediate goals attainable remains key. Unfortunately, once the symptoms go away, some people might not continue to work toward ongoing balance. Then the imbalance could surface in another way or even return again with the very same symptoms.

Success with the branch issue, coupled with an inspirational explanation of building overall health, gives us the chance to succeed fully with herbal intention. Matthew

Wood tells this story of a patient who happened to be a hospital administrator:

I took his pulse and said, "Have you been to a cardiac specialist?" He said, "Yeah, the doctor said nothing's wrong, I'm okay." Obviously he suspected something, and so did I. "The doctor's right, you don't have a heart problem, but you do have a circulatory problem." The old herbalists would have called this *unequal circulation*. Their phrase a hundred years ago in the treatment of heart disease was to first equalize the circulation. Meaning—if you drink too much, take too many drugs, consume too much fat and oil—there's an excess of blood around the liver. There's murkiness and stagnation. The same for the intestines and the lungs. In some circuits the blood is coagulating, while in other circuits the blood is tense, not relaxed, empty. All the blood is in one place, not in the other. This is hard to describe. Physicians don't even think this way nowadays. I explained this to this patient, just as the Eclectics would have described it. He said, "You're just like all the old doctors who died off in the 1960s." I knew exactly what he meant. The old doctors thought in terms of "what is the body doing." They would palpate the wall of the stomach to find out if it's prolapsing. They would palpate different circuits of the circulation, different organs, and could tell what was going on inside the body. My patient went on: "Those old doctors, that was the thing they were proudest of, that they knew how to diagnose, how to tell what was wrong by direct examination of the patient." Stagnation, liver problems . . . try to go to a doctor today and say you have a liver problem and you'll be laughed at. But for our great-grandparents, mention a liver problem, and their doctor would say, "Oh yes, we can treat that."[4]

The ability to beam our minds into the body is integral. Most people are combinations of the "constitutional types" and have more than one imbalance. So, so many factors go into determining who we are. And yet, as Phyllis Light pointed out in answering our diagnostic inquiries, the most important assessment technique available is really rather basic. "Our willingness to listen to and make a connection with the client counts the most. To open your senses, your energy field, and your heart, and to really look at the person. Nothing can take the place of this," maintains this sweet Alabama herbalist.

We emphasized at the beginning of this section how we make assessment skills our own through continual practice. Sometimes it takes a few good references to get the diagnostic ball rolling. *Tongue Diagnosis in Chinese Medicine* by Giovanni Maciocia is recommended highly by several respected practitioners. Margi Flint summarizes the likely areas of concern indicated by an array of assessment techniques in her handbook, *A Practicing Herbalist*. Complexion considerations, facial analysis, constitutional body types, energetics of the condition, emotional and physical reflexes, elimination analysis, eye appearance, and tongue analysis fit admirably in this good woman's toolbox.[5] A teaching manual put together by Michael Moore, *Principles and Practice of Constitutional Physiology for Herbalists*, superimposes whole-body thinking within a Western framework. Organ systems can indeed be analyzed from a constitutional perspective from the start. Matthew Wood's *Practice of Traditional Western Herbalism* is a contextual godsend for fitting all the pieces of differential diagnosis into a relative sense of order.

"We need to be able to visualize what's going on in the body," summarizes Matthew. "Getting a picture in your mind is an excellent start. Imagination is like the switchboard of reality, the images flip in and out, and pretty soon you're not making up these images, but getting them directly from the body. Another rewarding thing is being able to explain to a person so they too see what's the problem. Then, if your remedy helps, that's great. You don't always get those two aspects. If you get one, it's better to get the cure. But a good explanation that makes sense to them and to you is always helpful."

## GETTING STARTED

Today's urgent call for holistic healers reveals a very fundamental human need. People are looking for someone who will spend more than fifteen minutes with them, who will hold hands with them when appropriate, and who will give them a follow-up phone call. Caring means so much to a person. "You just have to do it," advises Rosemary Gladstar to starting-out herbalists. "You have to trust that when you begin you don't have to be good. You can't be good! You cannot get good reading books, and you cannot get good studying with the best teachers in this country. You cannot get good by learning all the best

# WHAT IS HOMEOPATHY?

Homeopathy and herbal medicine are sometimes incorrectly assumed to be the same thing. These two healing modalities do share the use of certain plants, but in a markedly different manner. A German physician, Samuel Hahnemann, developed homeopathy based on the philosophy that *like cures like*. Highly diluted remedies were used to treat illnesses that in larger doses would cause the illness or symptom. A strong dose of ipecac, for example, is used by various health care providers to induce vomiting, but it is used also as a highly diluted solution (often in tablet form) by homeopaths to treat nausea. Homeopathic remedies pose little safety concern. Many of the remedies are so dilute, in fact, that few actual physical molecules are left of the natural substance being used for medicine. Medicinal strength actually increases the higher the dilution due to an exacting potentizing process.

We know many people who use these remedies for their families, as well as health care providers who successfully prescribe them to clients. Certainly the healing energy in plants lies beyond what we can taste, smell, and even detect with a microscope. Homeopathic remedies are chosen for their ability to match the symptoms of a sick person, and thus go with the body's attempts to heal itself. Aiding the defenses of the body rather than suppressing symptoms makes sense.

Try them yourself, but do realize that there are some distinctions between the two healing systems. The following books offer more information, including long listings of specific ailments and their specific homeopathic remedies.

*Everybody's Guide to Homeopathic Medicine* by Ullman and Cummings
*The Complete Guide to Homeopathy* by Andrew Lockie, M.D.
*Materia Medica 9th Edition* by William Boericke, M.D.

"If you can read, you can do homeopathy," says Joe Lillard of Homeopathy Works in West Virginia.

formulas in your head. The only thing that will make you a good herbalist is practicing on yourself and other human beings. Relating directly to the plants, listening to them, and practicing. You have to go out and really be willing to make mistakes and to learn from them. You never start off wise—it takes you eighty or ninety years to be wise."

"It can be scary when you finally say 'I am an herbalist,'" observes Kate Gilday. "It's much easier to simply be learning about herbs, to still be a student. Yet the time comes when you are ready to say, 'I am an herbalist, that is my life, that is who I am. I know there is so much more to learn and it is a lifetime process, but I know enough to feel comfortable with what I am sharing.' When you do that, and offer your first care, it really gets fun. There is a tentative sweetness to it, and there is also an amazing strength. You are sharing who you are."

Having at least one other skill that goes along with herbal knowledge helps in being able to share with people. That may mean being a wonderful listener. Or a licensed massage therapist. Or a crafter of potent flower essences. Feeling comfortable with a community of healers to whom you can refer clients also bolsters any herbalist. A naturopathic physician, an M.D., a nurse practitioner, an acupuncturist, or a psychologist can offer sage advice to consider when you feel pushed beyond the familiar.

"I refer a lot," acknowledges Margi Flint, who has years of solid clinical experience under her belt. "A few times someone will call and I'll just say, 'This situation is too complicated with too many pharmaceuticals.' Or I will just get an intuitive hit that I am not the right person for this. I have no qualms saying to someone, 'I haven't had any experience with this condition.'" Work-

ing reverently and humbly, you will do no harm.

Integrating the practice of herbal medicine into one's life, of course, is more than just a matter of confidence. Where do you create a quiet space to meet with people? At what times are you available to take phone calls and at what times are you not? The ability to establish clear boundaries for yourself and your family ultimately will determine how well you are able to stay centered in this calling. The apparent casualness of a community practice out of the home can soon become a constant influx of demands often lacking in respect for one's privacy. People might not be prompt for an appointment, or might just drop in as you sit down for a family meal. They stay longer to chat. All of which may be fine with a few friends, until you realize that in pursuing a living as an herbalist, you suddenly have no time left for you.

Keeping an immaculate house can also get old for anyone comfortably inclined to random piling. Neat and tidy should be the rule wherever clients go, and not just in what you consider to be professional space. *Never trust a doctor who has dead plants in the office* is all the more apt for the herbalist. An organized desk and paperwork matter— people who give us their trust want to know that trust can indeed be found again. Intake forms and treatment plans should be kept in a separate folder for each client. Date all correspondence; jot down notes for phone conversations; record those intuitive impressions. Ideally, a room in the home can be set aside entirely for herbal work; otherwise you'll need to plan appointments when no other family members will be home. Two comfortable chairs, fresh flowers, and a pot of tea make a simple enough setting in which to listen and observe. Always turn off the phone during a consultation.

Planning to move out of the home as soon as possible will be motivation to grow your herbal consulting practice. Quite a number of the herbalists we talked with had arranged a separate space for consulting with clients one or two days a week. Others were able to delineate a section of their homes with a private entrance for their herbal practices. This astute compromise on laid-back availability works for good reason. People's expectations of the healing encounter have changed from several generations ago. An aura of professionalism doesn't have to work against the guiding partnership we promote

# THE PATIENT'S POINT OF VIEW

FORTY-TWO-YEAR-OLD men sometimes need to be reminded that bounding outside on a warm winter day to split wood ain't like it used to be.

I awoke the next morning sore. Nothing unusual in that. I had been swinging a maul into hardwood at a steady clip yesterday afternoon. Turning to get out of bed brought a sharp pain from my heart region up through the left shoulder. The pain lessened in certain positions but never quite went away. Some mighty powerful realizations come to the fore when muscular tightness centers in the chest. My health has always been so good. I want so, so many more years with Nancy and Gracie. Me? Heart problems? Come on.

Deep down a muscle strain hurts. Put that pain in the leg, the lower back, even the right shoulder, and you face a body needing rest. Put that pain near the heart and you turn pronto to the dire cautions of a first-aid manual: *Seek*

*medical treatment immediately*. Yet the obvious connection of wear and tear the day before suggests I'm okay. Maybe the pain will go away. Not having health insurance enters my thoughts . . . don't incur the big costs unless it's real, man. Nancy, reasonably, isn't so sure. The hospital route entails many choices we might decline.

The morning passes. I can't lie down comfortably. Ironically, the position most tolerable is in front of the computer, striving to meet the deadline for this book. Stress . . . now there's a thought. Maybe I better go see the doctor after all.

Then we remember our friend, Rachel. A nurse will have a good idea of the possibilities behind this pain. Rachel has the voice of a reassuring angel. My breathing is regular, my pulse steady, and, no, I'm not sweating. Inflamed muscle tissue hurts . . . why not try ibuprofen? (Talk about true confessions to the

herbal world!) Reducing swelling in the cartilage tissues should abate the aching pain if we're not dealing with more serious heart issues. It does. Now I face the days ahead with a truly appreciated muscle strain. It's invaluable when you hurt to talk to someone who knows.

I'm off one round of the anti-inflammatory after a reasonable night's sleep, ready to focus on the underlying causes behind yesterday's pain. Comfrey/lobelia poultices rapidly help the tissues in my shoulder regenerate. Ginger adds a soothing heat to the moistened herbs. Nancy brightens my outlook with calendula oil rubs. My herbalist and love feels quite capable with a muscle ailment, but in a clear expression of boundaries, acknowledges not yet being ready for hearts. Especially the big guy's. I understand. Experiencing the dynamics of healing from the patient's point of view teaches precious lessons. —M.P.

actively in the healing relationship. A meeting outside the home assures your full attention on the other person and a courteous regard for you as a practitioner. The possibilities are endless: a spare office above the natural foods store; room made available at a progressive hospital; using the facilities of a massage therapist on her mornings off; even sharing rent with other alternative practitioners amenable to a certain-day-of-the-week schedule. A multidisciplinary clinic may be ideal for community herbalists who eventually step into full-time clinical practice. Cross-referrals, a practitioner support group, an enhanced reputation, and splitting costs for a receptionist come with this territory. But our focus in this book is a bit more unassuming.

Wherever you may roam, take a moment to center before seeing a client. Prayer and meditation help us find that inner serenity so important for healing clarity. Request help from Spirit for both yourself and your client. Taking time to create sacred space in the room can be as simple as burning a smudge stick of sage or ringing bells. A spritz of lavender oil or opening a window between clients renews the air. The importance of clearing energy can be overlooked too easily . The dancing flame of a lit candle during a consultation can be purifying as well as comforting.

White-light visualization at the end of the day allows us to bask in good energy before we return home to our families. A walk after work to release stress rids us of any lingering negativity. Nurturing ourselves as healers keeps us renewed to give fully to our clients. Take a long lunch with friends. Schedule a personal massage. Get out with the plants as often as possible.

We need to get pleasure and satisfaction from our practice. Pursuing this desire to help others with herbal medicine and holis-

tic healing falls short if our spirit does not delight in the work. When we find the right balance of serving others and taking care of ourselves, we have more to give.

## INDIVIDUAL HEALTH PROFILES

Learning a client's physical, emotional, and life history creates a holistic profile of the human being before you. Health issues clarify more readily when viewing the whole story. A questionnaire specifically designed to draw forth such pertinent details can help here.

The range of individual health profiles, or intake forms, used by herbalists reflects personal style. Some practitioners rely on intuition alone to ask a few important questions, then maybe work with muscle testing and reading the pulses when herbs or tinctures are applied. Many prefer running down a list of questions designed to open up an encompassing dialogue with a client. The typical profile of three to eight pages serves as a springboard to the heart of the matter. The Health Inventory that Nancy put together for her practice addresses the reason a client has come and looks at diet, habits, individual and family health history, and emotional and spiritual well-being.* A diet diary extending over several days often reveals the biggest piece of the puzzle. Individual herbalists, however, should shape their own questions. "We ask the question only if we know what the different answers will mean," says Margi Flint.

Whether to have the client fill out the form at home before the actual consultation depends on how we prefer to orient the time together. If the form is filled out in advance and given to the practitioner beforehand, the

---

* A copy of Nancy's Health Inventory can be found at www.herbsandapples.com.

herbalist has a chance to research any pharmaceuticals or supplements the person may be using. The client begins to consider the whole story, and in that sense comes primed for holistic assessment. Some herbalists prefer instead to ask the intake questions during the initial consultation. Body language and tone of voice can be observed, and these often indicate areas that need further probing. Most important, the people coming to see us often want this chance to be heard by a compassionate listener.

An intake session can seem more about psychology and guidance when we delve into the emotional context of another person. Our job is never to judge these confidences, but rather to understand their significance in relation to overall health. We can give ideas to help as long as we are clear: Each person ultimately must take responsibility for his or her own situation. Some might need to be steered toward other therapists if psychological patterns warrant it. Creating an atmosphere of trust begins with reducing the other person's anxiety. People need to feel comfortable with the right chair, a cup of tea, whatever it takes. We're there to sweep aside the professional barriers that isolate human beings from one another. Eye contact and appropriate touch are simply normal ways of expressing care and concern.

More often than not, how we live lies at the core of how we feel. Well-worded questions about lifestyle and diet certainly point out the obvious—who isn't clear about his or her bad habits?—but more so educate and encourage. So many people really don't have a clue about wholesome foods. Fortitude and knowledge are more effective for doing right by our bodies than censure and guilt. Coffee might always taste good, but that caffeine kick comes at a cost. Taking

time for a daily walk should be an adventure. Work needs to be fun and rewarding in all aspects. People need empowerment in these matters, not value judgments.

"I ask the client, 'What are you willing to do to help yourself? What is your intent for this session?' I try to get it down to something they can really do," explains Candis Canton. "I want the client to take an active role. Some people come and they are so tired. They want more energy. I find out they are only sleeping four or five hours, I don't give them herbs, I tell them they need to sleep! I have had amazing results from encouraging people to do the simple things."

Family health history comes into play by revealing genetic disposition for certain diseases. How one chooses to live with this knowledge can determine whether one's hopes will be thwarted or resolutely claimed. People have a strong need to talk about their fears and what is realistic to expect. It helps to shift their mind-set in the intake session away from a specific disease to viewing the situation as a weakness or imbalance. Stories abound of beautiful people who have overcome the worst, not necessarily by becoming completely well, but by choosing a positive attitude. Illness can be as much an opportunity to find inner harmony as any other life situation.

The physiological basics that make up an individual's health history help us discern the whole picture. The details requested will reflect general patterns that can be correlated to our understanding of the organ systems of the body. Many of the questions are meant to reveal the person's view of his or her own health. A wide range of subjective response will be encountered. Some people will avoid any question that does not have an obvious bearing on their primary complaint. The all-too-common notion of *separating self from affliction* needs to be left behind if we are to get people to address constitutional imbalance. Others will check off practically everything or worry inordinately about providing the "right" answer. People who have taken many prescriptions can be the most difficult to evaluate. Years of routine medications for chronic disease can alter profoundly such a person's innate strengths or weaknesses. Herbalists need to develop insight that sorts through the confusion.

Putting these recommendations on paper helps set a holistic framework for each person to ponder and pursue. If during the session we mention exercise and diet changes as being helpful for a client's situation, but then he goes home with only an herbal protocol in writing, we are missing the boat. Clearly writing down what amount of sleep, how many glasses of water to drink a day, and the goal of a daily walk in Nature gives these things as much credence as the specific herbal teas and tinctures we might recommend. Having a form prepared for this purpose helps us achieve our primary goal as practitioners—to empower clients to take charge of their own health (see appendix seven). Encourage them with good questions when you review such an herbal recommendation form together:

- What do you think you can do the first week?
- What is going to be the hardest part of the plan?
- How can we make it more workable for you?
- Are you more likely to take your herbs as a tea, tincture, or in capsule form?

Let clients know you will call them in a week or so to check on how they are doing. It helps to schedule this phone call at a specific time. Set up a follow-up date at the end of the first session as well. People will perceive any changes brought about by treatment, and formulas can be adjusted accordingly. Those with long-standing chronic disease particularly need ongoing encouragement to stick with a program. An informal rule of thumb used by some practitioners is worth noting here: Allow three months of treatment for a problem of a year's standing and a month for every additonal year (or a week's treatment for every month with problems of shorter duration).[6] Correcting a constitutional imbalance can be achieved only when a person starts to trust his or her body's native ability to heal. Positive results with the right herbs may take time but eventually gets them to that place.

## BODY SYSTEMS

Understanding human anatomy and physiology as an awesome collaboration of organ systems—gastrointestinal, respiratory, reproductive, circulatory, nervous, lymphatic, musculoskeletal—helps us to understand the miraculous complexity of the human body. This system view of our bodies allows us to comprehend herbs in much the same fashion as any physician comes to understand conventional therapeutics in terms of bodily function. The Western approach, being home turf for the majority of us, is a reasonable place to begin. We don't have to lose sight of the whole by thinking of the body merely as the equivalent sum of its parts. Systems are just that much easier to grasp; herbs for systems are that much easier to remember.

When we learn about anatomy, we delve into the structure of the body and its parts.

The study of physiology animates these parts, so to speak, for this is the life science that encompasses biological function. These conventional dimensions of healing knowledge are most certainly a piece of the holistic puzzle. The key for herbalists is not to get stuck on a strictly mechanical view of the human body. Viewing biological dysfunction solely as a pathology indicated by symptoms limits healing options. Yet at the same time such an approach can be valuable in contributing to our overall understanding of what is actually going on. All herbalists become better practitioners by devoting time to learning the rudiments of anatomy and physiology. Dr. John Scudder put it this way back in 1870 in a classic Eclectic text, *Specific Medication and Specific Medicines:* "Anatomy and Physiology are the true basis of direct medication, for if we do not know the healthy structure and function, it is not possible that we can know the diseased structure and function."

A visual exploration of the human body coupled with a comprehensive understanding of how the organs work and depend on each other is a vast undertaking. Luckily, many resources are available for taking on such an assignment. Family herbalists desiring a visual guide to get started will find a good overview of key concepts in *The Human Body* published by Dorling Kindersley. *The Anatomy Coloring Book* by Wynn Kapit and Lawrence M. Elson couples a chance to use hands-on artistry with relevant detail. The EastWest School of Herbology recommends *Anatomy and Physiology in Health and Illness* by Ross and Wilson as both economical and relevant for the alternative practitioner. Used textbooks complete with chapter-ending assignments for the self-directed

student can be found at any campus bookstore meeting the needs of medical undergraduates. Continuing education courses in anatomy and physiology (regularly offered for nursing students), provide accreditation and cadavers, if so desired. Designating one evening a week to get together with other herbal students comes without any tuition payment—and yet commitment to the group motivates the inescapable home study needed to learn the names of connecting muscle tissues and the physiological implications of high blood pressure and the like.

Many herbal teachers link their presentation of herbal medicine to the systems of the body. Identifying herbs that have a specific role to play in any one body system enables our brains to grasp important basics. This is not to say that the synergistic action of an herb does not apply to other body systems as well, nor that our organs do not depend on the healthy functioning of all other organs. The actual journey will always be holistic, even if we contemplate one body system at a time. Blood circulation touches on vitality throughout the body. The digestive system acts as a major interface between our insides and the outer world—the total surface area of the digestive tract is a hundred times larger than our skin and comes populated with as many beneficial microbes as the total number of cells in our body. Properly assimilating food and disposing of wastes relates to every aspect of our well-being. The body extracts the oxygen it needs from the air and discharge carbon dioxide as waste from the blood through the respiratory system. The lymph system is contiguous with the whole inner ocean of the body: The water runs through the plasma to get to each cell, and this needs to be kept clean. If a problem

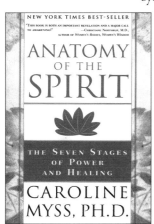

Anatomy of the Spirit *has been called the boldest presentation to date of energy medicine. Author Carolyn Myss has chosen an apt title to remind us that every illness corresponds equally to a pattern of emotional and psychological stresses, beliefs, and attitudes that in turn influence our physical anatomy.*

develops in any of these systems, the body compensates by increasing the load on the others.

We learn that nervine tonics, nervine relaxants, and nervine stimulants feed and strengthen the nervous system. Similarly, we know remedies to help the ears, nose, throat, and eyes. Herbs that aid the respiratory system act to loosen and expel excess mucus from the lungs, soothe irritated membranes, and tone circulation within the capillary-rich air sac. Problems that manifest themselves in the musculoskeletal system can be treated effectively with herbs, provided we bring the body back to a state of health and balance. Antirheumatic herbs, for instance, have different primary actions suited for different situations. Alteratives such as bogbean and devil's claw can be very helpful in improving rheumatic and arthritic conditions through the general revitalization and cleansing these herbs bring about. Long-standing inflammation of joints can be mediated with anti-inflammatory herbs such as meadowsweet and black willow. Weakened kidneys often lie at the root of bone and muscle degeneration, and here diuretic herbs such as celery seed and yarrow can be most helpful. The interconnectedness of plants for specific body purpose—analagous to the interconnectedness of body systems supporting the whole—makes the study of herbal medicine absolutely fascinating. Quite a difference lies between simply regurgitating these kinds of facts and truly understanding the whole of a situation to arrive at the best herbal recommendations for each unique individual.

Herbalists recognize that when the liver can't correctly detoxify everything there tend to be metabolic waste products drift-

# ADAPTOGEN HERBS

ADAPTOGENS help the body to *adapt* around a problem. The core of their action appears to lie in helping the systems of the body cope with stress and change. Many forms of illness can develop when external pressures overwhelm us. By supporting adrenal gland and possibly pituitary gland function, adaptogens boost our level of immunity. Ginseng, borage, licorice, astragalus, and nettles are among those mild herbs that help fortify hormone production and thus strengthen the body throughout. No analogues for herbal adaptogens exist in the allopathic apothecary.

ing around, which can eventually cause toxicity wherever they go. The liver—the largest internal organ in the human body—serves us incredibly well when we pay heed to supporting its vital work. It is involved in metabolizing carbohydrates and maintaining blood sugar levels. The synthesis of blood plasma proteins (such as globulins and clotting factors) happens here, as well as the breakdown of proteins and amino acids. The liver metabolizes fats and vitamins, with the vitamins A, D, K, and $B_{12}$ actually stored in hepatic reserve. The bile secreted by the liver, stored in the gallbladder, and subsequently discharged into the duodenum is essential to the digestive process. The liver helps protect our inner ecology from drug toxins, pollutants, and artificial food additives—all of which unquestionably stress modern-day livers with a constant workload. So often the root that underlies a branch symptom can be associated with improper liver function. Supporting a strong liver that can properly cleanse and tone the whole body begins with taking bitters. Liver stimulants such as dandelion, gentian, yellow dock, barberry, wormwood, and goldenseal were once considered vital. Folk remedies known as "spring tonics" were based on such bitter herbs. We just happen to need a spring tonic every day in these more contaminated times!

The organs of elimination are four: skin, kidneys, intestines, and lungs. The liver's job of disposing of metabolized wastes and toxins depends in turn on proper elimination. A pathway of herbal understanding develops as we learn to emphasize these vital interrelationships. An older person, say, whose skin is no longer supple and open, is likely to experience an additional elimination burden on the kidneys. More fluids have to go through the kidneys or somewhere else to get out of the body. The person may even have a lung problem, because excess moisture is trying to get out through the lungs. Or this may show up as diarrhea or mucus in the intestines. A core idea in Western herbalism is to keep the internal organs functioning cleanly so that the organs of elimination aren't overwhelmed.

A coherent ability to describe such physical reality inside the body directly benefits our clients. Clear language and physiological understanding can be incredibly helpful for people trying to visualize their own healing. A positive focus within can empowers miracles on the cellular level that transcend medical knowing. Immune function endowed with prayerful insight protects us. Appreciating the liver and the heart and the lungs and the thyroid and so forth—and here we mean actually visualizing their place and awesome purpose—strengthens any wellness meditation.

## HERBAL REPERTOIRE

Categorizing plant medicines by understanding their abilities to treat particular body systems makes good sense. To do this, herbalists have long recognized the types of bodily changes that occur as a result of taking any plant medicine. These *actions of the herb* may be due to a specific chemical in the plant, or they may be due to a synergistic interaction between various constituents of the plant. What ultimately matters is not the mechanism, but rather the results. *Alterative, carminative, demulcent, nervine, vulnerary,* and so forth are terms that describe the effects of different herbs. (A complete listing of the terminology used by herbalists to explain these actions can be found in appendix one.) Always keep in mind that herbs stimulate the body's own functions, whereas drugs tend to mimic or inhibit digestion, absorption, and the like. Many plants feature a spectrum of actions capable of assisting the body attain balance rather than providing a single solitary thrust. Some herbs even possess the mind-boggling ability to switch gears (so to speak) depending on the body's need. These herbs help normalize the system by adapting their actions to meet the conditions at hand. The alkaloids found in lobelia, for instance, produce apparently paradoxical effects: Lobeline is a powerful respiratory stimulant, while isolobelanine is a respiratory relaxant. Each aids in the expectoration of mucus from the lungs, whether or not a body is more amenable to a neurological reflex to loosen that mucus or an easing of tension to promote better mucus flow. The underlying intelligence for this function ties directly in the innate healing ability of the body itself, which chooses the assistance it needs where it needs it.

This whole classification scheme can be compounded yet again by synergistic interaction when two or more herbs are used together. Someone seeking help with seasonal affective disorder (SAD), for instance, might find that St. John's wort doesn't really work that well for him or her. The same holds true for lemon balm, another good herb for treatment of SAD. Yet if we combine these two herbs, we find they work better together than either did alone. We asked David Winston to elaborate a bit on the synergy of herbs. "Lots of people use black cohosh for menopausal symptoms. I might recommend chaste tree—I think it is better alone than cohosh—but if I combine the two together they are better than either one by itself. Then I like to add a third herb, dong quai. Used by itself, dong quai has no symptom use for menopause, but with the other two it improves the overall action of the other herbs. You get a sort of exponential action with all three herbs, a broader sphere of influence," notes David. "That is how I see synergy."

What might seem impossibly complicated biochemically is observed to be effective. What counts is that people get well. Each herbalist has a particular approach to determining which herbs are best called for in a given situation. Some have encyclopedic memories (it sure seems so to us!) in remembering the empirical understandings passed down in Eclectic materia medicas. We all learn from past healing experiences of our own, clearly recalling situations where whole-plant remedies either met our expectations or taught us anew. The art of formulation (which we'll briefly discuss in chapter 7) proportions targeted actions through the selection of the right herbs for the individual. Part of this discernment can certainly be intuitive.

"The first step is learning to connect with the plants," explains Rosemary Gladstar. "Then I listen to the person I'm treating—watch their skin tone, listen to their background and symptoms. All the time I'm thinking about the plant spirits. Then I turn around to the herbs and shut my brain down and watch where my hands go. I hope this doesn't sound too much like voodoo. There is that whole other approach to herbalism, but I think this is one of the most important parts."

A wide-ranging knowledge of specific herbs for healing purpose is essential for a master herbalist. Firsthand knowledge of the plants in one's repertoire goes without saying. Just how many plants you need in an effective materia medica is debated hotly. The American Herbalists Guild has suggested a working knowledge of 150 plants as requisite for professional affiliation with the Guild. Yet quite a few herbalists insist that the majority of their practice rests on about 25 plants. Some find healing satisfaction in far fewer, treating the gamut of disease with 4 or 5 herbs and common sense dietary rules.[7] "To attempt to learn too many is to fail in all," says Stephen Buhner. "I would rather have an herbalist who knows 5 plants than one who has information on 150 plants."

Intimacy qualifies our work with the plants. The actual number of herbs we come eventually to know and use isn't nearly as important. "If I studied only one plant for the rest of my life I would never know it. It is just the tip of the iceberg when we learn about plants for food and medicine," observes Oregon herbalist Cascade Anderson Geller. "There is so much more to learn about the energetics of each herb." Depth of knowledge is as important as breadth.

*Energy, plant spirit, medicine power.* These words describe that distinguishing line that carries herbalism into the holistic sphere. The mechanistic view of Nature that drives modern medicine seeks a very common denominator: Everyone who receives the

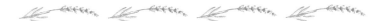

# TOP TEN HERBS IN 1921

THE LLOYD BROTHERS company in Cincinnati, the leading distributor of botanical extracts to physicians in the first part of the twentieth century, compiled an annual list of their best-selling herbs. The exact species was not necessarily indicated.

Echinacea, *Echinacea* spp.
Fringe tree, *Chionanthus virginicus*
Black cohosh, *Cimicifuga racemosa*
Hawthorn, *Crataegus oxycantha*
Pulsatilla, *Anemone pulsatilla*
Gelsemium, *Gelsemium sempervirens*
Thuja, *Thuja occidentalis*
Poke, *Phytolacca decandra*
Cactus (night-blooming cereus), *Cactus grandiflorus*
Passionflower, *Passiflora incarnata*

All these herbs remain in use in naturopathic medical practice in the United States. Echinacea, hawthorn, and black cohosh continue to be highly favored by the general public. Valid questions suggest themselves: Why these herbs? Have we lost sight of something? Which stresses of modern life caused a change in what we most need?

same diagnosis gets the same cure. Just as we have spelled out many factors that determine our constitutional uniqueness, the same holds true for the plants. Far more is afoot here than mere chemical analysis.

"In working with clients in my psychotherapy practice," reports Mary Pat Palmer, "I teach them to meditate on the herbs that they are taking. Those who report success in connecting with the plant on a spiritual level recover from depression much better than those who simply see herbal medicine as equivalent to allopathic, but safer. Without the essence of herbs there is nothing. It is a great tribute to the

power of herbs that they have such strong spirits that they can heal even those who don't see them, although not as well as those who do."

"One summer I was very ill, bleeding [menstrually] for six to eight weeks at a time. There were days when I could barely drag myself out of bed, let alone go to work, keep house, and run my business," says Julie Manchester, a Vermont herbalist. "Sometimes I was so weak and tired, I literally crawled into my garden—not to take care of it, though I tried—but to lie among the plants and feel their healing energy surround me. It was like being hugged and caressed. I could feel them offering me their strength and could feel it sink into my body. There is no way you can tell me the chemicals that make up plants are more important than the plants themselves. They are sentient beings and respond to us as we respond to them."

Choice of herbs in a repertory will vary widely. An emphasis on local plants (responsibly wildcrafted or ably cultivated) will meet the general needs of local people. Personal style establishes our palette, so to speak. "An herb by itself," says Michael Tierra, "is like a color to an artist. It has little meaning until it is combined with other herbs in complex formulations to accommodate the complexity of individuals." Michael's conception encompasses the vast nuance taught in traditional Chinese medicine. We can all respect complexity designed to reflect the energetics of both the individual and the medicines as *good stuff*. And yet it's worth remembering that all combinations of hue eventually trace back to the primary colors. The Eclectics often argued against polypharmacy for the simple reason that botanical subtleties can be lost. The art of herbalism can shine just as vividly for those herbalists who offer that primary connection with the plants that we all agree is the true power behind this medicine. Even when we work with just a few plant friends.

The real purpose of an herbal repertory is to assemble the herbs we have available to best treat the range of health situations that came before us as community herbalists. A series of manuals put together by Michael Moore of the Southwest School of Botanical Medicine (and available to be downloaded gratis from his Web site) provides very useful insight. A manual of differential therapeutics for the health care professional, *Herbal Repertory in Clinical Practice,* gives a constitutional and patient-specific approach to using herbs based on distinct symptoms. A known condition—according to the nature and stage of the disease—points to a range of remedies. The botanicals, preferred preparation, and doses are outlined in his definitive reference for every medicine maker, *Herbal Materia Medica. Specific Indications for Herbs in General Use* highlights Michael's opinions about the best applications for each herb. Similarly, specific indications for tinctures are outlined in *Herbal Tinctures in Clinical Practice.* Peruse these gems to get some idea of the range of plants you might find yourself called to work with in the years ahead.

The situations we feel comfortable treating with herbs are reflected in our repertoire as well. Margi Flint, for instance, is tuned in to issues concerning cardiac care: "I feel very comfortable using a formula based upon hawthorn, linden, and rose hips to support the heart. This beautiful triangle of herbs is nutritive, tonic, and has tons of bioflavinoids. If the person is not on major medications—which of course changes the story for everything—then I am very com-

fortable giving people those three herbs. I shift the formula a bit depending upon their individual constitution." Margi has her tried-and-true herbs for many general conditions. Somebody with a viral condition will receive lemon balm nine times out of ten as a major part of a viral formula. She may add elder or eyebright, although, as Margi is quick to point out, she shies away from herbs such as eyebright now listed as at risk by United Plant Savers. "I went through gallons of elderberry cordial last year," observes Margi. "It's a very delicious way to clear up a virus."

"I often make up the formula right in front of the person," explains Kate Gilday. "We talk about everything that is going into the formula and what each herb will do. People want to know, they want information." How many times going to the doctor did we get all the information we really wanted? Sharing the thinking behind the chosen herbs empowers the formulation decisions for that client.

Our training begets a philosophy that enters into our herbal choices. David Winston has a strong foundation in a number of approaches to healing. "The way that the Cherokee perceives a human and disease is different than that perceived by traditional Chinese medicine or Western medicine. I do the regular case history and all the diagnostics when someone comes in to see me. The person usually fits into one of these models better than the other," notes David. "If someone comes in and really fits the Cherokee model, I will use that. I approach the patient usually from one perspective, yet, on the other hand, the way I use herbs is extremely eclectic [and David doesn't mean Eclectic medicine], because I draw herbs

*Text continues on page 152.*

# David Winston

IF YOU ARE LUCKY enough to catch David Winston at home, you are likely to find him engrossed in an antiquarian book at an old rolltop desk in what is a bit like a huge cave—his personal library filled with more than eight thousand books on all aspects of herbs and medicine. Shelves of books line the walls, sectioned neatly by topic: botany, pharmacy, ethnobotany, women's health, Thomsonian medicine, seemingly ad infinitum.

David has been studying, practicing, researching, and teaching Cherokee, Chinese, and Western herbal medicine for the past thirty-two years. He is the one called on to drum and offer prayers at the opening and closing circles of many herbal gatherings and symposiums. David speaks passionately for the plants from the experiences of his heart. This person who encompasses so many herbal facets turns out to be a warm, personable guy.

"I actually have four companies. Herbalist & Alchemist, Inc. manufactures more than three hundred products. I do product consulting as David Winston, Inc., for other companies, both grassroots herb businesses and giant pharmaceutical corporations like Bayer. My third company is Herbal Therapeutics, Inc. (HTI), which is basically the enterprise that sponsors all of my teaching. I travel all over the United States and Canada and occasionally Europe to teach at herb conferences, medical schools, and herb symposiums." HTI also handles any writing David does. *Saw Palmetto for Men and Women* joins the informative herb series put together by Storey Publications. His next project is a professional manual for nurses and physicians on using herbs, and a weed herbal is in the works.

"Then finally I have Herbalist & Alchemist Books, which sells antiquarian, out-of-print books on herbal medicine and pharmacy. I talk about these wonderful books wherever I teach, and naturally people wanted to know where to get them. They of course are not easy to find, so I began buying duplicates and selling them to my students. I put out two catalogs a year of books on herbal medicine with more than three hundred titles on just the kind of material herbalists are looking for."

Community can be widely defined in this well-traveled age. The call to join one's people brings David back to family in North Carolina often. His uncle is the last full-blooded medicine man of the eastern band of the Cherokee. David leaves the busy world behind to focus on being a Cherokee medicine priest in his own right. "We have no word for 'healer' in Cherokee medicine. Two terms describe what I am to my people. The first word, *didahnvwisgi,* means "medicine priest." The second term is more of a verb, *dasgi,* which means "provoker." My job is to provoke somebody to move beyond where they are stuck. It could be their diet, their relationships, or their job. I help to provoke the inner doctor.

"Cherokee medicine is a fas-

> *Medicine is being able to look at somebody and help them understand why life is not working for them.*
>
> —DAVID WINSTON

cinating system that is at least five thousand years old. *Nvwisti,* our word for 'medicine,' doesn't just mean herbs, a surgical procedure, or body work. Anything that has power is medicine. So to us ceremony is medicine, dreams are medicine, songs are medicine, herbs are medicine, water is medicine, fire and the earth are all medicine. Western medicine has not completely embraced the holistic model; the body is still the main focus. Allopathic medicine is still trying to integrate the mind, but has forgotten the spirit altogether. The Cherokee perspective considers the body, mind, and spirit in looking at a person's health. Well-being is also strongly connected to the family, community, and what we call the Great Life. The Great Life is the sum of all the parts and more."

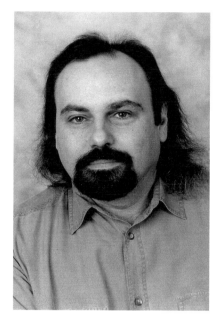

Cherokee ceremony revolves around Earth, the seasons, and cycles of life. People come for doctoring during these times. Days of preparation take place before the actual healing ceremonies. "We don't just doctor the individual, we treat the whole family. We just assume that if a family member is ill, there is a problem in the family as well. Illness flourishes in imbalance, disconnection, and disharmony," says David. "There are no spectators in our ceremonies. Nobody sits there and watches this happen."

One powerful ceremony is based on the woman's moontime. David radiantly relates how often gynecological problems have cleared up when women learn to work with their moontime energies. "The menstrual power is one of the most powerful energies in the universe. Women—when they are in their moon—are the only ones who have the power to heal the planet.

"Medicine is more than giving somebody herbs. Medicine is more than massaging somebody, more than surgery, more than pharmaceuticals. Medicine is being able to look at somebody and help them understand why life is not working for them. Helping them to see what they need to do to reconnect in this Great Life so they can move in harmony with everything else. If you are doing that, you are alive. If you are not doing that, you are dying. There are only two states in life: living and dying. Either your spirit is growing and getting stronger or your spirit is withering away."

The Cherokee have one of the largest materia medicas of any native people in North America. Traditionally the average Cherokee person intimately knew at least 100 to 200 plants for food and medicine. A *didahnvwisgi* knew 600 to 800 different medicines. We find similarly huge materia medicas in Chinese medicine and Ayurveda. We asked David why.

"Because the more materials of medicine you have, the more tools you have to make change. The Cherokee concept of the plants is broader than the dominant culture's concept. To the Cherokee, a plant is much more than its chemical constituents. Each plant has a personality, which includes its physical constituents, but also abilities to heal the mind and spirit as well. Every herb has a quality of its personality that is unique and gives insight into the subtle use of the plant. An example would be wild grapevine's ability to cling; it is used to bind broken hearts and relationships. When a plant is gathered in the proper season and dried, you preserve the chemical constituents. Only by ceremonially harvesting a plant—asking permission, offering tobacco, and always leaving a viable community behind—do you preserve the subtle healing abilities."

"The Cherokee use a great variety of medicines, not only to prevent overutilization of species, but also because they believe that every plant has its specific use in relationship to human ailments. To the Cherokee, the use of herbs is only one tool of many necessary for regaining health. We believe it is crucial not only to heal the body, mind, and spirit, but also to reintegrate the ill person within the family, the community, and with Earth herself. This is a holistic perspective beyond our culture's limited understanding. None of us can truly be well unless we recognize our connection to the rest of the Great Life." ✌

from my Cherokee tradition, Chinese medicine, and Ayurveda."

"I have found that, underneath them all, they are all the same," says Phyllis Light. "Underneath the Ayurvedic is the same thing that is underneath the traditional Chinese, which is the very same thing that is underneath Appalachian folklore. Underneath the *trappings of a system,* what you learn about the plants is all the same, and how you use the plants is all the same."

## THE MÉTIER OF HEALING

Effective herbalists come in many shades. Botanical depths can be hidden behind personable warmth; thoroughness can cut to the quick; wisdom may find root in earthy humor. Yet each and all possess qualities that radiate a strengthening grace to those seeking healing.

"I have known some incredible healers in my life," says Rosemary Gladstar. "They have personalities that are all different. You see these really prickly ones, these really arrogant ones. You see these passionate, loving ones that everybody speaks about. I think the key is inner connection to spirit. The power that comes with this is absolutely recognizable. It doesn't matter if you're a scrawny old lady or a handsome young man. There's this open channel that spirit works through. Almost always these people really know suffering to the core of their being. It doesn't mean their life has been rougher than anybody's, but the experience scorches them. There has to be an ability to know pain deeply. And to know joy also. Healers can touch this when they go into other people. Knowledge—your bag of tools—is important as well, but not nearly as important. Your knowledge is your language, what you use to administer that depth."

People reasonably expect an herbalist to walk their talk. Encouragement coming from someone following the same lifestyle guidelines being advised can be respected. Philosophically speaking, a healthy connection to spirit and the good life would be expected to show. And yet we all have our human frailties to face. *Striving to do well ourselves* perhaps expresses this reality best: Those personal struggles and temptations come regardless of holistic insight. The virtue of being real more often strikes the first chord in the healing relationship.

"I've seen many great teachers and healers who are tremendously out of balance," continues Rosemary. "People who eat horrendously or people who are very ill or have terrible addictions. Yet they have amazing ability to heal other people. They may not have good relationships, they may be crabby or very arrogant, and yet without a doubt they have affected people. Spirit doesn't always choose perfect vehicles. I think spirit chooses whoever is open, and a lot of times, the most damaged are the most receptive. I know in my own experience I would not want to emulate the life of many people I respect and admire. And yet their power, their ability to transform other people's lives, is awesome. Sometimes people go down to that grieving place so deeply, they are not able to heal themselves. I don't believe this concept that you have to be a perfect vehicle to do this perfect work. I think you can be very crippled, incredibly crippled, both emotionally and physically."

The question of arrogance versus humility is worth examining. The medical axiom to *present one's self as certain* expresses legitimate intention. Confidence in the therapist/therapy by the patient is deemed as crucial for the cure. Expressing any doubt in a recommended course of action is held to undermine this confidence. The so-called placebo effect hinges on optimistic expectation. The rub comes when we invest too much of our ego in our personal power to act against disease. Arrogance loses sight of the true source of healing within each human being. Arrogance ignores the generosity of the plants in guiding us to that place. The greatest doctoring advice will focus on the positive in any situation. Being upbeat differs considerably from knowing it all. Our work becomes that much more satisfying and pleasurable when we can openly acknowledge that inevitable unknowns accompany our certitude. The most meaningful answers lie within one's self.

A large part of the distress accompanying an illness comes from uncertainty and fear. A healer reassures and comforts. The sincerity of our care supports a client's desire to get well. Apprehensions about treatment and fears of the unknown lie within every patient. The art of medicine will be found in a shared empathy with the people before us. More often than not, a loving nature proves to be as vital as technical prowess or any herbal repertoire.

"Almost anybody that comes to me from a place of being treated through the Western medical model and hasn't really gotten better," says Kate Gilday, "cries by the end of their story. It is the first time anyone has ever taken an hour or two, sometimes three hours, to really listen to them. I think that is probably the most important part of my practice, just really hearing people and then next introducing them to the plants. It comes back to me. I feel their gratefulness and then I see their connectedness to the plant world and I know that I have planted a seed for them that will grow."

# QUESTING FOR A HEALER

ALL OF US should invite anyone looking for medical help to seek out the level of our experience. The terms *clinical herbalist* and *master herbalist* are used by people with very different depths of experience. This makes self-proclaimed titles somewhat meaningless. Trust and confidence are vital to the healing relationship.

The following are some questions one should ask or find out about an herbalist. As responsible health care providers, we should have all of this information readily available in our brochures or handouts:

- What did your training entail? What type of studies, how long, etc.?
- How long have you been seeing clients?
- How many clients do you usually see in an average week?
- Tell me your personal philosophy about health and healing.
- Where do the herbs and products come from that you recommend?

The range of healing choices available today is mind-boggling. All of us know on some level of consciousness what we need to heal. Each individual is ultimately in charge of his or her own healing. Finding the right person(s) to help on that healing journey should be encouraged by every herbalist.

---

Individual attitudes play a large role in what we deem appropriate health care, and, even more important, what we believe to be effective medicine. So much returns to our beliefs. Michael's father's ending days with lung cancer placed him between an unwavering commitment to allopathic medicine (given his medical training as a dentist in the late 1940s) and a surefire conviction that chemotherapy and radiation would serve no purpose. Accordingly, any alternatives were out of the question. He went through the conventional treatments to please his family—a not atypical reasoning—but rued every declining moment. He died almost to the day all too audaciously pronounced by the oncologist four months before. Working with people on their unique paths toward wellness and the inevitable transition beyond this life foremost involves respecting their parameters.

Many lessons come with the death of someone you love. Some are immediate, others await the fading of acute grief. This passing over to the next realm should by all rights invoke our tenderest affection. Healers have a special call to embrace death in order to fully embrace life. The ending of bodily time is a sacred part of our ever-continuing journey. The experience of losing a parent, a child, or a loving partner requires personal healing at the deepest level. And yet we now grasp mortality in a way that transcends illness and wrought emotion. The real priorities of life become ever so clear when Spirit takes back its own. Every day is a blessing. A healthy body is a most precious gift. Love is the all within all. A perspective filled with such

heartfelt meaning—however we come to this divine place—compels every healer to be of service to others.

We must not be afraid or reluctant to touch and be with the sick. People get overwhelmed by illness. The ability to step in and provide direct care is at the core of what we do. Taking time to breathe deeply with sick people focuses mutual intent. Using touch in our work—a hug, a massage, or simply holding hands—lets love be shown. Connection to the plants and their healing purpose completes this circle of care we can offer as herbalists.

"It's absolutely our responsibility to use the gifts offered by the plant spirits. Part of being a good healer," says Pam Montgomery in concluding our talk on healing intimacy, "is taking on the responsibility of these gifts. When people are sick—regardless if they don't have money or we're too tired or whatever it is—our primary responsibility remains to help. These gifts are given to us because we make a deal with the plant spirits to serve."

## NOTES

1. *The American Heritage Dictionary* (Boston: Houghton Mifflin, 1992).

2. A handful of states recognize naturopathic doctors. Licensed acupuncturists find legal leeway as well.

3. The penalties differ slightly state by state. The punishment mandated by California law regarding this misdemeanor is a fine of not less than $200 nor more than $1,000, or imprisonment for a term of not less than 60 days nor more than 180 days, or both fine and imprisonment. A separate clause in California law makes the unauthorized practice of medicine a felony if it results in or creates the risk of great bodily harm. Loss of license accompanies an incompetence ruling.

4. Matthew Wood, speaking at the 4th International Herb Symposium at Wheaton College in Norton, Massachusetts, in June 1998.

5. She's a modest gal, our Margi. If you'd like to get a copy of the self-published handbook, contact her at EarthSong Herbals, 10 Central Street, Marblehead, MA 01945.

6. Simon Mills and Kerry Bone, *Principles and Practice of Phytotherapy* (London: Churchill Livingstone, 2000), 83.

7. Roy Upton wrote about one such herbalist. Leah Conners used four herbs predominantly when working in her health foods store in Clearlake, California. The herbs she used were the fluid extracts of echinacea, goldenseal, hawthorn berry, calendula, and, once in a while, valerian. See "Profile of a Community Healer," *American Herbalism,* Michael Tierra, ed. (Freedom, Calif.: Crossing Press, 1992), 60–64.

# CHAPTER SIX

# Growing and Drying Medicinal Herbs

CATNIP
*Nepeta cataria*

*T*he yarrow seed in my palm has presence. These tiny specks contain the biological map of a steadfast medicinal helper. The energy caressed between my fingertips sifts slowly downward. A continuity flows between these seeds, myself, and the living soil. I no longer merely start seedlings in our greenhouse. Today, with this yarrow, I initiate a conscious act of healing. ❧ Many medicinal plants remain in the ground for more than one growing season. Time enough to get to know each plant, if not individually, then as a returning row or cluster each spring. Earth awakens. Stout garlic tips emerge, bronzed in anticipation of an ever warming sun. Valerian, marsh mallow, and elecampane follow in turn. Out in the woods, goldthread, black cohosh, and ginseng push aside leafy blankets and stretch delightedly in the widening day. Hawthorn trees break bud, crooked behind arrays of formidable thorns. Blue vervain, borage, and angelica seedlings volunteer without so much as a whisper on my part. I have reversed my good farmer's impulse to weed out every dandelion, to hoe asunder the lamb's quarters. Stewardship of boundless diversity deepens my craft. I am a grower, a keeper of the soil, the artist of a farm. ❧ The high sun calls us to harvest. I breathe fully the scent of soothing lemon balm. Resins of calendula blossoms fill the soil cracks in my fingers and palms. Perhaps this year the nettles won't sting . . . my awareness grows, insistent teacher of the green. I'm infused with righteous joy as St. John's wort flowers crest the rim of each gathering basket. To the tunnel, to the tunnel, to dry *more herb for the healer's call! Milky oat heads waft in a breeze without respite for a grower's sore wrists. Summer's end at last offers sweet repose. ℘ Roots are dug after pervasive autumn frosts send plant energy fully back beneath the ground. My own roots have touched a thousand friends. The land has nurtured us in preparation for the coming winter. We give thanks— mother, father, daughter—for an Earth so rich, a life so loved.  —M.P. ℘*

GROWERS AND GATHERERS of the healing plants provide the green matter with which practitioners and herbal pharmacists work. The allure of creating a living with medicinal herbs hinges on niche-marketing specialty crops that, acre for acre, return more than twice the value of vegetables. The reality, however, remains much the same as for any grower: Building a reputation for high quality takes time. You need to heed the prompting of plants that aren't obliged to follow the rules of domesticated tilth, harvest for maximum medicinal value, and be committed to drying good herb. Some herbalists are growers themselves, achieving the majority of their apothecary needs in home gardens and through wildcrafting in their bioregion. But many herbalists don't have the time to grow what a knowledgeable farmer or wildcrafter can supply.

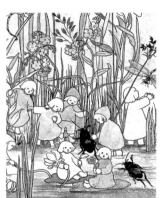

*An illustration from* The Root Children *by Sybelle von Olfers, originally published in Germany in 1906.*

The plants most needed are the ones willingly growing nearby. Sometimes common blessings are too readily overlooked in our haste to find a satisfactory niche. Growing local medicine means we can branch off from the wholesale recommendation to specialize in large amounts of a few herbs. The focus shifts from contracting for 1000-pound lots to meeting the health needs of our surrounding communities. *Echinacea purpurea* might well be on its way to being over-cultivated in North America. But that doesn't mean neighbors shouldn't be encouraged to tincture fresh root on their own. Herbalists can arrange with farm friends to custom-grow the medicinals they need in their practice. Non-native species shouldn't be entirely ignored—herbs such as ashwagandha and spilanthes can be grown in the temperate North, on a small scale, to offer even more fresh healing diversity to the community medicine chest. Tim Blakley did a particularly generous favor for the rest of us by detailing the plant-by-plant possibilities in his section of *Medicinal Herbs in the Garden, Field and Marketplace.* Our thrust in this book will be more on what it takes to be a successful grower on the local and regional level. Meeting the needs of our own communities is paramount. Responsible gathering of wild plants and organic cultivation of both native and introduced species are the only ways we can ensure that herbal medicine will be sustainable.

## NURTURING THE ROOT CHILDREN

Any plant can tell you: Life begins in the soil.

Basic soil science addresses the physical needs of plants. The concept is much like the science of discerning which constituents in a plant appear to provide its medicinal potency. Good knowledge can be learned and applied to advantage, but the sense of the whole can be overlooked too easily. Soil reductionists have touted NPK—the nitrogen/potassium/phosphorus trinity of chemical agriculture—just as medical reductionists focused on hypericin as the standardized constituent in St. John's wort. Learning how chemical elements and specific minerals bring about healthy plant growth matters. In fact, good production depends on it. But only when we venture deeper into the world of Fairie—whether imaginative or dashedly real—do we begin to dance with the soil microorganisms that enable all life.

Our daughter, Grace, has a fun book, *The Root Children*, published at the turn of the previous century in old-world Europe. Mother Nature awakens the flower fairies in early spring to make their colorful costumes anew. Ground beetles and bees are groomed to emerge into the warming day. Finally comes the morning of the grand procession out into the world. The root children carry their flowers and waving grasses splendidly from beneath the soil, each blessed in turn by Mother Nature as they go out the door. The fairies frolic. The earth is filled with quickening chorus. Summer passes. As the days shorten and frosts nip the air, Mother Nature calls the children and insects back home for a long winter's rest tucked in among the roots. Mother resumes her knitting, the children yawn, the world rests both above and below.

What's so wonderful about that story is the imagery of the earth alive. Of soil pulsating with life-forms. Of a space within the ground where fairies and insects can move as easily as if in air. Certainly we don't have to embody Nature spirits to understand that more is afoot in living soil than meets the eye. Past cultures have embraced the wee folk in both legend and sincere recognition. The ethereal realm indeed touches those who have this desire.

A hundred years ago humans could not have imagined the inroads of understanding waiting to be unveiled beyond the physical world we normally see. We started with bacteria, stripped apart the molecule, found energetic quarks, and engaged in microscopic stewardship. A small leap of faith opens similar doors into the ethereal realm—a world intuitively comprehended by our ancestors. Elemental beings likely do fill the terrestrial sphere as much as we suppose angels inhabit the celestial sphere. We each possess the latent faculties necessary to become aware of a many-dimensioned universe. The plant world beckons a mutual consciousness that takes the art of agriculture far beyond the mere science of agriculture. Sometimes we can trust our hearts to proceed where only the best fools have gone before. Sometimes we can say thank you to the plants and the Nature spirits that attend them. Sometimes we can simply believe in what we might never see.

**The Living Earth**

Scoop up a handful of rich earth. Piled in your palm are more microorganisms than there are human beings living on the planet. Boggles the mind, no? The teeming trillions of bacteria and other microscopic flora and fauna in the top few inches of our soil are the very engine of our existence. Organic agriculture begins with the recognition that these microbes feed the soil, which feeds the plant (which feeds the animals), which feeds our bellies. There is no chemical shortcut to this existential truth.

The miracle of life that began with a single-celled bacterium coexists with and will end with single-celled bacteria. Our bodies rely on the microbes lining our intestines to assimilate the nutrients in our food. Similarly, raw organic matter from plant and animal tissues can't become humus until metabolized by soil organisms. Even rocks, ground to fine dust by time and weather, yield their elements to the minuscule feeders in the soil. This degrading of mineral and organic molecules into a soluble form that can be readily taken up by plants is the basis of our being.

The foundation of medicine farming lies in stewardship of the soil. Building humus is always the goal. Feeding a population of thriving microorganisms a diverse blend of organic matter results in a continuing humus. Nature's perfect fertility plan loops round and round on itself to the utter chagrin of the fertilizer companies: There are no profits to be made in a self-enriching soil. Plants and algae create organic matter through the process of photosynthesis. Animals eat plants and so on up the food chain, consuming what amounts to the stored energy of the sun. All plants and animals eventually die, and their bodies return to the soil by the action of microorganisms. Bacteria, fungi, and actinomycetes secrete different enzymes that begin the decomposition process. These microbes absorb the soluble nutrients first released—especially carbon and nitrogen compounds—and use them to reproduce. Decomposition proceeds rapidly as each microbe multiplies by as much as 300 million a day. The resulting humus satisfies the nutrient needs of our plants in more ways than one.

Humus—the residue left after the extensive decomposition of organic materials—contains 60 to 70 percent of the total organic carbon in soils. It also contains chains of sugar molecules that help cement soil aggregates together, as well as the countless billions of bacterial bodies whose proteins will be further reduced into soluble plant nutrients. Stable humus is resistant to

further microbial decomposition, thus holding the soil carbons somewhat in place. These form active chemical structures known as *humic acids,* which provide for long-term nutrient storage expressed as *cation exchange* capacity on soil tests. Positive ions such as calcium and potassium latch into place until such time as they are taken up by the root hair of a plant (in exchange for a hydrogen ion). Chemically speaking, the humic acid has become a humate. A dead soil requires applications of soluble fertilizers to make up for its lack of humates.

Chemical fertilizers cannot begin to rival Nature. Hers is a twofold process by which plants draw their nurture from the soil. And again, microorganisms are at the heart of the matter. Living fungal threads, called *mycelia,* that invade young roots and are gradually absorbed in turn provide organic nitrogen directly to the root system. The mycelium's proteins, digested by enzymes in the root, soon enter the sap current of the plant as soluble nutrients. In soils where humus is lacking, this symbiotic feeding does not occur. Plants are then limited to the absorption of soluble salts.

Mycorrhizal fungi enhance disease resistance by warding off pathogenic organisms with antibiotic secretions. This living friendship helps explain why some medicinal plants, seeded far from their native habitat and thus bereft of native mycorrhizae, never actually thrive, even though the test climate may well be agreeable.

Farmers who understand this big picture know that soil audits serve only as a rough guideline to what's going on in a living soil. Pooling together the dynamics of chemical elements and trace minerals and striking a desired average for each never successfully describes the unique vitality of humus. A soil with good biological activity transcends the numbers soil scientists have worked out to define viable reality. Biological farmers don't rely on the NPK incantation. The "cation waltz" better indicates actions to consider in choosing soil amendments. Humus holds calcium, magnesium, potassium, and sodium in colloidal saturation. Our job as growers is to respect the proper proportion among these alkaline cations—a regard too often lost in myopic adjustment of pH (hydrogen acidity) alone—so that base saturation values of Ca-Mg-K approximate a 65:15:3 ratio. Too great an excess of one cation will inhibit uptake of the others by the roots. These nutrient elements have a lot to do with maintenance of hormone and enzyme systems, healthy plants, protection against insect and fungal attack, weed control, and medicinal effect. Soil pH becomes self-adjusting when calcium, magnesium, potassium, and sodium are in proper equilibrium. Other nutrients such as nitrogen, phosphorus, and sulfur exist as proteins and carbon compounds in organic matter. These are mineralized into available plant food by bacteria at a slow and sustained rate.

Most microorganisms rely on the carbon in organic matter as their prime energy source. Available carbon correlates directly to a larger and more diverse microbial population. Biological equilibrium achieved through diversity resounds with health across the board. When all is said and done, creating organic matter and shepherding the microorganisms are what lead to self-sufficient soils that are quite capable of striking elemental balance on their own.

## The High Art of Building Soil

Soil improvement works from the surface down in Nature. Leaves fall from the trees to the ground, joining last year's dead grasses in a decomposition feast for earth-worms and microbes. The rains wash released nutrients down into the soil to roots and mycorrhizal fungi in the humus layer. Root tips secrete a weak acid that chemically breaks down some of the surrounding soil particles. Subsoil cycling takes place as well, with roots accessing minerals made soluble in groundwater. Tree roots go the deepest of all, as the pump of photosynthesis takes minerals from deep within the earth high up into the leaves, which eventually renew the soil from above.

We build soils best by keeping this model in mind. Tearing open the living Earth—whether by hand spade or tractor-powered spader—has a long tradition in agriculture, one that we should apply with reverent discretion. Tillage accomplishes an open seedbed while incorporating organic residues from previous crops. Stable humus is biologically resistant, so earth-turning can stimulate the microbial soil dynamic as well. Every good farmer knows that soil organic matter is consumed by aerobic bacteria in the very act of plowing under new organic matter. Northern growers have slightly more leeway to work with tillage as a cultivation tool than warm-climate growers, with soils that decompose organic matter at accelerated rates. A sustainable agriculture will find ways to reduce reliance on opening Earth's surface in order to integrate natural soil health into the balance. A winter-killed cover crop of oats, for instance, leaves a field mulched and ready for direct transplanting in spring without further soil preparation. A light scratching of the soil surface to set back germination of unwanted species (what we used to call "weeds" before we became medicine farmers) not only gives crops a jump on early competition but shows regard for top-down soil dynamics. Many perennial medicinals—those with a flair for finding the right spot—move about in weedy fashion, inviting us to change our notions of proper agrarian order. Interestingly, when we allow ourselves to embrace such plant consciousness—which comprehends soil interaction far more intimately than humans ever will—we often reap more potent healing from the herb.

Matured compost rates high in any organic grower's plan for renewing soil organic matter. (The use of raw manure, however, comes rife with concerns, ranging from high nitrogen levels that shift microbial focus to gut pathogens such as *E. coli*.[1]) Compost that has properly ripened over time is an amazing soil conditioner. Only 3 to 5 percent humus will transform lifeless sand into a rich loam. The plant and microbial mucilages in humus reduce the size of pores between sand particles, increasing the moisture-holding capacity of soil and reducing the leaching of dissolved nutrients. With added humus, more plant species and microbes can thrive in the once barren sand. This newfound diversity, in turn, spurs on the creation of additional humus. Wow! In clay soils, humus formed from the organic matter in compost couples with the clay particles to form complexes that increase the soil's overall cation exchange capacity and lighten the cohesive nature of pure clay. Compost adds essential carbon matter to the soil that soluble chemical fertilizers lack completely (and carbon, as we learned earlier, fuels the microbes themselves). The organic principle of feeding the soil relies on these many circles of life that are constantly in renewal.

We find an intriguing reciprocity among the selected medicinal herbs used in biodynamic agriculture. All life pulsates with spirit, and it is this spirit that biodynamic farmers and gardeners seek out in a healing partnership that reaches far beyond merely curative organic agriculture. The biodynamic compost preparations originally described by Rudolf Steiner[2] involve the florets of wild white yarrow, German chamomile, stinging nettle, the outer bark of the white oak tree, dandelion blossoms, and the extracted juice of valerian flowers. These herbs are combined with animal substance in specific recipes in certain seasons of the year and then placed in compost piles. These energetic preparations in turn are thought to abet the composting process. Some biodynamic friends have described their involvement in these ways as *pleasing to the elemental beings who arrange the chaotic elements of Nature into living plants.* Regardless of how one approaches such matters, working deliberately with healing intent resonates with the pulse of the land.

Let's take an open-minded look at the first biodynamic compost preparation, known as BD 502. The yarrow florets are enclosed in the bladder of a stag (usually dried from the previous fall hunt) at the height of bloom, and hung in the air through the summer and fall. The filled bladder is then buried in the top foot of fertile earth to age through the winter and spring, completing a full year's cycle of exposure to cosmic and earthly influences. Yarrow, through its association with the sulfur element, encourages potassium to be brought into the organic processes of the farm. Each of the preparations is buried separately within a working compost pile to enhance the vital energy of humus renewal. More generally speaking, yarrow (*Achillea millefolium*) helps purify the soil, while chamomile (*Matricaria recutita*) speeds up the release of nutrients from soil organic matter. Stinging nettle (*Urtica dioica*) gets forces flowing. Remember that herbal adage to give nettles when in doubt as to which herb to use? White oak (*Quercus alba*) builds immunity (disease resistance) on the farm; dandelion (*Taraxacum officinale*) helps crops fill out, and valerian (*Valeriana officinalis*) serves to regulate plant metabolism.[3]

"Steiner chose yarrow [and the other herbs used in the preps] through divine inspiration," says Rob Wooding, a biodynamic herb grower in Virginia. "No chemist will say yarrow balances the cosmic influences of sulfur with the other mineral elements. It's a leap of faith, but, nevertheless, biodynamics gets results." Perhaps herbalists are best poised to ponder the connections between these plants that heal our bodies and apparently actualize Earth-healing energies.

The physical structure of soils certainly affects cropping results. Heavier soils benefit from the addition of sand. We have changed the composition of sodden ground here at our farm over the years by spreading sand and compost in equal proportion, followed by shallow tilling. Coarse sand provides excellent drainage and is a good source of minerals. Soil-building isn't just about nutrient levels or increasing organic matter content. Drainage tiles (perforated pipes laid in gravel trenches) have been used to carry excess groundwater away on other farms. Those medicinal plants that like wet feet provide a nice way to wild-crop such ground without paying for drainage. Near our brook is a perpetually soggy area that we have planted to boneset, nettles, marsh mallow, and joe-pye weed.

Cover crops bring us to a zenith of understanding in guiding soil renewal. These plants retrieve soil nutrients and make them available to the plants that follow in turn. Legumes such as clovers, alfalfa, and bell beans fix nitrogen on their roots. Cereal grasses such as rye, oats, and barley create vast quantities of green organic matter and fibrous root systems to decompose. Fast-growing buckwheat smothers sod in newly turned ground and sends taproots far below to access subsoil phosphorus and break up clay hardpan. We try to keep our garden ground planted throughout the growing season to both protect and enrich the soil. Garlic will go where oats waved in the breeze until early September, when the grassy cover is cut and rough-tilled into the soil surface. Annual rye is sown in late summer wherever a planting bed or pathway opens up, growing long into the fall before succumbing to the cold of a New Hampshire winter. We plant a patch of red clover each year within an oat sowing for successive medicinal harvests over the course of the next two or three summers. Beneficial insects groove in buckwheat flowers planted along tilled garden edges to keep creeping sod at bay. All cover crops absorb the energy of the sun, releasing it in the fullness of time to new generations of crops and microorganisms.

Rock powders and soil amendments help to address immediate fertility needs as well as long-term requirements of sustainable growth. Flakes of granite weather slowly, releasing potassium without altering soil pH. Greensand from eighty-million-year-old marine deposits provides more than thirty trace minerals needed by plants in minute amounts. Azomite, mined in Utah, more than doubles this ante of minerals, along with a 5 percent flush of calcium. Dried kelp meal is an excellent source of chelated minerals, enzymes, and amino acids. In addition to adding it directly to the soil, our sheep and goats love it. We know this goodness from the sea gets

*Text continues on page 164.*

# Richo Cech

HORIZON HERBS in Williams, Oregon, is a seed company dedicated to preserving the diversity of medicinal plants from around the world. The Cech family grows more than five hundred species of herbs for seed, with about three acres under intensive cultivation. Richo Cech acknowledges that keeping these gardens looking good and productive are a full-time occupation. "We work really, really hard to provide our customers with viable seeds for improving their environment and their health. Cultivation of medicinal plants from seed is of absolutely imperative importance," observes this Earth steward, "if we are to turn the global tide of degradation of native medicinal plant resources."

The ways to do just that are shared liberally throughout the Horizon catalog, which includes a thorough description of germination requirements for each herb. This seed information covers all the essentials: light-dependent germinators need to be sown shallowly; some species do best started outdoors in nursery beds; certain seeds require scarification of their impermeable coating. Richo encourages gardeners to plant at-risk species such as arnica, *Echinacea tennesseensis,* and yellow gentian. The concept of plant conservation through organic cultivation rings clear throughout the catalog. Advice on how gardeners can incorporate herb use into their lifestyle is included. Marsh mallow root, for instance, can be cut into cross-sections and dried, later to be used as "tasty pills" that can be chewed as treatment for gastric ulcer.

Early on, Richo developed a bent toward ethnobotany while doing anthropological research on the coast of East Africa. "I came back home to Iowa and started doing the back-to-the-land thing with Mayche," recalls Richo. "We focused more and more on medicinal herbs when we moved out to the West Coast. I was heavily influenced by Maude Grieve's book, *A Modern Herbal,* right from the start." He worked for Herb Pharm (a well-respected manufacturer of liquid herbal extracts) for a decade, first as the production manager in the fields, then as the staff herbalist in charge of making medicines. Horizon Herbs was conceived in 1985. "Our first catalog was basically a one-page list of seeds that we had harvested from our gardens. My mom saved a copy of that first list and sent it to me recently in a scrapbook. I had to laugh when I read the ordering details. Instead of the usual rundown of specific shipping and handling charges, it just said, trustingly, 'send extra for postage.'"

Horizon Herbs will never stray far from the family vision on which this lovingly tended farm began. "Our kids were all involved with the seed work from the get-go," Richo says.

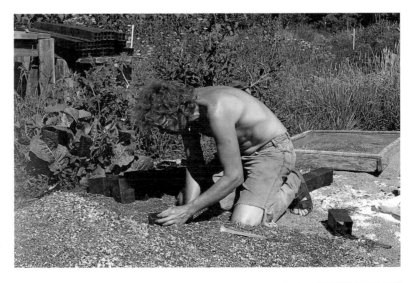

"They've illustrated our packages and catalogs, worked in the gardens, and are especially good at hand-winnowing. Herbal roots like these remain even after our children move on to other things," explains this proud father. "Nadja is pursuing her Ph.D. in chemistry at the University of New Mexico, researching analytical techniques in mass spectrometry, using goldenseal as the subject for some of her

*You just have to have the openness to hear the message from the plants and the right attitude to use it well.*

—Richo Cech

investigations. Sena continues to be our botanical illustrator and cartoonist. She invented Cheesie, the little mouse cartoon character who demonstrates things like straining St. John's wort oil through a cheesecloth. Jeb has stayed close to the land, homesteading and gardening on the coast of California."

The family gathers together for the yearly seed harvest. "We shake plant tops into buckets each fall to gather the seed," says Richo. "We do this with plants like motherwort and mullein that have open capsules holding the dry, mature seed. The buckets of seed are brought into the winnowing area, where we lay out clean sheets, then dump the seed slowly onto screens so the

wind can blow away the chaff. It's a nice method, because not only are we using the elements at hand, but we separate out the mature black seed from the lightweight empty seed capsules that wouldn't germinate. Those blow away on the wind, leaving the heavier, viable seed behind. About 80 percent of our seed is collected this way."

Many traditional food plants are also good medicinal herbs that can be integrated into the daily diet regularly to improve health and prevent disease. Richo offers seed of select food plants in his catalog to help reinforce this kind of thinking. "Traditional vegetables like artichokes, beets, and creasy greens are both foods and medicines. Several medicinal herbs brought in from other traditions are also good food. Astragalus and codonopsis jump to mind. People may consider these to be medicinal herbs, but the reality is they are excellent nutritive foods that can be incorporated into soups made in every household. The mystique about medicinal herbs having very specific actions and potential contraindications and side effects needs to be dissolved in areas where it's appropriate to do so. Obviously there are herbs that need to be treated with much greater respect, like pulsatilla, herbs that would never be appropriate to include as part of an everyday diet."

Simple common herbs work so well. "If I was stuck with three

herbs," states this passionate grower, "I'd choose to have burdock, dandelion, and nettles. We need to learn to live with local plants and make use of them on a small scale. Why use commercial herbal preparations when we could just as easily go out with a shovel, cut off a lateral root of echinacea, wash it off with the garden hose, and chew on it? This would cost literally nothing, and probably do a hell of a lot more good.

"There are untrammeled spaces in the plant-person relationship. We've only really scratched the surface. I think there are vast depths still to explore. You just have to have the openness to hear the message from the plants and the right attitude to use it well," says Richo. The true power of medicinal herbs correlates directly to an intimacy with the whole plant: root, stem, leaf, flower, seed, and spirit. In the face of increased standardization and isolation of plant constituents for mass-marketed herbal medicine, people like Richo keep the faith in medicine derived directly from the land.

"Every good gardener knows that grass roots grow the fastest. We need to encourage our own grass roots to take over and make herbalism meaningful." Richo wrote his latest book, *Making Plant Medicine,* to help people learn appropriate ways to use homegrown medicinal herbs. Good seed, backed by a wealth of knowledge, can do powerful things. ✃

returned a hundredfold in the manure they provide for garden compost piles. Dolomite lime can be used in soils needing both magnesium and calcium, but crushed oyster shells will supply cation balance where calcium needs are proportionately greater.

## Medicinal Notions

Rich soil produces lush vegetables and fruits, but is this necessarily what we want with healing herbs? Many of the medicinal plants have developed their strengths in response to rugged reality. Levels of active constituents in these plants depend somewhat on approximating natural conditions. We know all too well the health ramifications of "pumping up" vegetables with soluble NPK fertilizer. Organic nitrogen fertilizers such as corn gluten meal and blood meal can be overdone, too. Soil health flows from moderation and diversity. Constituent levels may well change in response to the plant being placed in a human's perception of soil paradise. The active saponins in American ginseng (*Panax quinquefolium*) can differ among plants from the same seed stock being grown on opposite sides of the hill. Protopanaxadiol has a sedative effect; protopanaxatriol has a stimulating effect. The same genetics but different soils lead to different therapeutics. Good ginseng contains a balance of these two constituents (and other active substances as well), but you get the idea. We can analyze plant chemistry in the lab and estimate optimal growing conditions from such studies, but we must keep a sense of the whole. Choosing one active constituent as a guide is far different from hiking up Mount Everest with a community of tending Sherpas.

The incredible range of growth habit and therapeutic effect in any herb species tells us that nuance is important. Herbal pharmacists and practitioners may eventually determine that certain variations are medicinally significant as a result of laboratory analysis. Stinging nettles reportedly increase angelica's oil content by 80 percent when grown side by side.[4] Growers can work with such knowledge as it develops. Our focus will remain on the whole-plant dynamic. Matching conditions preferred in the wild will likely remain a good guide for how to grow each herb. The strong-tasting roots of wild ginseng are smaller, having closely spaced growth rings. Cultivated roots under shade cloths grow larger, but the taste is weaker and pronouncedly less complex. Growing the plant from seed in prepared beds under the natural shade of hardwood trees strikes a workable middle ground. A balance of active constituents, size, and flavor results from cultivating woodland ginseng. We need to be as mindful of ecology in growing these herbs as we are in selecting desired traits in parent seed stock. Do replicate desert rain patterns in watering dryland plants. A thick mulch of soft wood bark or rotted sawdust increases acidity well beyond what the plants may experience even in the acid rain soils of the Northeast. Mountain plants face altitude extremes with perseverance, not pampering. Black cohosh has its reasons for growing in woodland shade and forest duff.

## PROPAGATION

This short primer on starting herb seed, taking cuttings, dividing parent stock, and *walking on the wild side* will fill your fields and gardens. The nuances of propagation vary widely among the many herbs, of course, but more often than not hinge on emulating Nature. By successfully cultivating medicinal plants for local use, we also tend to the bigger picture of protecting diversity in regional ecosystems. Replenishing and preserving native species can be an offering of restoration that transcends commercial intent.

## Seeding

Almost all of the medicinal plants we grow at Heartsong Farm are started from seed. Our growing season begins in early March in the 10 × 16-foot greenhouse attached to the southwest end of our 1880s farmhouse. A small woodstove makes the greenhouse a toasty place to be on a blustery day. Some seeds get their start in ten-row planting trays kept atop electric propagation mats in a poly tent that Michael rigs on the planting bench. Quick germinators are planted in rows in the same flat to keep the transplanting schedule on an even keel. Small seeds with a longer germination period and needing more frequent misting are planted in separate flats. Seeds requiring early spring stratification—species from areas with cold winters need some chilling-off time—go out to our growing frames planted in four-inch-deep wooden flats. The slanting frame covers are propped open on stacks of bricks to lessen any solar gain by day and ensure a freeze by night. These deeper flats retain moisture longer than a row tray by virtue of greater soil volume (we prefer not to have to check on these cold-frame plantings every day). Other seeds, planted in nursery beds back in late fall, await the thaw cycling of true spring. Only a handful of medicinals are seeded directly in the field, such as deep-rooted burdock, dainty German chamomile, and anything-but-dainty milk thistle. Transplanting seedlings into the field gives us much better charge of weed management and is the only way to ensure a full, evenly spaced row.

Any good seed supplier will list the germination requirements of each medicinal plant. Catalog codes indicate which species require light to germinate, which species require scarification, and so forth. Keeping a moist planting surface for angelica and valerian works best away from the drying light of direct sun, so these spend time under our planting bench.

Recommendations for cold-conditioning certain species often stress relying on refrigeration: Plant seeds in a moist medium, enclose in a plastic bag, and stratify for anywhere from two weeks to several months in the fridge. Richo Cech puts all this in plain language in his Horizon Herbs catalog and provides a great deal of detail for successful seeding. The same processes by which each species germinates naturally will ultimately work best for us as growers.

Consider those seeds needing extended cold stratification, for example. Overwintering such seed (see table 6-1) in outdoor nursery beds works best. Let the weather work for you, not the refrigerator. The rain and snows, the sunny days and deep cold nights, create a rhythmic awakening in the seed as the ground begins to warm come spring. Nursery beds need to be protected from foot traffic. We use 2 × 6 wooden frames to clearly delineate where winter seeds have been planted. Where cats roam, consider creating wire mesh covers across the frames, as kitty scratching wreaks havoc on species-precise rows. Frames should be on the order of three to four feet across (wide enough to straddle a raised bed) and a manageable six feet long. A permanently established seeding bed can be as long as desired. These nursery frames lessen the effects of drying winds on the soil surface as well. Seeds are planted in very shallow furrows, about eight to twelve inches apart,

TABLE 6-1. *Herb Seed Benefiting from Extended Stratification*

Many species are partially if not entirely dependent on the freezing and thawing cycle that occurs naturally outside. Their seeds sprout in the spring after this cold-conditioning. Garden nursery beds work well for us, or you can plant in flats in the fall to bring into the greenhouse early the following spring. Consider ordering seed of these herbs for such autumnal planting:

| | |
|---|---|
| Agrimony | *Agrimonia eupatoria* |
| American Ginseng | *Panax quinquefolium* |
| Angelica, Giant Purple | *Angelica atropurpurea* |
| Arrowleaf Balsamroot | *Balsamorrhiza sagittata* |
| Barberry | *Berberis vulgaris* |
| Bearsfoot | *Polymnia uvedalia* |
| Blue Camas | *Camas camassia* |
| Blue Vervain | *Verbena hastata* |
| Cowslip | *Primula veris* |
| Echinacea angustifolia | *Echinacea angustifolia* |
| False Unicorn | *Chamaelirium luteum* |
| Lemon Balm | *Melissa officinalis* |
| Lobelia | *Lobelia inflata* |
| Lungwort | *Pulmonaria officinale* |
| Oregon Grape | *Mahonia aquifolium* |
| Pleurisy Root | *Asclepias tuberosa* |
| Schizandra | *Schizandra chinensis* |
| Senega Snakeroot | *Polygala senega* |
| Spikenard | *Aralia californica* |
| Stinging Nettle | *Urtica dioica* |
| Stoneroot | *Collinsonia canadensis* |
| Turtlehead | *Chelone glabra* |
| Tansy | *Tanacetum vulgare* |
| Wild Quinine | *Parthenium integrifolium* |
| Wood Betony | *Stachys officinalis* |
| Yellow Gentian | *Gentiana lutea* |

running across the width of the bed in late fall. Clearly mark each row with an indelibly inked wooden stake to be sure what's what four to six months later. Cover the seed with finely sifted soil and tamp down lightly. A thin smattering of organic mulch (finely shredded leaves work great) across the entire nursery bed tucks our seed children in for their winter's rest. Spring should bring a higher rate of germination with these naturally stratified seeds than any chilling spell in the refrigerator has achieved in past greenhouse endeavors. Thin the seedlings early to allow each plant to develop a somewhat autonomous root system. These can be transplanted to the garden when they are a few inches tall.

Choose a damp, overcast day for moving seedlings. A narrow-pointed hand trowel works well to lift each plant into an empty flat. We try our darndest to leave as much soil clinging to the roots as possible. Watering beforehand helps hold dry soil together. Any plants left in place in the nursery bed over the summer will have a jump on their exiting cousins. The temporary frames surrounding the bed can be removed and stored until fall seeding time again. One can up the brilliance of working with Nature's cycles yet again by maintaining small patches of mother herbs to drop their seed in late fall onto nearby open ground. We've come to count on the blue vervain and motherwort transplants that sprout as a result of natural stratification over the winter.

We avoid damping-off disease in the greenhouse by avoiding overwatering. Many medicinals don't need as much water as faster-growing vegetables. The soil surface needs to be moist, but far from puddle-saturated. We mist light-dependent seeds that have been gently pressed into the soil surface, but not covered. For seed that does get covered, fine vermiculite makes an excellent germination surface, as its moist golden hue will lighten when it's time to water again. Annuals started before their natural germination time tend to have a greater damping-off problem, as do any seeds that are planted too thickly.

Take this next advice to heart: Avoid sterile growing mediums. Such "soil" is essentially a blank slate open to any kind of fungal attack. Living compost, on the other hand, is filled with organisms that protect plants symbiotically. Just as the human intestinal tract lies exposed after taking antibiotics, natural balance in the soil is lost in the quest to be sterile. The organisms responsible for producing root rots, primarily *Pythium* spp. and *Rhizoctonia solani,* never need become the dominant culture in an unsterilized potting soil. Some growers offset heat treatment (soil is sterilized at 170°F or more) with the purchase of beneficial microorganisms watered into the soil surface. A good idea, but expensive. We prefer using living compost, blended with greensand, peat, vermiculite, and a touch of lime. A handful of worm castings and kelp in the mix adds a full spectrum of nutrients. Germination will be enhanced by compost and sifted topsoil, due to the release of growth hormones in the cycling of beneficial fungi. A good preventive medicine with seedlings susceptible to damping-off (make note of past experience!) is Mother Cottontail's remedy of chamomile tea. Served cool, please.

The progression of transplanting suits limited greenhouse space. Home gardeners have the option of deeper planting trays and pots with room for each seedling to grow without becoming rootbound. Many commercial growers prefer plastic cell trays to start seeds, knowing the resulting "plugs" can be timed to be put out in the field without delay. The larger the cell size, the more days a seedling has before it outgrows its space. Constraining tiny seedlings in a soil base too small is the worst mistake one can make in a production greenhouse. Ideally, the roots should just begin to encircle an allotted radius before the seedlings are "potted up" to a larger cell or container. Spiraling roots beneath the soil reveal the time to act, or rather, having waited a mite too long to act. Wee sprouts transplant quite readily, with whittled-down chopsticks making an excellent soil dibble. If necessary, tiny starts can be thinned with tweezers so each little herb develops bushy stature rather than gangly posture before transplanting. Learn to seed lightly to save this thinning step.

Our tool of choice for transplanting is the Ladbrooke soil blocker made in England. Moving away from plastic in the greenhouse strikes us as Earth-friendly. Soil blocks can be placed on three-sided wooden trays that allow easy access when the time comes for setting seedlings out in the garden or field. The block maker we use forms four soil blocks at a time. These measure two inches on a side, thus a flat measuring nine by twenty by three inches overall has room for thirty-six plants. Table 6-2 shows the relationship between number of flats

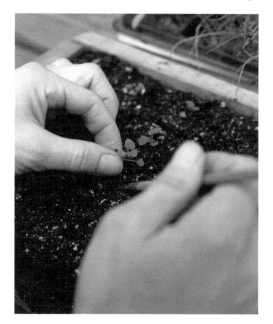

*A simple wooden chopstick (whittled to a point) is great for transplanting seedlings into soil blocks.*

**TABLE 6-2.** *Correlation of Soil Block Flats to Row Spacing*

| | |
|---|---|
| 2 flats | 16-inch spacing |
| 3 flats | 12-inch spacing |
| 4 flats | 8-inch spacing |

Each flat holds 36 blocks; row length is 100 feet. A double-row bed would be 50 feet long.

(give or take a lost plant or two) needed to plant a 100-foot field row at various plant spacings. The real beauty of soil blocks shows in the surprising lack of root interaction between seedlings. The air space between blocks is as tangible a barrier to root tips as any wall. Each plant can thus be separated with little root damage, which is not the case in an integral flat of soil containing an equal number of seedlings. Transplants experience less shock when root systems are least disturbed. A hand-snipped piece of heavy gauge sheet metal, six inches wide by as many tall (with upper corners rounded), makes a good dividing trowel for lifting three rows of blocks at a time from the flat. These can be broken apart easily

and set at the desired row spacing. Always be sure to give seedlings coming from the greenhouse several days to acclimate to the unsheltered day. Placing flats along garden paths hardens the young plants to wind, rain, sun, and cooler nights. Tender plants may be less stressed by a two-week stay in a semiprotected cold frame before this final transplanting.

Blocks allow you to create the containers for your seedlings from the soil itself. Success depends on a righteous soil mix. Peat fibers play a big role in holding blocks together (and the eventual root system even more so). Our mix consists of peat moss, well-aged compost, and coarse vermiculite in roughly equal proportion. We sift the compost to remove rocks and coarse organic debris. Some gardeners substitute topsoil for half the compost. Sand can be substituted for half the vermiculite. Azomite, kelp, granite flakes, and paramagnetic rock dust add essential trace minerals. The collective pint of such amendments that we sift into approximately ten gallons of soil in a plastic mixing tray has purpose beyond immediate soil blocking:

*Making good soil blocks requires using soil that is wet enough to come out of the press neatly.*

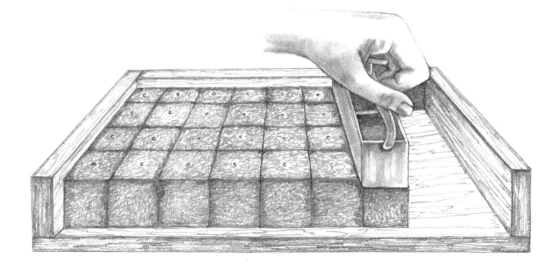

The minerals added will be available in the garden for years to come. A dusting of lime helps to neutralize the acidity of peat, on the order of about one tablespoon per gallon scoop. We prefer using foliar fish emulsion as a supplementary source of nitrogen (if needed) rather than using a high-nitrogen source such as blood meal in our mix. Elliot Coleman's excellent book, *The New Organic Grower*, gives precise soil mix recipes for those of you challenged by our sense of home cooking measure. Adding the right amount of water to the soil mix makes all the difference between a sloppy mess and pristine blocks that glide out of the soil press with perfect regularity. A quick push into the soil, followed by a twisting motion to fill, seats the soil mix in the block maker. A spring-loaded handle ejects four blocks at a time onto the flat. Grace shines at making these "cakes" for her daddy's seedlings.

Certain perennial seedlings begun in early August in the greenhouse can be set out in September to get a jump on next year's planting. Echinacea or St. John's wort can follow a milky oat harvest where the cover crop residues have been chopped and tilled to prepare individual planting rows within the field stubble. Ground where garlic has been harvested also becomes available in early fall to set out such perennial seedlings. Come spring, crops in place can be counted on to take off rapidly as second-year plants. German chamomile can be seeded directly in the fall with an Earthway seeder, using the smallest seed plate, set for a two- to four-inch spacing. Plants grown by this direct-seeded method produce more medicinal blossoms than those grown from spring transplants.

You experience the full beauty of seed when you start to save these precious gifts from plants lovingly tended. Such continuity brings our growing efforts full circle. Local selection now enters into play as we gather seeds from particularly noteworthy mother plants. But unintended crosses of similar species let the air out of such genetic promise. Seven species of *Angelica* are pocketed throughout the land at Elixir Farm Botanicals, intentionally distanced to keep each strain isolated from the others. Despite such thoughtful care to preserve species integrity, the culver's root patch shows traces of lilac shades among the white flower spikes, indicating that another strain of *Veronicastrum* in the upper far corner of the land has crossed desired bounds. Needless to say, these unruly aberrations are weeded out quickly. Any seed curator will try unfailingly to maintain species integrity. A gardener, on the other hand, could find promising new strains by not deterring pollination crosses. At Johnny's Selected Seeds in Albion, Maine, hundreds of *Echinacea purpurea* plants were individually evaluated for winter hardiness and medicinal potency, then the top dozen of these were sequestered together to cross-pollinate the year we visited. The resulting seed stock will carry the vigor of open genetics, yet should show a selection tendency toward higher levels of cichoric acid. Similar work with valerian targets higher levels of isovaleric acid and lower levels of valepotriates.[5]

Out in the woods, Don Babineau of Woodland Essence has learned seeding lessons of his own with ginseng. He's tried transplanting peat pot starts into raised beds, only to have to resort to wire cages to protect young ginseng plants from mice. Don now prefers tilling his planting areas eight inches deep (enough to chop up the finer tree roots) and then scattering his own gathered seed in the fall. "Come spring, I uncover the plants buried beneath the autumn's leaf mulch, transplanting those that need thinning. The mice, for whatever reason, let the seeded starts alone." Score another point for natural succession.

## Cuttings

The vast majority of medicinal plants to be grown in the field will be started from seed. Some of these—lemon balm, catnip, hyssop, bergamot, horehound, and sage—can be propagated by vegetative cuttings as well. Seeding or root division works more easily for us. Herbs that do not do as well from seed include gotu kola and wormwood. Select strains of lavender, lemon verbena, and rosemary are often maintained by avoiding the genetic variability of open-pollinated seed. A grower looking to produce a substantial crop of any of these might consider snipping off tender plant stems and getting them to root in an appropriate medium. Sand or perlite works well for many species. Cuttings can be made at any point from late spring through the summer when the parent plants are flush with new growth. Herbalists in more temperate climes have a longer opportunity to root successfully and then transplant these stem clones out in the field to get established before winter. Obviously, frost-sensitive perennials need to be able to survive that very same winter. You won't find us pumping out gotu kola in New Hampshire until global warming really kicks into high gear. Tender-rooted cuttings can be potted up to wait out the dormant season in a heated greenhouse prior to spring planting.

The key to propagating herbs by cuttings is maintaining high humidity, ideally by misting within a vapor-containing environment. Bottom heat helps, from either electric mats or hot water pipes in a designed planting table. Thomas DeBaggio does an excellent job of presenting all the nuances of propagating cuttings in his book, *Growing Herbs from Seed, Cutting and Root: An Adventure in Small Miracles*. We recommend it highly for those of you so inclined.

Organic growers will choose to decline the chemical rooting hormones in which stem cuttings are conventionally rolled before being inserted in rooting medium. In truth, these are products more for the propagator's peace of mind than they are vital to the process itself. Most herbs root rather easily if the environmental conditions are right. Tim Blakley observes that bearberry (*Arctostaphylos uva-ursi*) is the one plant in the vast depths of his growing experience that actually benefits from the use of hormones. A diluted honey dip (one part honey to three parts water) is used by some to sweeten the success rate with cuttings.

## Root Divisions

Dividing parent stock by the roots pertains more to home gardening. One plant that can be cleaved into three or four sections, say, isn't necessarily field-scale propagation even on a small farm. Nevertheless, plantings of certain medicinal herbs are increased readily by root division. Incredible ease—you couldn't eradicate this plant if you tried—and challenging seed germination set the two stages of feasibility.

Short pieces of comfrey and horseradish root invariably become new plants in their own right. This tends to be frustrating if your aim is to move these plants to a new locale, for any rootlets left in the ground will grow their way back to the surface. Increasing the size of one's comfrey patch couldn't be easier. Root cuttings about the size of a thumb work well, providing the new plants with enough reserves to get a vigorous start. We harvest the majority of the mother plant's roots for medicine and get root stock for fall planting at the same time. Michael continually spreads comfrey throughout our orchard each spring (this herb makes an excellent living mulch beneath an apple tree) by shaking a spadeful of earth free of the sod and merely inserting comfrey root pieces to do their thing. Agrimony, alkanet, elecampane, and marsh mallow can all be propagated by root cuttings as well. These fleshy roots sprout many buds atop their crown; each chunk should be left with at least one bud to sprout anew. Root division is also worth trying with black cohosh after fall harvest—just be prepared to give the buds that do survive two springs to appear. We'd be wise to try replanting root crowns of other species as well. Michael Pilarski, a wild-crafter in Washington state, has reported *Lomatium dissectum* will reestablish from replanted crowns.[6] We take pleasure in continuing the life of any plants we can. Those that readily reseed, such as *Echinacea purpurea* and *Althaea officinalis,* do seem to produce a larger root from a fresh start, however.

Members of the mint family are often propagated from below, though technically speaking these root divisions are actually divisions of the plant's stolons. These underground runners look like roots at first glance, but you'll see hairy roots dangling from the jointed nodes along each stolon if you're mindful. Each node is in essence a new mint plant, so break apart the stolons accordingly for spring planting. Larger sections (two or three nodes' worth) will experience less transplant shock. The stolons on mature licorice plants can be replanted in the fall. Certain herbs such as gravel root *(Eupatorium purpureum)* and sweet flag *(Acorus calamus)* send out horizontal stems along or just below the soil surface. The nodes on these rhizomes send roots downward and leaf shoots upward. Again, snip these apart throughout the growing season to increase the mother plant's reach. Goldenseal (*Hydrastis canadensis*) also spreads by rhizomes, leading to those dense forest patches that perhaps made it seem we could never overharvest this precious root. People have, of course, and thus the call to commercially cultivate it. Fall planting works best with the rhizome of goldenseal. Radiate the rootlets out into the soil, covering the upper bud just below the surface of the soil. A thin layer of shredded leaf mulch (whole leaves will tend to mat together and, if thick enough, can prevent emergence) tucks the babies away until they pop up first thing in the spring.

Most plant people think of true root division as the cleaving apart of the parent plant into new sections. The best candidates

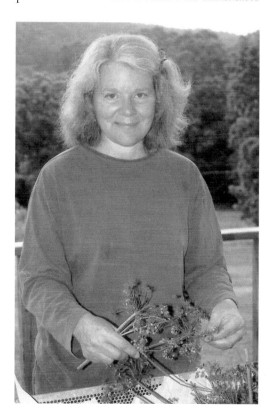

*Vinnie McKinney of Elixir Farm Botanicals sorting angelica seed*

# A MODEST GARLIC GROWER REVEALS ALL

TURNING CUSTOMERS on to garlic as a great food is that much easier once you share its medicinal uses. Growing large bulbs gives the farmer a shot at earning an earthly profit. Intensive hand-cultivating and harvesting methods limit the amount of garlic one can tend, but that's okay . . . the garlic receiving a premium price will always be those bulbs grown with intimate care.

*Modest*, when we use that word to indicate our garlic-growing efforts here at Heartsong Farm, means modest. We currently have a crop of 3,000 plants set in the ground back in mid-October. Eight varieties are represented in this planting, all hardneck rocamboles, with cloves selected from approximately 70 pounds of seed bulbs. Growers in the successful hand-scale range work with anywhere from 50 to 250 pounds of clove stock. The subsequent harvest amounts to 300 to 1,500 pounds of marketable bulbs. Saving your own seed stock favors a strain increasingly suitable for your specific soil type—select moderate-size bulbs with a diameter of 2 to 2½ inches for seed—although this reduces the amount of garlic you have to sell by a factor of six. (Different varieties vary as to the number of cloves per bulb. Our favorite, Russian Red, averages seven to ten cloves, of which six usually meet our planting standard for singularity and heft.) Custom garlic growers receive anywhere from $4 a pound wholesale for eating bulbs to as much as $12 a pound for biodynamic seed stock.

We're big on the concept of medicinal food, and perhaps no vegetable or herb is more representative than garlic. Anyone who wants to be well listens closely when we explain its healing properties. You can literally lose a sore throat overnight after sucking on a crushed garlic clove. Fresh garlic has strong immune-boosting and antibiotic properties. Immediate cooking destroys the allicin released upon cutting the clove. Chopping cloves up ten minutes before throwing them into the frying pan allows the allinase enzyme time to produce the cancer-fighting allyl sulfur compound. In truth, more than one hundred compounds give garlic its synergistic abilities as a healing herb. Allixin reduces the infection stresses imposed on the body by disease itself. Ajoene (produced by macerating fresh garlic in olive oil) helps prevent blood clots and works against certain cancers. Diallyl trisulfide is liver-friendly and antiviral. These compounds together help reduce blood pressure and blood sugar, relieve asthma and bronchitis, and improve circulation and heart function. No pill company will ever be able to deliver the whole-plant potency of fresh organic garlic.

As a grower, Michael's appreciation for garlic begins with planting in the second half of October. Each clove initiates root growth in the compost-enriched earth through late fall, poised to send forth some of the first greenery of spring. We rely on snow cover in northern New England, so we forego any mulch. Garlic tops make a great addition

---

for division are the herbs that die back each winter to return in the spring larger than they were before. Such perennials grow from a number of stems as opposed to a single central stem. Choose the more vigorous of the potential parent crowns to divide. Carefully dig up the root ball—enough to reveal the physical structure, yet leaving some protective soil in the root crevices—and then cut the crown vertically with a sharp knife. The buds at the top of the root clumps are guides for where to cut.

to dandelion greens, so plant the smallish cloves separately for a spring tonic harvest.

Shallow hoeing in the presence of these powerful healing plants is more meditative pleasure than work. The scapes (these nonflowering stalks are topped with miniature bulbils) get clipped off when they begin to uncurl on the rocamboles. Removing this scape allots more energy into the sizing bulb, although leaving them on until a week before harvest can result in a longer storage life. Each leaf above ground represents a papery sheath around the cloves. Once the leaf tips begin to yellow and die back, it's time to dig the garlic. Optimal harvest time is indicated by the lower six leaves still being green: This allots five or so protective wrappers after cleaning the bulbs. Our harvest is completed by early August. The bulbs cure upside down in 2 × 4-inch mesh fencing frames that hang from the rafters of our harvest shed. Good air flow ensures good results.

Growing large garlic bulbs makes a tremendous difference when it comes time to sell the crop. Spacing cloves 6 to 8 inches apart in rows one foot apart (four rows to a bed) works well in the gravelly loam of this farm. Sandy

GARLIC
*Allium sativum*

*If you understand the uses of garlic, you understand 50 percent of all herbal medicine.*
—Steven Foster

soils require drip irrigation, but have the advantage of bulbs that are easier to clean. Control of white rot disease and assorted botrytis molds is best achieved by crop rotation. Garlic ground should have a minimum of four years between crops. Onions and leeks, which are more susceptible alliums, should be grown in another field entirely. Penicillium molds result in rotting cloves, and the infection is spread at planting whenever you handle bad seed.

Dusting the cloves with sulfur before planting can help limit penicillium mold.

Effective marketing comes down to educating customers over the long haul. Display your garlic proudly at farmers' markets and herb festivals by arraying your bulbs openly in a wire mesh rack, leaving the drying tops intact beneath. (Offer to cut off the tops with sheep shears once you clinch a sale). Varieties add to the allure—spicy Yerina obliges a fiery yelp; porcelain types such as Georgian Crystal yield better-keeping cloves; and lab tests have indicated a higher [allicin] content in the Romanian Red and Siberian strains. Peeling off the outer skins results in prettier bulbs that sell best. Here, in truth, is "the rub" that keeps a garlic grower like Michael ever so humble.

---

Each section ideally will have two or more buds left to face its new tomorrow. Cut only as far as necessary to reach the intertwining roots. Once free of the crown circumference, these often can be untangled with less overall damage to the rootlets left in each section. The bludgeoning method of driving a well-honed spade into the root crown results in fewer new plants, simply due to the lack of surgical finesse. The recovering plants hardly break stride when divided in early spring before leaf growth.

Fall division, after the plants have gone dormant, works equally well.

Division offers us a good way to increase plantings of vital forest medicinals such as black cohosh, blue cohosh, goldenseal, bloodroot, wild yam, and stone root. Many of these present germination challenges that not every grower might choose to struggle with: a rather short viability hinging on extended stratification; aerial parts not appearing till the spring of the second year; exceedingly delicate seedlings ending up trampled. However, plants can be propagated readily from the roots (or rhizomes, as the case may be). Sensitive forest plants are best dug and transplanted in the fall, after the energy of the growing season has returned to the roots. Firm the growing tip into deep, loamy soil and cover with mulch wherever a deciduous forest canopy will provide dappled shade throughout the summer. Mark the site. Return many times. Offer prayers. Provide water if necessary. Watch miracles unfold.

"It's getting to be harder and harder to find ginseng, black cohosh, and goldenseal in our Ozark woods," reports Vinnie McKinney. Overzealous wildcrafting has taken a toll on many stocks of such forest medicinals. This plant conservationist has taken to moving forest plants to shaded garden beds to secure her seed stock from another person's root harvest. "These black cohosh [about twenty plants thriving beneath a shade tent] are all from a single plant I moved from the woods and root-cloned," says Vinnie. "And here they all are in flower on their way to being seed bearers."

### Take a Walk on the Wild Side

A lot of advantageous reproduction takes place in our fields once we've established medicinal herb crops. Plants start to move out and find their own nooks. Our work in the perennial fields around early spring is to identify what has endured from the year before in terms of returning mother plants and volunteer seedlings. Is the valerian patch not as strong, for instance? Or is it moving out by way of rhizomes, or showing up in a moister area from seed carried on the wind? The job of the grower then becomes to isolate these plants: weeding around the preferred species, perhaps composting and fluffing up the soil around each, marking areas where tilling can be done. "You don't want to till in valuable reproduction of medicinals that short-circuited the cycle of coming out of a package, being planted in flats, and then transplanted out to the field. These labor-intensive techniques," says the ever observant Richo Cech, "can all be skipped by taking advantage of natural reproduction in the field. Such volunteers tend to make really good medicine because they found their ideal location versus trying to make do within the confines of a flat, then transplant shock, then being in a place that you chose as appropriate." Oftentimes growers see this in plantings that languish. Crops clearly communicate when the human/plant interrelationship is lacking something. We eventually find how to live in harmony with each particular plant so all can thrive. Stewarding the natural course of events ultimately brings us to that place where the plants can best do what we need them to do for us.

Don Babineau has intentions of just this sort with skullcap. He's seeding *Scutellaria lateriflora* where Mill Creek takes sharp bends in the meadows beyond his woodland home. We follow the swath of previous passings through the high grasses, carefully stepping over hidden canals the beavers have created in dragging countless poplars down to the brook. "See that mud flat on the inside bank? The flats facing to the north thaw last, so I'm expecting the ice pack to protect the soil surface beyond the spring runoff. These are the kinds of places I've seen skullcap in the wild." Following Nature's lead serves several purposes here. Fall seeding paces the germination just right for spring thaw. Naturalized skullcap in a mud flat will grow in thick clumps that won't require the usual garden hand-weeding. This herb thrives on water, so positioning couldn't be better. Last, come harvesttime on a sweltering summer day, the swimming hole is a mere plunge away.

Such connection of agriculture with Nature fascinates us. We've instilled thousands of years of cultural effort to domesticate the plant world to field notions of order. How fitting that the healing herbs never acquiesced to this insistence. But now times have changed. Only by cultivating that which once ran abundantly wild will we ensure a sustainable supply of vital plant medicines. Some species propagate readily to our agrarian whims. Others—notably osha and blue cohosh—resist such attempts. Each plant teaches us its particular reality quickly. Many will only be partially tamed. We've begun our lessons by thinking like a seed.

## SOUND FARMING

Those who toil in the soil create a palette where the diversity of Nature melds with human intent. Plant sense, timely cultivation and mulching, equipment appraisal, and common sense are the skills on which sustainable farming thrives. Producing robust healing herbs is an intuitive agriculture in many ways. The plants tell their secrets to those who listen and observe. Our techniques evolve as we come to understand the big picture of what is taking place in the fields and woodlands.

### Plant Sense

The stinging nettle patch at Healing Spirits Herb Farm lies at the far end of the roadside field. The first harvest of *Urtica dioica* leaf came in the second summer. Compost had been spread atop two-foot-wide beds in spring, the pathways between cultivated with an occasional pass of the tiller. Yet new runners continue to claim the paths. Undomesticated plants can vex a farmer's scrupulous standards—*Thou shall have order in thy fields*—yet they provide us with an opportunity to think better. Matthias Reisen debates whether to let this patch go wild, and thus invite back other species that will make harvesting less efficient, or to switch the pathways back and forth with the growing space. A cover crop could be rotated into this latter approach—planted in the current year's pathway and tilled under come midsummer—to help replenish the soil. Ultimately, only moving the patch every three or four years will address the need for renewed vigor. Regardless, Andrea doesn't believe the nettle leaves here in the field are as dark green as those they gather in the wild. We've seen tremendous caterpillar assaults on nettle started in the greenhouse and subsequently planted out on our farm that just don't seem to affect its untamed cousins. Soils can be rich, nurtured with compost, and fed judicious mineral amendments. Yet nettle's nature will always be to roam and sting any harvester who misses her teachings entirely.

"The happiest plants are the plants growing between the rows in communion with others. Then it goes beyond that—the plants are telling us that we shouldn't

*Text continues on page 178.*

TABLE 6-3. *Crop Recommendations*

Horizon Herbs recommends these potentially profitable crops, because they are currently experiencing moderate to strong demand. Other herbs are included because they are increasingly rare in the wild. The bioregions listed here include crossover herbs, such as valerian, which grow well both in wetlands and at higher elevations. The exclusion of a given medicinal herb from this list does not mean you can't make a go with it.

**Wetlands:**

| | |
|---|---|
| Boneset | *Eupatorium perfoliatum* |
| Bugleweed | *Lycopus americanus / europaeus* |
| Calamus | *Acorus calamus* |
| Cramp Bark | *Viburnum opulus* |
| Eclipta | *Eclipta alba* |
| Elderberry | *Sambucus* spp. |
| Gravel Root | *Eupatorium purpureum* |
| Marsh Mallow | *Althaea officinalis* |
| Meadowsweet | *Spirea ulmaria* |
| Mint (Peppermint) | *Mentha* spp. |
| Plantain | *Plantago major / lanceolata* |
| Skullcap | *Scutellaria lateriflora* |
| Stinging Nettles | *Urtica* spp. |
| Sundew | *Drosera rotundifolia* |
| Valerian | *Valeriana officinalis* |
| Wood Betony | *Stachys officinalis* |

**Arid Regions:**

| | |
|---|---|
| Astragalus | *Astragalus membranaceus* |
| Black Seed | *Nigella sativa* |
| Cactus grandiflorus | *Selenecereus grandiflorus* |
| California Poppy | *Eschscholzia californica* |
| Catnip | *Nepeta cataria* |
| Chaparral | *Larrea tridentata* |
| Chaparro | *Castela emoryi* |
| Chaste Tree | *Vitex agnus-castus* |
| Epazote | *Chenopodium ambrosiodes* |
| Ephedra | *Ephedra sinensis* |
| Horehound | *Marrabium vulgare* |
| Hyssop | *Hyssopus officinalis* |

| | |
|---|---|
| Indigo | *Indigofera tinctoria* |
| Lavender | *Lavendula* spp. |
| Morman Tea | *Ephedra nevadensis* |
| Oregano | *Origanum* spp. |
| Peppers | *Capsicum* spp. |
| Psyllium | *Plantago psyllium* |
| Red Root | *Ceanothus americanus* |
| Rosemary | *Rosmarinus officinalis* |
| Rue | *Ruta graveolens* |
| Sage | *Salvia* spp. |
| Syrian Rue | *Paganum harmala* |
| Thyme | *Thymus* spp. |
| Wormwood | *Artemisia absinthium* |
| Yerba Mansa | *Anemopsis californica* |
| Yerba Santa | *Eriodictyon californicum* |

**Mountain Regions:**

| | |
|---|---|
| Angelica | *Angelica archangelica* |
| Arrowleaf Balsamroot | *Balsamorrhiza sagittata* |
| Arnica | *Arnica* spp. |
| Dong Quai | *Angelica sinensis* |
| Echinacea | *Echinacea angustifolia* |
| Gentian | *Gentiana lutea* |
| Juniper | *Juniperus communis* |
| Lady's Mantle | *Alchemilla vulgaris* |
| Lomatium | *Lomatium dissectum / nudicaule* |
| Osha | *Ligusticum porteri* |
| Pulsatilla | *Anemone pulsatilla* |
| St. John's wort | *Hypericum perforatum* |
| Yarrow | *Achillea millefolium* |

## Temperate Hardwood Forests
## (herbs of the understory):

| | |
|---|---|
| American Ginseng | *Panax quinquefolium* |
| Black Cohosh | *Cimicifuga racemosa* |
| Bloodroot | *Sanguinaria canadensis* |
| Blue Cohosh | *Caulophyllum thalictroides* |
| Siberian Ginseng | *Eleutherococcus senticosus* |
| Goldenseal | *Hydrastis canadensis* |
| Goldthread | *Coptis* spp. |
| Helonias Root | *Chamaelirium luteum* |
| Lady's Slipper Orchid | *Cypripedium* spp. |
| Partridgeberry | *Mitchella repens* |
| Stoneroot | *Collinsonia canadensis* |
| Trillium | *Trillium* spp. |
| Virginia Snakeroot | *Aristolochia serpentaria* |
| Wild Yam | *Dioscorea villosa* |

## Temperate Forests or Open Land Trees:

| | |
|---|---|
| Black Haw | *Viburnum prunifolium* |
| Black Walnut | *Juglans nigra* |
| Fringe Tree | *Chionanthus virginica* |
| Ginkgo | *Ginkgo biloba* |
| Hawthorn | *Crataegus oxyacantha* |
| Horse Chestnut (European) | *Aesculus hippocastanum* |
| Linden | *Tilia europea* |
| Prickly Ash | *Zanthoxylum clava-herculis* |
| Sassafras | *Sassafras officinale* |
| Slippery Elm | *Ulmus rubra* |
| Wild Cherry | *Prunus virginiana* |

## Tropical or Semitropical Herbs and Trees:

| | |
|---|---|
| Aloe | *Aloe* spp. |
| Ashwagandha | *Withania somnifera* |
| Damiana | *Turnera aphrodisiaca* |
| Ginger | *Zingiber officinale* |
| Gotu Kola | *Centella asiatica* |
| Henna | *Lawsonia alba* |
| Kava Kava | *Piper methysticum* |
| Neem | *Azadirachta indica* |
| Noni | *Morinda citrifolia* |
| Pau D'Arco | *Tabebuia impetiginosa* |
| Passionflower | *Passiflora edulis/incarnata* |
| Sandalwood | *Santalum album* |
| Spilanthes | *Spilanthes* spp. |
| Tea Tree | *Melaleuca alternifolia* |

## Additional Recommended Herbs,
## Adapted to Many Gardens:

| | |
|---|---|
| Bergamot | *Monarda didyma/fistulosa* |
| Blessed Thistle | *Cnicus benedictus* |
| Burdock | *Arctium lappa/minus* |
| Calendula | *Calendula officinalis* |
| Dandelion | *Taraxacum officinalis* |
| Echinacea | *Echinacea purpurea* |
| Feverfew | *Tanacetum parthenium* |
| Garlic | *Allium sativum* |
| German Chamomile | *Matricaria recutita* |
| Hops | *Humulus lupulus* |
| Lemon Balm | *Melissa officinalis* |
| Licorice | *Glycyrrhiza glabra/uralensis* |
| Lobelia | *Lobelia inflata* |
| Milk Thistle | *Silybum marianum* |
| Motherwort | *Leonurus cardiaca* |
| Pleurisy Root | *Asclepias tuberosa* |
| Poke | *Phytolacca americana* |
| Red Clover | *Trifolium pratense* |
| Sheep Sorrel | *Rumex acetosella* |
| Uva Ursi | *Arctostaphylos uva-ursi* |
| Wild Indigo | *Baptisia tinctoria* |

Reprinted with permission from Richo Cech, *Finding Your Niche— Making a Living with Medicinal Plants* (Williams, Oreg.: Horizon Herbs, 1995).

segregate ourselves from each other either. We shouldn't put the old people here and the young people over there, and the disabled over there. We, too, need to live in community and in harmony . . . like nettles and cleavers do well together. Some places in our fields have two or three herbs that have naturalized together, and we just manage the cultivation around them. Catnip doesn't like to grow in a row, but comes up everywhere else with the other plants. Some of the farmers around here tell us that we have the worst-looking gardens," Matthias laughs, "but it doesn't bother us."

The plants are quite willing to tell us many things when we truly listen. Even practical details such as expected yield. The business-plan approach promotes a thorough analysis before starting a medicinal herb venture: Dedicate so many acres to the popular herb of the day, find the expected yield in some book, reckon the dollars to come. Any farmer knows reality paints a far different picture. Land, climate, and grower experience influence the average yield any plant species will produce. Monica Rude of Desert Woman Botanicals suggests new herb growers try out the twenty or so medicinals that have a natural habitat similar to where they live. "Learn how many plants it takes to grow ten pounds dried of each herb so you can extrapolate crop yields for your farm. Then you can focus on doing a quality job with the more promising ones. Find out not only what grows well in your area but also what you like to grow, and all that is involved in actually bringing the crop to market. Chamomile has a high pound price, for example, but what you have to do to get a pound of dried flower heads is insanity."

Cayenne suits this highly charged woman well. The heat of the New Mexico desert certainly goes into her peppers. "Normally, cayennes register around 40,000 Scoville heat units. Ours have hit 77,490 . . . almost starting a fire at the analytical lab," jokes Monica. "The desert heat and dryness stresses the plants and intensifies their heat. It is an ideal crop for this climate and so has become our specialty." Growing in the desert isn't like growing in other areas of the country where there is lots of rain and cooler temperatures. Monica, understandably, is big on growing the right plants for this place. Ashwagandha, an Ayurvedic herb used much like ginseng, succeeds as another prime cash crop. Her first-year harvest of ashwagandha averaged about 4 ounces a root, with these mostly going to herb shops. The second year saw a big increase in size, with one or two plants producing a pound of fresh root, which she dried and sold readily. Yerba mansa, "used by everybody in the Southwest," finds a home in the lower corner of the field where clay abounds. "Yerba mansa will actually alter the soil chemistry and improve that clay soil for the better. Eventually plants will grow there that wouldn't before," says Monica, a nurse-turned-farmer, who is very much attuned to the lessons plants reveal in the wild.

Growers are innovators too. We can sense which non-native plants might be useful to suit local medicine and are willing to absorb the extra expense of a modest planting. Far northern New Hampshire does not offer the growing season required by tropical perennials. Only green tomatoes were assured, not red, until we erected field tunnels to protect sensitive crops from frost. Vegetable economics worked for once—the $1,000 investment in a 14 × 50-foot galvanized pipe frame, greenhouse plastic (the four-year film) to cover, and framing lumber for the rails and ends was recouped in one season of homegrown tomatoes. Now we integrate warm-climate herbs into those same tunnels, including ashwagandha, whose fresh root extract helps with chronic fatigue and tonifies the nerves, and spilanthes, whose antibacterial influence nicely complements the immune-enhancing activity of echinacea. Spilanthes reverses degenerative gum disease and ousts infections of the urinary tract. The beat goes on. Certainly our costs are higher to produce these crops than in warmer climes. We're not going to plant the back forty to these herbs any time soon. But we do have very effective medicines not otherwise available for the community in which we live.

All this assorted plant savvy eventually brings us to the plants we do not plant. "People should let more weeds grow around their vegetables," councils Faye Burtch from her medicinal backyard in State College, Pennsylvania. Weedy taproots reach down into the subsoil, helping to break hardpan and accessing minerals for other plants. Weeds provide neighborly shade, which helps especially in times of drought. Purslane makes an excellent living mulch. Faye thins her rampant volunteers to allow starting room for planted crops, yet gives lamb's quarters, dandelion, and amaranth their due. "These weeds are really good foods and medicine. How much broccoli can you eat without getting bored anyway? The sours, bitters, and natural sweets in the wild garden have so much more diversity of taste." Sounds sensible to us.

## Cultivation, Mulching, and Irrigation

The basic tenets of sustainable farming are much the same no matter the crop. Medicinal herb or vegetable, fruit tree or root crop, farmers and gardeners seek to provide optimal growing conditions for each plant. Soil health results in plant health. Our work in the field centers next on the interplay of species and maintaining adequate soil moisture.

This business of weeds becoming our friends requires further perspective. Growers cultivate to maintain a friable soil around herb crops, knowing that by midsummer the medicinals will become self-mulching. Once plants have grown to the point that they're shading the soil, weed competition becomes less relevant. We have two rules of thumb to apply to weeds. First, shallow-hoe early on. Any unwanted seed in the soil surface will germinate if conditions are right: Don't introduce additional seed potential by turning the soil deeply. Young sprouts don't have the reserves to reestablish connection to the ground: Cultivate to eliminate tiny seedlings as they sprout. A weekly pass with the hoe over the course of a month should get the bulk of the seed load in tilled ground. Choose late mornings on a sunny day to ensure good results. Also, vigorous transplants provide a much better jump on weeds than direct seeding because the crop reaches adequate size more quickly. The second rule of thumb is never let unintended crops mature seed. This doesn't mean you can't reap a nutritious lamb's quarters lunch or plan a dandelion leaf harvest from summer volunteers in the garlic field. But only by preventing vast quantities of new seed do we eventually reduce weed pressure to more congenial levels. Cover-cropping pathways between beds—or interplanting a low-growing cover such as white clover among established calendula rows— lends us a say in which plants mature. Paths can be mowed if annual rye threatens to go to seed, or even tilled if wild weeds rule, but now is the time to knock back seed potential.

The planting beds at Cate Farm are standardized at 44 inches wide, which corresponds to the distance between the tractor tires. Single, double, or triple rows are set out in each bed, depending on the area requirements of each crop. The ground gets disked, chisel-plowed, and then formed into 660-foot-long beds. Roller pins behind the bed shaper mark where plants will be set at a predetermined spacing. Keeping ahead of field weeds goes smoothly when the tractor—with cultivator hoes and sweeps adjusted manually to the row layout of each bed—fits the farm throughout. Medicinal herbs in the same planting bed are grouped by row patterns and by when the crop will be finally out of the ground.

Ditch irrigation of crops is essential in arid New Mexico. Rights to the flow of the Gila River are established in Monica Rude's lease. A narrow canal feeds the precious water flow into a series of furrows running parallel to the field rows. The plants are set in the ground along the edge of 4-foot-wide beds to enable a good soaking of the root zone. The middle of these beds serves as a footpath. Straw mulch along the ditch side of each plant row slows down the flow of water over the carefully crafted slope of this apparently not-quite-flat field. "I'm a big advocate of mulching," says Monica. "It's one of the best things you can do to improve the soil, add organic matter, stabilize the temperature of the soil around the roots, feed the worms and soil microorganisms, and minimize weed growth."

We take full advantage of the mountain stream flowing down through our farm. A gravity-fed water line brings water down to our fields with enough pressure to turn two pulsating sprinklers at a time. Drip tapes are set up in each growing tunnel, fed by hoses from this same natural source. Irrigation can be much more critical early in the season until plants get established, even in a moisture-retaining loam like ours. Perennial herbs in their subsequent years have more resiliency in handling the start of a drought period. Still, mulch or no mulch, it's good to have a watering system in place when you base your living on the land.

**Righteous Scale**

The scale of one's farm is an individual decision based on many considerations. The lay of the land determines arable acreage. Equipment investment—and this includes the choice to work entirely with hand tools—points to how much ground we can cultivate and harvest efficiently. A medicinal effort can focus on wild areas as well. Intimacy matters, both in the heart of the farmer and the soul of the farm. Our culture has been driven too long by the concept that bigger is better. Centralized economics pivots on producing more and more for seemingly less and less cost. The problem is, we don't reckon the full extent of the costs. We have been exhausting our planet home, our local communities, and ourselves for a fantasy lifestyle sorely lacking in respect for beauty. Any sensible discussion about the size of our farms begins on the side of the line that recognizes happiness is more about balance than about abject materialism.

Others before us have suggested that farming the smallest possible acreage so as to get it right will do the most good. We agree wholeheartedly. Small diversified farms provide satisfaction when we can keep up with the work to be done. Farmers will always push the bounds of what's considered a normal working day. The height of the growing season demands it. Getting up with the first light of a summer day to cultivate and not coming in till the last rack in the drying shed has been filled is okay. This flow of energy is balanced by the deep rest of winter. But it is another thing entirely to be running constantly and frantically throughout the growing season trying to crop enough to barely cover the bills. Much of society today will not pay the value of nutrient-dense food that would make small farms viable. Broaching consciousness in people is a longer-term crop than most root medicinals.

We didn't agree initially to work with cultural reality in our dreams for our farm. Fifteen years ago what struck us when we first walked down the driveway to this abandoned place was the lay of the land. We could visualize where gardens and an orchard would go once we cleared the overgrown fields. We would rebuild the barn (that had burned down forty years before) to house our animals, fence in pastures, have a greenhouse, and make the sagging farmhouse proud again. Idealistic youth learns, of course, that over time you can get about half that done while working outside jobs as a carpenter and a teacher to pay for it all. Our first marketing ventures were filled with enthusiasm: a CSA in a paper-mill town, an organic orchard leased in conjunction with a water-powered cider mill down the road, connections with summer chefs and natural foods stores. We toiled with commitment, we grew beautiful crops. But we only made our living because we still worked out. Obviously we needed to get bigger! We planted more orchard. We tried to get more than twelve families interested in community supported agriculture. We schemed how to buy a tractor. Michael went through the angry phase social activists eventually face. Our lives were anything but harmonious.

Now the dust has settled. Fears of *E. coli* shut down the cider mill, bringing Michael fully home to our land with a realization that a large homestead orchard has community merit. We grow fresh vegetables (beyond our year-round needs) for appreciative customers who purchase their intentions at planting time with farm reserve notes. Nancy's patient desire to study herbalism and teach others has opened doors. Our marketing thrust has turned to healing herbs that have a prolonged vitality both dried and in tincture. The pace of these days suits our need to work off the farm occasionally. We are out of debt, thankfully, having maintained a fiscal prudence from the beginning. We have blended financial reality in a sparsely populated area with the deep contentment of living on the land.

A grasp of potential markets is a big determinant of how much time can be allotted to producing crops that in turn will provide your living. All the calendula in China won't add up to a plug nickel if no one chooses to buy it. Not every blossom needs to be sold ahead of time, of course, but do plant with a sense of whom you can market to. Early years on a bioregional medicine farm are about making yourself known as a quality grower, learning cropping systems, and networking with other growers and herbalists. All this takes time to establish. Grow with your farm at a pace that keeps you out of debt. Tooling up with labor-saving equipment makes sense only when you have a firm grasp on what it takes to grow a volume crop and who will be buying it. The herbs we eventually focus on will be those we love most. Our relationship with a particular plant will resonate in its healing energy well beyond the boundaries of the farm.

*The BCS two-wheel tractor serves multiple needs on a small farm. We can rig a brush hog–type mower, cutter bar, and rotary tiller on this versatile farm machine.*

Because we crop slightly more than the mythical acre, it's fitting that we talk about equipment scaled to medicine farms of this size. (Actually our property amounts to 58 acres, mostly wooded, nestled up against state and national forest lands.) A family can cultivate only so much ground when intimately involved with dozens of different herbs for direct sale. We're learning more and more about cultivating woodland medicinals, knowing that the thriving forest around us has purposes far more splendid than stumpage value. Plants such as hawthorn and wild raspberry on the orchard's edge, goldenrod and horsetail in the sheepfold, and white ash stump sprouts in forest clearings don't need our growing involvement at all. Good hand tools are the ticket for much of this work. Quality not only lasts but has a heft and finesse to appreciate over decades of use. An English digging fork (with tines forged from one piece of metal) can turn planting beds and compost piles alike, lift roots at harvesttime, and even help secure a bulging wheelbarrow load.

Felco hand clippers are designed with the ergonomics of the human hand in mind, and the anvil blade can be replaced. Avoid the bypass-type clippers. Hedge shears work equally well to harvest the aerial tops of many herbs. Michael seems unable to resist a good hoe. Shallow hoes—whether the curved onion, the sharp collinear, or the pivoting hula—slice just beneath the soil surface to dislodge sprouting weeds and scratch compost into the active soil layer. Different width blades fit assorted crop spacings. A wheel hoe with offset stirrup blades makes cruising down the sides of lengthy herb rows a joyride.

We use a 10-horsepower BCS walking tractor with a 26-inch rototiller attachment to open ground for planting. Tillers churn organic matter into the soil. Ideally, we like to prep the soil weeks ahead of any anticipated planting. A cover crop shallowly incorporated breaks down faster when the active soil layer remains on top. A rough tilling can be smoothed out with a subsequent pass of the tiller a week or two later, or forked free of any extant clumps of the previous crop to give transplants a congenial start. The advantage of the BCS lies in having a power take-off to which attachments such as a brush mower can be interchanged for the tiller; the disadvantage lies in paying big bucks for pricey Italian-made parts. Give Joel Dufour of Earth Tools in Frankfort, Kentucky, a call if the BCS line might avail on your farm: United Plant Savers members receive a 10 percent discount, plus Joel contributes another 15 percent of his profit to the work of UpS.

Vintage tractors suit practical farm budgets provided you have the temperament to do basic mechanical work. Tractors give more horsepower and thus ability in the field than a walk-behind machine. Useful attachments include a tiller, a spader for rock-free ground, harrows, assorted cultivators, a root digger, and a cutter bar. Hydraulic tractors with a front bucket loader have inestimable worth in turning compost piles and getting that "black gold" spread across planting ground. Don't overlook bartering with a neighboring farmer to handle certain fieldwork if your overall farm needs don't warrant purchasing a tractor. Shared ownership arrangements, however, rarely work out in the long run unless maintenance responsibilities are clear to everyone involved.

Scale, ultimately, is perhaps best understood as a harmony where we can let our spirit join in the song of the land. And that may well be the reason many of us find our way back to the dirt. "I don't want to become an agribusinessman," says Rob Wooding of Southern Virginia Herbals. "I want to be a farmer in touch with the earth. The key is to have enough where you can make a living. Farming can seem pretty difficult. You do have a quality of life if you learn not to get too overwhelmed or in debt. I'm pretty much a one-joe show, just hiring out for help at harvesttime. I'm in control of the farm, so I can guarantee quality and integrity. I like to work the land that I have. I couldn't do a huge acreage anyway with my equipment. I'm funny about getting into debt. That's the difference between having freedom and not having freedom. I may be a stick in the mud, but I have a sense of freedom."

"Doing a good job with what we do do," muses Matthias Reisen, "probably means we should cut our production back to three acres [from the current four]. Last year we put in six rows of calendula, only weeded two, and ended up mowing down the others." Every honest farmer has stories of crop intentions lost to disarray at one time or another. The agrarian urge to plant an ever increasing harvest often does not result in increased income. On the contrary, knowing what you can handle, and sticking to it, tends to be the more profitable route.

## Common Sense

A friend recently told us that the Japanese word for farmer translated as a "hundred jobs." Certainly we have many things to consider: building healthy soil, the germination requirements of varied herbs, the best way to peel cherry bark, the diverse interactions of perennial crops, remunerative pricing, networking with herbalists, constructing a drying space, shredding roots, and so on. Our work has many constituents, you might say. And much like the synergy of the whole herb, no one task runs the farm. We need this holistic perspective of the farm as an entity. Integrated understanding emerges from probing the depths of what once may have appeared to be isolated events.

A core value of biodynamic practice is striking a balance within the circle of the

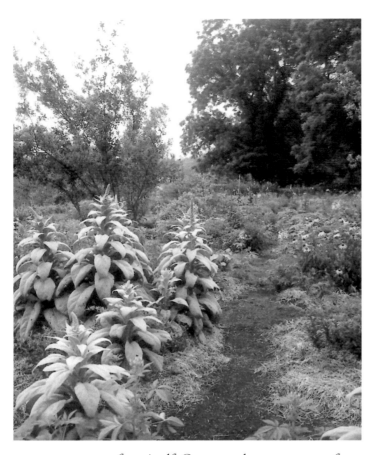

*Garden diversity provides answers that sometimes simply lie beyond our ken.*

"Look at all those insects," says Vinnie McKinney, pointing to a stand of *Veronicastrum virginicum.* Indeed, beneficial insects hover in profusion over the blossom spikes of these culver's root plants, darting between the bass riffs of the nectar-gathering bumblebees. Such diversity and abundance of the insect world at Elixir Farm in the Missouri Ozarks—as anywhere else—indicates a garden and a gardener in harmonious balance. "Everything here takes care of itself," Vinnie notes. "We never have any [prolonged] bug problems." Plant health flows from a vibrant soil, of course, and the community here worked hard to build up the creek sand that now makes up the medicinal seed gardens. Tons of leaves were mixed with composted manures, sheep were intensively grazed, biodynamic preparations were bestowed upon the land. "Rudolf Steiner's agriculture lectures are hard to penetrate," says Vinnie, smiling, "but biodynamics is foremost about spirit. I don't need to understand why biodynamics works as much as see that it does work. The Demeter certifier [of biodynamic methods] told me, 'You have the most highly developed sand I've ever seen.'" The belief runs strong here that cosmic connections support the microbes that in turn fuel the health of the plants and the people. "It's a different kind of agriculture when you let the land lead you rather than [the mind]," Vinnie observes, pointing to her head. "The pace is slower, more intimate."

Good growers are both innovative and intuitive, constantly thinking through the purpose of each task and the interrelationships among plant, soil, and human. What works for one may not suit another at all. Direct-seeding possibilities in early spring include angelica, blessed thistle, calendula, marsh mallow, and valerian. All are frost-

farm itself. Composted manure comes from a pastured cow that provides whole milk for the family. There should be just the right number of animals to provide manure for fertility, and these animals should in turn be fed from the farm. An oat sowing interplanted with nitrogen-fixing red clover gives ground a vital two- or three-year rest from tillage, medicinal harvests along the way, and good fall grazing. Communities drawing health and sustenance from such farms need to commit to providing a viable living for those who toil there. Seeds from selected mother plants become next year's crops. The extracted juice of homegrown valerian flowers activates the phosphorus element.[7] We come to see and work with people, plants, animals, earthworms, microbes, and minerals as one.

resistant enough. Preparing seedbeds in fall to lie fallow under a thick winter mulch allows time for microbial symbiosis to come back into balance long before planting.[8] Rows can be parted in the mulch for seeding not long after snow melt rather than waiting for the ground to dry out to till. Vigorous germination comes after expansion and contraction of the seed coat as the ground alternately freezes and thaws. Seedlings developing in close proximity to other broadleaf plants in Nature appreciate the hovering protection of mulch nearby. The resulting plants have an assured sense of place and better resistance to climatic extremes. A bigger crop may very well ensue without the effort of transplanting. Spacing and thinning issues fall to the wayside for growers who can assimilate these kinds of advantages. Integrated thinking can apply to every aspect of our humble efforts to make a living from the land.

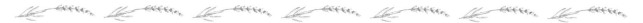

## AUTUMN MUSINGS

Shortening days and pervasive frost signal plants to shut down for the coming winter. Many gardeners choose to clip away perennial tops neatly; the particularly fastidious even rake up leaves fallen from the trees above. A farmer does much the same driving a brush mower down beds of elecampane and astragalus. All is neat and tidy for the first shoots of such plants to rise in the spring. Straw mulch spread over tender perennials completes this approach to autumn cleaning.

And should this instinct toward order be put aside? The birds feed well on seedheads left for those migrating travelers. Echinacea seeds receive rave reviews. (This intelligence of boosting immune systems in preparation for flight serves equally well those of us sharing the recirculating air of a plane.) Chickadees and finches that stay through the cold months will have an ongoing food source standing above snow cover.

Whether windblown or deliberately placed, leaves enrich the earth. Tree roots reach deep down into the subsoil, pulling up minerals that in turn become the leaves shading us all summer long. The fall to earth marks the beginning of decomposition—the minerals are converted into rich humus, available for another plant's benefit the next growing season. Let this circle of renewal happen in your gardens! The leaves form an insulating layer beneath which both earthworms and microbes continue to work their composting magic until the ground freezes solid. Michael likes to take advantage of people's inclination to rake up this valuable organic matter into plastic lawn bags. We bring pickup truck loads of bagged leaves home to the farm each fall to spread atop field stubble. The leaves in turn are anchored by a light smattering of composted manure. Our soils continue to improve even as the first snowflakes gently touch down.

The plants themselves get to harden off fully when tops die back completely to ground level. Clipping early may result in winter injury to the roots. Dead stalks become a mulch to catch drifting snows. Lavender is one plant we do shear back to woody twigs (in late November), as its slender leaves, by remaining green this far north, can literally suck the life force from the plant by desiccating cold winds. Needled branches of evergreen make an excellent winter blanket for lavender, lemon balm, and other tender plants. Fields and gardens get a more beneficial spring cleaning once the snows melt and new growth begins to reappear.

*We return thanks for all herbs,*

*which furnish medicines for the cure of our diseases.*

*We return thanks to the corn, and to her sisters,*

*the beans and squashes,*

*which give us life.*

*We return thanks to the bushes and the trees,*

*which provide us with fruit.*

—An Iroquois Prayer

Richard Wiswall and Sally Colman do their "winter homework" well, constantly evaluating the profitability of each crop at Cate Farm and deciding where to direct the coming year's marketing thrust. Richard sagely shares this tenet on which family balance hinges: "You need to subtract something [from that infernal unending job list] when adding on something else. It can be hard not to pursue an increasing market share when making money already on a particular crop." Farm families need and deserve a certain income for the vital craft of producing good food and medicine. Yet there needs to be balance. Time to play and relax. "We live in a fishbowl here," says Richard. "Look out any window and all you see is Work."

All of us start out farming with enthusiasm. That initial drive understandably dwindles with the toil of years not always redeemed by an erratic market. Yet experience refines us—it toughens our roots—and we temper deep passion for this good Earth with a surer judgment of the direction in which our farm efforts need to proceed. Common sense lies in finding a harmony between the work we think we need

to do to make our living and the pure joy of being alive in this incredible place. We all tend at times to miss the obvious on this spiritual journey through life. The plants teach an eternal rhythm that can help us stay attuned to ourselves, our families, and our communities. The deepest healing of all on a medicine farm may well happen in the heart of the grower.

## HARVESTING POINTERS

Each herb has its moment in the sun (and moon!) when its medicinal content is optimal. Root diggers may face the more daunting task, but no one starts the day before the clover blossom pluckers. The following collection of grower's best tips will make a difference on your herb farm.

We start by approaching the plant world with gratitude and loving respect. Putting intent and thankfulness into each and every leaf, flower, and root can only increase the healing energy. Always gather with reverence. Some choose to honor the plant with an offering of tobacco or cornmeal or even powdered seaweed. A song or simple prayer works equally well. We have smudged whole areas of the garden, singing and offering prayer before harvesting a large quantity of plants. Wassailing the apple trees on Old Twelfth Night (January 17) is a tradition rooted in such mutual respect. We give, we receive. Taking these moments to acknowledge this partnership that makes our lives possible embraces the spirit in all.

### Picking Herbs

We've been using the word *herb* in the inclusive sense when we refer to medicinal plants as healing herbs. This focus narrows as we temporarily leave roots and tree barks behind. Everything above ground that may be picked from a fleshy-stemmed plant (one that generally dies back at the end of each growing season) for medicinal or culinary use is the definition of the word *herb* in Webster. Being botanically precise here— leaf, flower, seed, or fruit—takes away the ambiguity. The words *aerial parts* refer to the upper portion of the plant, with flowers, buds, leaf, and tender stem intact.

Each herb has an appropriate growth stage for hand harvesting. Many flowering tops are cut when the first blossoms open in tender perfection, prior to maturing seed. The desired essential oil content of most herbs peaks as the plant comes into bloom. Peppermint has been studied in depth in this regard. The constituents in young plant tissue are aromatic pulegone (which we also appreciate in pennyroyal) and menthofuran. The latter tastes quite bitter. Just before flowering, harsh-flavored menthone is the predominant element in peppermint oil. Menthol becomes the oil's primary constituent once the mint blooms. This offers the clean, biting peppermint essence we expect in our favorite tea herb. Methyl acetate replaces the menthol once flowering ceases, giving the mint an acrid, slightly fruity taste. The timing of harvest certainly matters for peppermint. We lack such constituent tracking for most medicinal plants, relying instead on intuitive understanding to point the way.

A plant continues to have specific photosynthesis needs in order to build root reserves once the aerial parts have been harvested. Understanding cutting height works to bolster subsequent harvests and enables perennials to return the following year. Hardened stems lack the constituents we find in the leaf, bud, and early flower. However, the upper portion of the stem—still succulent, tender, and growing—contains active constituents that woodier portions below no longer have. Aerial parts are clipped off with this division in mind. Often we read advice to take the upper third of the plant. We do this with mints, understanding full well the importance of waiting to harvest until flowers are initiated. The stems below the point we shear are woodier, their leaves less green. New mint shoots will grow from the upper node points where leaf attaches to stem for a subsequent cutting. When a combine is used to harvest mint on a large scale, it cuts much lower to the ground, relying on mechanical thrashing to remove woodier stem and a hammermill to pulverize what stem remains. We cut our lemon balm heavier than the dense-growing mint, gauging where by the greenness of the leaves, yet still above any woody stem.

The focus shifts to potent bud when aerial harvesting the top four to six inches of St. John's wort. Wild raspberry leaf can be stripped off the canes in the field or dried on the canes and then garbled. Blossom buds on the raspberry (these look like pointy hats) add to the potency of the medicine.[9] First-year canes (primocanes) can be leaf-harvested throughout the summer months. Ryan Drum points out that dormant raspberry canes with fruiting buds—think about the Doctrine of Signatures here—makes an excellent male tonic for improving circulation, lessening pelvic tension, and stimulating sexual desire.

Each herb gets harvested with attention to where the medicine will be found. Additional cuttings depend on shoots sprouting from basal buds or leaf nodes. We respect plant integrity by not clipping the entire plant off at ground level. Older leaves still connect the roots to the sun. Rosettes of certain plants (yarrow, plantain) are an exception: A neighborhood of *Achillea* spp. shares an established root system that will persist despite some of its members being basal-harvested in late spring, while the corm bases of *Plantago* spp. left in the ground regrow successfully by midsummer. The possibility of multiple cuttings in warmer growing zones has to be weighed against the need of the plant to prepare for the dormant season.

Removing the woody portion of the stem while harvesting out in the field is difficult. Since we aren't necessarily planning to dry the stem in most cases, on some plants we use this handle to advantage. Certain leaves bruise readily prior to drying, so stripping catnip, for instance, ahead of time lessens quality. Aerial parts turn easily on the solar drying racks with a quick flip of each stem. Crisp leaves on bristly motherwort and hairy nettle strip off far more easily dry than moist. We do remove yellowed leaves that have died back low on the stem, either in the field or in the process of placing the herb across the drying racks. Once dry, leaves can be hand-stripped from slightly moist stems in whole form to dry a wee bit longer (borage and comfrey come to mind) and for the simple beauty of still being whole when sold. Garbling the dried stalks across wire mesh is quicker—leaf pieces are left relatively intact, and any stem pieces getting through tend to be the less wiry portions, which have some medicinal worth.

Wait until after the morning dew has dried to harvest most aerial tops for drying. (Harvesting for fresh tincture is another matter entirely, as dewdrops may well enhance the alchemy of the medicine.) Drops of moisture on newly harvested leaves can cause rust spots or browning. Yarrow stalks in mixed stages of flowering are an exception: A coating of morning mist seems to protect hydraulically the leaves from bruis-

*Harvesting yarrow with pruning shears*

ing trauma. The high heat of day can alter the chemical content of some essential oils, so harvest aromatic herbs by midmorning. Be aware that herbs heaped too deeply in the gathering basket or wheelbarrow can heat up rapidly and actually begin to decompose. Frequent trips to a shaded garden edge to strew full baskets atop cotton sheets helps avoid this problem.

Harvest tools include a good sharp knife (preferably with a curved blade that pushes through handfuls of bunched herb), anvil clippers for snipping woody-stemmed tops, and a pair of pruning shears for bulk row harvesting. The silica-rich stalks of the horsetail (*Equisetum arvense*) quickly wear a honed knife edge to dullness, but fingernails recover from such abrasion by simply regrowing. We forego all mechanical picking, such as the cutter bar rig available for a BCS walking tractor, simply because intimacy feels like a vital part of our process. Healing

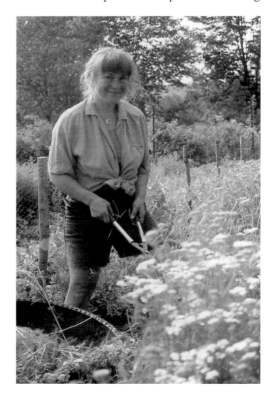

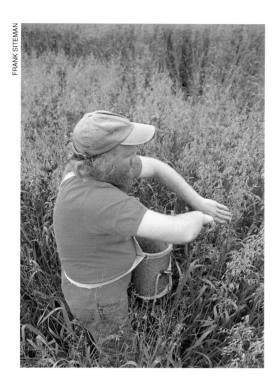

quarter acre yields roughly a hundred pounds of dried milky oat seed), depending on whether the hot sun discourages Andrea and Matthias from gathering their third sowing. These all-day efforts come when the oats say "now is the time," regardless of other needs on the farm. Stripping with gloved hands prevents cuts and chafing. Matthias, often harvesting the oats on his knees to spare his back, daydreams about developing a taller strain of this dual-purpose cover crop.

*An inverted wrist position works well in stripping milky oats off the grain stalk from the bottom up.*

intent flows clearer when we are bent over each plant in silent communion rather than when we walk behind the exhausting hum of a machine. Quality suffers as well: A machine harvest is much more likely to pick up other species of plants, a greater proportion of woody stem and yellowed leaves, and severely bruise sensitive plant tissues.

The milky oat harvest will always be a crop that defies machine efficiency.[10] Hand-stripping the succulent heads of *Avena sativa* requires an intense effort as the harvest window lasts five days at most. The fresh green seeds are picked when they are plump and a whitish milk oozes out when squeezed. Planting three rounds of this crop, rather than a one-shot block, breaks up the intensity of stripping off the forming seed heads before they harden. The milky stage is desired as medicine for soothing the nervous system and helping with withdrawal symptoms. The milky oat crop at Healing Spirits amounts to 200 to 300 pounds (a

Some herbalists will request that a particular herb be harvested according to the waxing or waning moon. Folklore holds that the vitality of aboveground plants is enhanced by an increasing moon—drawn up by the tidal pull, if you will—but that root energy centers best when the moon is on the wane. Nancy always waits to harvest echinacea roots until just before the new moons of September and October. Aboveground crops planted in the first and second quarters of the moon are said to do better, while seeds of all plants that bear food or medicine below ground are said to do better if planted in the third and fourth quarters of the moon. Increasing our awareness of plant energies from a planetary perspective makes intuitive sense to us. Still, aerial plants reach an optimal point of harvest that may not wait for the apt advice of a waxing moon. The biodynamic planting calendar, *Stella Natura,* published by the Kimberton Hills community in Pennsylvania, clearly shows which days are best for working with leaf, fruit, flower, and root from a slightly broader perspective. Zodiac influences are cross-referenced with the position of the moon. We try to choose a leaf day in harvesting lemon balm, a flower day for adding to a St. John's wort oil infusion, a root day for planting elecampane. The weather—and our own busy lives—needs to be in accord with these intentions as well. Conscious harvesting uses the moon and seasons as guidelines, but the overriding rule of thumb is to use our intuition and connection to the plants to determine when each plant is at its prime—when it is full of life force and vibrancy. This moon chat would not be complete without the mention of nighttime magic: Don't forego spending time in your gardens or walking in the woods at night. All of us—plant, human, animal, fairy—feel the pull of the moon and the aura of the stars. *Lunar constituents* will really give the rational medicos something to think about!

### Plucking Blossoms

Numerous flowers can be gathered for medicinal effect. Pruning shears work well for flowers such as goldenrod, arnica, and lavender, which come into bloom somewhat evenly. A mix of developmental stages of yarrow blooms provides a medicine with different protective chemicals from the same plant. We like to snip elderberry blossom clusters off stem by stem with hand clippers. The chamomile rake (available through Johnny's Selected Seeds for $65) works much like the traditional Maine blueberry rake, but it is modified to cut the spry stalks at the base of each tiny flower of *Matricaria recutita*. Less stem results when we choose to hand-pick chamomile meditatively, but this gathering tool has proven itself for getting in the majority of sweet blooms on busy summer days. True plucking by hand comes into play with red clover, calendula, mullein, and St. John's wort.

Red clover blossoms picked from among dawn's protecting dew retain a deep mauve color after drying. Doing a consummate job of harvesting flowers of *Trifolium pratense* means getting outside at first light before the bees fly. Big bumblebees stress the flowerets in getting to the clover nectar. The blossoms in turn begin to brown on the edges after pollination and are no longer as desirable for medicinal harvest. Morning dew in this case helps to protect hydraulically the blossom from bruising. Our ideal is to harvest without actually touching the clover blossoms, gathering them within gliding fingers from below. An experienced picker can gather 2½ to 3½ pounds of ready bloom in an hour,[11] leaving only the lightly pink blossoms behind that will color (and sweeten!) up perfectly for the next round of morning ritual two days hence. Red clover has a dry-down ratio of 4.5 to 1; thus, an hour's effort amounts to ½ to ¾ pound of marketable herb. The blooms can be poured gently across cotton sheets or nylon screens, layered no deeper than three high, placed in the house at 70° to 90°F, to dry in four to seven days with regular stirring. Good air flow hastens the drying process. The resulting color puts to shame the brown, tasteless "red clover" found commercially.

Choosing flowers that are brimming with life force gives full advantage to the hand-gatherer who plucks one bloom at a time. Selecting bright calendula blooms on this basis keeps our patches of *Calendula officinalis* ready for picking every two days or so. Plants that don't achieve seed maturity will continue to bloom anew. Sally Colman at Cate Farm found a triple-row bed at 660 feet long yielded a substantial 65 pounds of dried calendula blossoms in one season.

The common mullein (*Verbascum thapsus*) with its large, drooping leaves has flowers that cling tightly to the tall stalk and bloom slowly over the summer months. The advantage here goes to the medicinal leaves. The

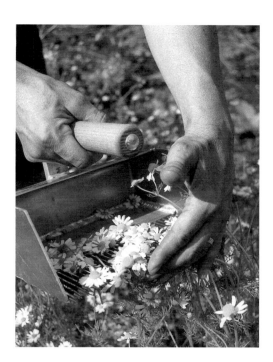

are sunny and dry. You can rake through flowering tops of St. John's wort using your fingers like tines to snag the plump buds. A surprisingly scant amount of leaf mixes in once you get the hang of this method. Ryan Drum charges $50 a pound for such dried flower buds; dried aerial tops (the upper 4 to 6 inches of the plant gets clipped off en masse) from bioregional medicine farms bring anywhere from $16 to $24 a pound, and whole plant powders wholesale at about $6 a pound. The depth of red in the medicine comes from the hypericin in the flower buds. The intensity of color affects the pricing accordingly. Jars brimming with red vigor line our stone deck each summer where St. John's wort oil infuses in the warmth of the sun.

*A modified blueberry rake (available from Johnny's Selected Seeds) speeds up the harvest of chamomile blossoms considerably.*

best mullein for flower production, Greek mullein *(Verbascum olympicum),* has blooms that adhere loosely to multiple upright branches. The yellow blossoms are stripped off the stalk in the early part of the morning before the bees make harvesting a daunting act. Being able to stand upright while picking justifies producing a pain-relieving ear oil with mullein flowers, but no profit with dried bloom.

Nancy crushes the flower buds of St. John's wort between her fingers to know when to harvest *Hypericum perforatum.* A violet/blood-red smudge indicates these potent blossoms are ready. Joyce Wardwell reports that plants growing on the sunny, north-facing slopes often produce a deeper red extract than plants harvested on a south-facing slope. The potency of these bright yellow flowers depends on the warmth of the sun, as cool wet weeks before harvest result in tinctures much muddier and without the distinctive sharp flavor that is produced when gathering days

Seeds are the end result of matured flowers. Echinacea seeds are burly enough to knock loose by rattling ripe flower heads inside plastic buckets. Burdock burrs (balls of tiny, recurved spikes which cling to fabric and fur alike) need to be shattered to release their hold on the blood-cleansing seed. Milk thistle—en garde!—involves a highly tactical approach. The flower heads are snipped off by hand when the white pappus tuft starts to develop. Seed maturity is uneven among the spiny plants in a milk thistle stand, and only the hand-harvester can compensate for this by going out every week to gather ready flower heads. Store the gathered seedheads in untreated burlap sacks, hung from a rafter in an open-air shed, to ripen. These can be run through a one-inch screen on a hammermill when the harvest is complete, or broken apart tediously by hand-garbling. All chaff gets removed by hand-winnowing on a breezy day. Nettle seeds are an exhaustive affair: Terminal clusters of the ripe fruits (each with a seed within) are stripped off with a bare hand while a gloved hand holds the stalk below. These are dried on shallow racks for several days, and stirred every twelve hours. Leaves and other debris are picked out by hand, as too many of the lightweight seeds can be lost in a winnowing process.

Fruits go round the seed. Hawthorn flowers, leaves, and berries rate highly these days as a cardiovascular tonic. The thorns on these small trees ensure that there will be sustainable crops of all three. Elderberries are a far moister fruit that proves difficult to dry. We opt for elderberry syrup and wine. Fresh berries can be frozen for processing during cold and flu season.

## Digging Roots

Root work is sacred. We are asking the plant for the very essence of its life in this act of harvesting. The human side of the bargain begins with honoring the plant spirit and ends with responsible use. We often find ourselves singing a simple yet powerful song as we dig roots:

> To you I give,
> From you I receive,
> Together we share,
> From this we live.

Root crops give us some leeway to complete the harvest. Leaf dieback in the fall indicates that stored reserves are once again centered in the root. Anytime between the first heavy frost and the ground freezing solid suits this gathering of subterranean medicine. The tall stalk of ashwagandha can even be found in the snow if need be. Roots can be dug in spring as well, before the growing energy commences. Spring-dug roots generally have more moisture than fall-dug roots, and therefore take longer to dry.

Nothing tones the stomach muscles better than digging out deep-seated roots by hand. This is plant communion at the basic gut level. We dig down beside burdock's long taproot to pull it out laterally. Nancy loves *following these roots to the center of the earth* with a narrow tree spade that once belonged to her Kansas grandpa. Many other root medicinals can be freed by circumferential prying with a garden fork. Forest roots growing in moist, soft soil take little effort to dig once they've been located. A "senging stick" (used by ginseng diggers in the Appalachians) consists of a hardwood sapling about the diameter of a broom handle, whittled down to a chisel-shaped edge.[12] Definite mechanical advantage abets sizable root harvests on many bioregional medicine farms. Tractors can pull a root digger that unearths plants up to the soil surface. Richard Wiswall modified a rusty potato digger (widened for a double-row crop) to do precisely this in his echinacea beds. Alternatively, a shank can be run alongside long rows to at least loosen adjacent soil for successful tugging. Joel Dufour of Earth Tools can set up BCS owners with a root-digger plow for walking tractors.

Harvesting roots by hand is very labor intensive. "I need to take this into consideration when setting my prices," says Monica Rude. "A small grower digging by hand cannot compete with the big operations who use machines and accomplish a lot quickly. But the quality and the energy of the herb cannot compare."

Timing will always be relevant, too. Marsh mallow has a greater mucilage content in roots harvested during the growing phase than in full dormancy. The optimal harvest comes anytime after flowering in late summer and through the fall. Spring-dug roots certainly still have some demulcent and emollient effects, as the mucilage content of *Althaea officinalis* varies between

25 to 35 percent year-round.[13] Such knowledge doesn't necessarily allay our spring efforts to complete harvests frozen in at the start of a New Hampshire winter. Spring gives us a chance to increase our supply of fresh echinacea tincture for early fall delivery of home medicine share orders as well. Elecampane tends to get pithy after two full growing seasons, so an April harvest aimed at cleaning up a planting of *Inula helenium* will save us some root-shaving work.

One full growing season produces marketable roots of valerian the next year, just before the plant flowers. The longer *Valeriana officinalis* continues as a basal rosette, the more root mass it puts on. Seedlings transplanted out as soon as possible in spring tend to go through the first year without bolting to flower. Plants set out in the heat of early summer tend to bolt. This urge to produce seed won't be denied valerian in its following year; clipping away the developing flower stalk, however, will keep its root mass undiminished.[14] (Be fair here. Letting a few plants flower pleases many pollinators, and any seedling volunteers that result next spring make the best transplants of all.) Valerian can be dug throughout the summer when the matted stolons give the highest yield. Valerian stolons actually die back by midwinter, leaving only a base root with high concentrations of essential oils and valepotriates. The stolons fatten up again by the time green growth starts to show. Rock and gravel always lodge in valerian's tangled roots—as will perlite from a greenhouse soil mix—so planting in choice ground avoids much cleaning hassle down the road. Large root masses are cut into sections before washing to help access the most ornery crannies.

Cleaning roots as soon as possible after harvest is a must. A field shakedown will get

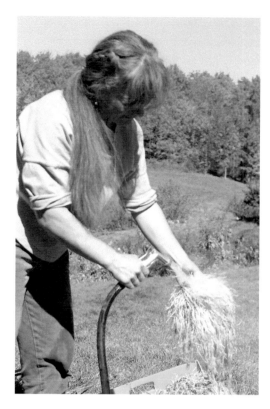

*Be thorough about washing roots no matter what your method.*

rid of the majority of clinging soil. A woodland harvester can take advantage of a mountain brook for a quick root rinse. Soaking roots for an extended period is not advised, however, as water-soluble constituents will leach out. A hose rinse, preferably pressurized, is the best most home herbalists can muster. A barrel washer (originally designed for vegetable crops such as carrots) tumbles the roots back and forth, shooting jets of fresh water, which cascade any mud out openings in the side and bottom of the barrel. We're most intrigued by the bioagitator—a high-tech sounding term for the wringer/washer machine of yesteryear—used at Healing Spirits (see the profile on page 204). Halving roots prior to washing can be a big help both in getting them clean and in drying them faster. A stiff brush helps get off any dirt that might still remain after the moisture is gone.

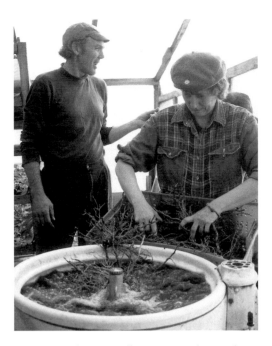

*A wringer/washer machine becomes a "bioagitator" for washing roots in the hands of Matthias and Andrea Reisen of Healing Spirits Herb Farm in central New York state.*

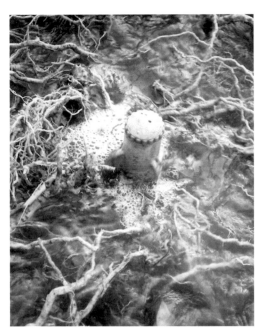

As much as small growers take pride in doing a job right, contract growers are held to measurable standards. Ash testing at Frontier Co-operative's quality assurance lab tells an undeniable truth about how well roots have been cleaned. A representative sample of each root purchase is literally burned at 400°F for three hours to get rid of carbon structure. Only dirt and the minerals found in the original root remain. The latter are soluble in acid. Placing such an acid slurry back in the oven for thirty minutes results in only acid-insoluble ash left behind. A 2 percent standard by weight allows for some minerals that arguably might not have gotten dissolved. A larger ash pile than this means dirty roots and reputation alike will be returned to the sender.

### Barking Up the Right Tree

Many medicinal barks can be gathered throughout the winter months, but any earnest harvester will wait for spring sap flow. Bark is best harvested when it slips or peels away from the heartwood of the tree or shrub. We test for optimal harvesttime by slicing free a small square of bark. The outer layer gets scraped away, and ideally the inner bark lifts readily from the moist wood. The outer barks of trees such as slippery elm, white ash, and wild cherry are discarded, as it's the inner bark that has the desired medicinal properties. Thin barks from shrubs or roots are dried without this delayering. Timing varies for different species, but generally speaking March through June are prime months to be considering bark work. Eventually the tree sap flow lessens as a new growth ring establishes itself and then hardens off.

People do take bark directly from living trees. This harvest need not be fatal to the tree if bark is taken from lateral branches. These branches are best pruned off the tree, leaving only the branch collar to heal over properly. Scraping the north side of the trunk (bark growth here tends to be more constricted and dense) may seem charitable from the human perspective. This scarring of the living cambium can indeed heal, but the larger the bark area taken, the less likely the wound is to callus over completely. We don't recommend this potentially harmful technique of barking. Demise follows quickly once rot organisms enter the tree's vascular system. Coppicing works far better for all concerned.

A copse of trees is a dense thicket. Black cherry thrives in the egregious clearcuts of the northeastern forest and where once-pastured fields are left to return to their native state. Young saplings, on the order of ten years old, approach several inches in diameter at the base. Thinning such a copse lets us harvest medicine and at the same time provide necessary growing space for nearby saplings of all species. An even broader understanding of coppicing applies when mature trees are harvested. Stump sprouts result from the root system left behind in the cutting of many deciduous trees. The herb gatherer by no means needs to be the logger in this case, as much as follow in the footsteps of the logger five to ten years later. Latent buds in the remaining trunk and root runners vigorously respond to the opened sunlight. The ensuing sprouts quickly become a dense coppice of saplings, growing much faster than if independently seeded. We can choose as herbalists to saw down a twenty- to thirty-year-old tree (in the process of selective thinning) to initiate a deliberate growth response. A series of such harvests over many years seems more tree-appropriate and renewable than bark scarring. As we should not use chain saws to cut trees intended for medicine—bar and chain oil contaminates the bark, to say nothing of the noise and exhaust being an absolute violation of healing intent—our coppicing efforts will never exceed the pleasure we derive from bow saw work on relatively young trees.

Ryan Drum is a good man to turn to whenever considering the nuance of a wild harvest. He points out that willows growing in drier environments tend to have more salicin (the glucoside that forms pain-relieving salicylic acid in the body) than their lowland counterparts. Young willows have a very thin layer of corky outer bark and nice green photosynthetic cells close to the surface. The cambium layer transfers the heaviest concentration of nutrients and medicinal constituents from the roots to the developing leaves following bud break. The bark of *Salix* spp., taken from cut sprouts one to three inches in diameter, is a very aggressive curler, akin to cinnamon sticks. Ryan recommends that knife-peeled strips of willow bark are best kept in widths of one inch or smaller to keep the inner surfaces from molding before they are dry. These strips are hand cut with scissors into two- to four-inch lengths, and then dried at 60°F to 70°F before storage in airtight, opaque containers. Higher drying temperatures degrade some active constituents in willow bark.

The nuances for cherry are much the same as for willow. Young barks, about the thickness of leather, have the best medicine: Twiggy branches haven't developed bark bulk as yet; mature wood has a much flakier outer bark. Cut a longitudinal groove with a sharp razor knife from the butt of the sapling all the way up to the smallwood, about one inch in diameter. The corky layer of outer bark gets peeled away and discarded. A bark spud (a long-handled chisel with a slightly upturned cutting edge) peels off the green inner bark in long strips. These in turn are hand cut into three- to six-inch pieces to dry at 70°F to 90°F for about a week. Such medicinal bark retains a green color and flexibility for up to three years as opposed to the wholesale junk that big botanical suppliers obtain through sawmill debarking and subsequent powdering.

### Yields

The past only reveals lessons if we have accurate records to look back on. Keeping track of germination times, days to maturity, and yield per plant make it possible to plan crop timing and volume. Jotting down daily observations during the growing season in a garden journal eventually makes the nuances of cultivation at your farm location clear. A good grower turns knowledge into livelihood. Bed uniformity and consistent row length can help in calculating yields. Each *Echinacea purpurea* plant may well produce ⅓ to ½ pound of fresh root, washed and trimmed, after three growing seasons, but it's much simpler to plan on a 500-foot-long, double-row bed producing 400 pounds of fresh root. It takes time to develop harvesting and processing techniques that work for each crop. How you sift dry herb or clean gnarly roots certainly affects yields. Dry catnip with stem intact might tally up more than 3,000 pounds to the acre; a quality-oriented contract grower may end up with 1,000 pounds of meticulously sifted dry leaf with stem removed. Book yields are at best averages that may or may not reflect the climate and fertility of any given farm and the thoroughness of the farmer.

## ETHICAL WILDCRAFTING

Native medicinal species that get overharvested, or face loss of habitat, are endangered. Gatherers of wild plants—and especially the people creating a misguided demand in the marketplace—have a responsibility to future generations to harvest without species devastation. Ethical wildcrafting implies this long-range concern for the continuation and health of each plant species. Humans are not alone in interacting with plants, and our needs are not necessarily paramount from the earth's perspective. Still, people have gathered their medicines in the wild for thousand of years. So why are we now facing a crisis with the herbs chosen for United Plant Savers' At-Risk and To Watch Lists (see pages 308 and 309)?

Popular culture does not know how to relate to the healing plants. The mass marketing of herbal remedies, from nutraceutical soft drinks to misconceptions about phyto-silver bullets, creates a demand for herbs that is out of line with the wise use of herbs. Glossy magazine ads promote pill popping and secure bottom lines. Lifestyle be damned: Take these eight supplements and discover the new you. We seem unable to make the mental link that how we live our lives affects the quality of our lives. And so we look for the fix, the cure, the miracle in a bottle that will turn things around. Naturally enough the herb industry offers a laudable alternative. The public responds with enthusiasm, spurring 20 percent a year sales growth. People who gather the herbs happily meet the rising demand. Herbs that are increasingly harder to find soar in price. The bounds of wildcrafting reach farther into back mountain hollows and across the windswept prairie, along state highways and deep into the swampy mire. Medicinal plants—these precious, precious friends—are a hot commodity too many people only know through a passing glance at a supplement or tincture label.

High-profile herbs have caught our attention. In the wild the overharvesting of ginseng roots, goldenseal roots, *Echinacea angustifolia* roots, black cohosh roots, and saw palmetto berries has made people understand the damage that can be done. The call for sustainable cultivation partially addresses the issue. Abandoning the wild harvest for local use does not. "Most wildcrafters harvest wild herbs because they need the money, not because sick people need the herbs. Most personal herb consumption is a waste of herbs at about the 80 percent level," says Ryan Drum. "What is usually needed is personal lifestyle change. Wildcrafters are relatively innocent, supplying demand created by those often more economically advantaged."

We have reached the apex of today's ethical wildcrafting debate. We know of no herbalist who would mindfully harvest the whole of a stand of healing plants. But our impact is collective, and where one ventures, others surely follow. Consciousness can be collective as well, and the herbal movement has crafted a code of ethics for the gathering of wild medicinals. What has long been apparent intuitively to indigenous people needs to be learned by generations too long out of touch with the living Earth.

Ideally, we harvest the right plant part from the right plant at the right time. Plant identification comes easier to some, but whether you learn through botanical keys in a field guide or on weed walks with experienced herbalists, practice is the only way to master this skill. Poisonous look-alikes of useful plants (poison hemlock closely resembles Queen Anne's lace, for instance) give reason aplenty to be absolutely sure you know plants well. Optimal medicinal effect correlates to which constituents are found in the plant at the moment of harvest. Let a thorough understanding of traditional use be your guide with each herb you encounter.

Awareness of the particular ecosystems favored by each plant helps immensely in locating a good stand of the desired species. Never assume one vigorous stand is replicated throughout an area, but rather, search around and know this isn't the only cranesbill geranium (*Geranium viscosissimum*) that grazing cattle have left in the valley. Pale purple coneflower (*Echinacea pallida*) is common in eastern Kansas, but is very rare in North Carolina at the eastern extreme of its range. Herbalists are not alone in affecting ecosystem change: Livestock, all-terrain vehicles, and rotational logging all indicate the need to tread exceptionally lightly around any native species that manage to survive. Old-growth plants such as goldthread (*Coptis* spp.) and wild ginger (*Asarum caudatum*) have far fewer acres on which to grow in these days of supposedly sustainable forestry. Not all environments are meant for the human foot. Marsh thickets rife with bugleweed (*Lycopus americanus*) should be harvested from the edges where nesting birds and amphibian croakers will be least disturbed. Pipsissewa (*Chimaphila umbellata*) grows ever-so-slowly in mossy, soft soils that readily compact under each footstep.[15]

Ethical wildcrafting above all else implies stewardship of the plants. We should always harvest with thoughts of beauty in mind. Our goal is to leave an area better off than when we first set foot on it. Tending and propagating stands of herbs ensures a mutual coexistence. Ginseng harvested after it matures seed can grow anew if that seed gets planted. One rule of thumb is never harvest more than 10 percent of a given stand. Not that you have to count: Any noticeably visual change in flora density means you took too much. We need to take equal care not to introduce invasive plants into pristine native ecosystems. One burdock burr can carry a long way from home. Plants can, however, be rescued from areas slated for development. Faye Burtch spent many days moving goldenseal from a forest glen decreed to be bulldozed for a state highway project in central Pennsylvania. Untended stands of plants can serve as good indicators of how we are doing elsewhere with the same species of plant. Many medicinals need the protection of remaining obscure, which means wildcrafters should lie equally low with respect to being seen by a curious passerby.

Appreciating the wild harvest fully means avoiding exothermic spoilage due to mishandling or delays in processing. Metabolic heat will build up in any pile of organic matter. Polypropylene grain bags work well as a protective girdle wrapped around leafy stalks, with the open ends allowing the harvest to breathe during the hike home. Five-gallon plastic buckets are good for moist root harvests and seaweed, provided containment is short-term. Our ash pack baskets work best of all, being light but sturdy, quite breathable, and snugly positioned on our backs. Once home at the farm, unbundling herbs and rinsing roots takes first priority. Fresh tinctures should be made that day to capture the highest medicinal quality.

Good books abound that help herbalists to identify and understand plants. *A Field Guide to Medicinal Plants* by Steven Foster and James Duke covers plants of Eastern and Central North America, using visual impressions of leaf and flower to key in on plant identification with line drawings and color photographs. The authors surveyed the medicinal uses of each plant, past and present, to provide an inkling of healing possibility. Michael Moore's books are a must for

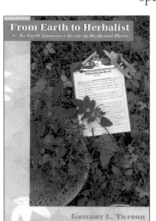

Greg Tilford profiles fifty-two species of wild medicinal plants in From Earth to Herbalist. *Our connection with Earth as herbalists strongly suggests we understand the impact we can have on wild plant populations. This field guide does just that.*

anyone using the *Medicinal Plants of the Mountain West* and the *Medicinal Plants of the Desert and Canyon West.* The plant knowledge included by this herbal guru was garnered firsthand over many years: exacting descriptions of each species, harvesting instructions, constituents as related to therapeutic use, cultivation, and potential side effects. In short, a complete herbalist's herbal for the stated ecosystem. *Medicinal Wild Plants of the Prairie* by Kelly Kindscher does much the same, probing deeply into Native American use of prairie plants. Detailed instructions for gathering sixty wild plants of the Pacific Northwest were assembled by Krista Thie of Longevity Herb Company in *A Plant Lover's Guide to Wildcrafting.* Gregory Tilford brings the precepts of ethical wildcrafting to full light in *From Earth to Herbalist.* The alternative remedies, plant-animal interdependence, and suggestions for treading lightly offered in this book are vital perspectives we need as herbalists.

Wildcropping is wildcrafting done on the sanctified ground of a certified organic farm. This distinction provides bureaucratic certainty that said wild herbs are indeed organic. Still, the odds are slim that someone sprayed or chemically fertilized crampbark shrubs (*Viburnum opulus*) harvested in the wild. Alfalfa or red clover gathered from a neighboring hay field likely has seen only the manure commonly spread on dairy ground. (Such would not be the case with cover crops gathered from a commercial potato field dosed with pesticides.) Goldenseal planted on the farm side of a property boundary might seem no more organic than goldenseal growing wild in the neighboring state forest. Yet encouraging all such herbs on the herb farm itself is the only way to legitimately make a certifiable claim, regardless of how far up the mountain you climbed to gather organic lomatium.

Two Idaho wildcrafters, Jim Flocchini and Meryl Kastin, come to Silver City, New Mexico, annually on their loop of the Southwest to both gather and sell herbs. Richard McDonald of the Desert Bloom Herbs shop asks them to bring along *Lomatium dissectum* for his antiviral formulations. This western cousin of wild parsley can only be found farther north, in dry, rocky, steep soils. Lomatium has a low germination rate and may be fifty years old before it becomes a sizable root. All involved here know and respect the integrity of this plant. Mountain harvests are confined to the bottom of slopes where the stand can be renewed by the distribution of seeds from the upslope plants.[16] Richard does not sell this herb in bulk on the store shelves, choosing instead to reserve its medicine for compounded tinctures should a viral remedy be indicated in consultation. "Other herbs often can serve the situation nearly as well as lomatium," he points out. "Spilanthes and echinacea are better options to boost the immune system and initiate tissue repair. I like using osha root, yarrow, and wild oregano for respiratory infections of bacterial origin."

We impact local ecology most by taking roots and rhizomes. Respect for continuity should always point the way: Seventh-generation thinking applies not only to our kind. We can sense if a harvest at this time in this place befits all the beings involved. Making a living is a legitimate need, as is supplying an herbal remedy to people in need. Choosing the larger of plants growing closely together and from the center of patches (that will readily fill back in) helps. Some people say you should never harvest the Grandmother plant—the very biggest, the most vibrant. We should replant pieces of blue cohosh rhizomes and lomatium crown buds even though the regrowth won't result in as strong a plant as one started from seed.

Conscious wildcrafting will not offset the current culture. Ethics for some will never go beyond a base profit motive. But plant medicine is far more than treasure lying about on the ground to be gathered and sold to the highest bidder. Only responsible demand will alter the market's call, and until then more plants will likely become endangered. The push for sustainable cultivation of goldenseal by the larger herb companies recognizes that as more people dabble with herbal medicine, our culture has poised itself to decimate the wild.

"Some environmentalists believe that to protect biodiversity you must exclude people. In their view you either have production or you have protection. I have seen farms as beautiful as a native forest," says Vandana Shiva, a world-renowned environmentalist. "I feel it is important to bring ecology and biodiversity into the heart of production rather than keeping it outside." We sustainably cultivate, we ethically wildcraft. Behind both efforts to gather good medicine is love. And that may well be what the plants have been asking for all along.

## THE ART OF MAKING "GOOD HAY"

Just as horses know good hay when they see it, herbalists know when the harvest from our woodlands and gardens abounds with life force and vibrancy. Drying and storage techniques are invaluable skills for any healing herb grower whose livelihood depends upon preserving medicinal potency. We prevent molding and chemical reactions that alter constituent levels by removing the moisture from the herb. Whatever the method, consistent drying at a moderate

80°F to 110°F temperature is best. Cell wall integrity breaks down when herbs go from wet to dry to wet to dry. Attempting to dry herbs in an open-air shed doesn't cut it. "Each night the enzyme systems of the plant get reactivated once wet," says Ryan Drum. "The secondary metabolites are the first to degrade, being the most fragile, unless they are resins or waxes." A good drying system must offer steady heat, lots of air flow, relatively low humidity, and grower savvy to work well.

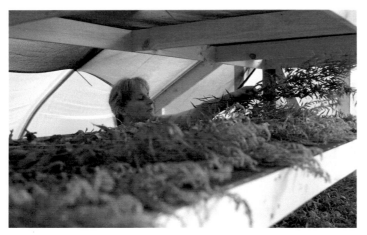

*Nancy gives the stems of goldenrod a flip in our solar drying tunnel.*

The percentage of water content varies greatly in herbs. Leaves and flowers range from 65 to 95 percent water content. Roots range from 45 to 75 percent water content. A plant with 75 percent water content is composed of three parts water and one part substance. Thus it has a dry-down ratio of four to one: Every 4 pounds of fresh herb will yield 1 pound of dry herb. Absolute moisture reduction isn't possible, of course, without reducing the plant to ashes, so in actual fact dried herb still has about a 5 to 8 percent water content. Think *crisp* (as opposed to *fried and brittle*) when judging your results. Thicker roots generally dry more slowly than leaves and flowers, even though less moisture may be present at the start.

Larger roots such as elecampane need to be split lengthwise to facilitate drying without molding.

### Solar Drying

The art of drying medicinal herbs in a solar greenhouse in the Northeast has proven itself in the hands of Matthias and Andrea Reisen. Our profile on this couple (see page 204) details how they carried the know-how of making good alfalfa hay into a prospective herbal livelihood. Solar drying very much depends on understanding the dynamics of moisture exiting the leaf or root. Experience will prove an uncompromising teacher. Each plant differs in the subtleties of care; each day's weather calls for adjustments to the system. Grower involvement is integral: Solar drying requires continuous engagement to work successfully. Supplemental heat at night and on overcast days makes all the difference in the world. A small wood fire is solar energy one step removed. We love the irony of lighting a fire in a twilight-cooled 80°F greenhouse on a midsummer's eve to make dried-in-full comfrey leaf a medicinal reality in two days' time.

The costs are practically nil for the Reisens' homegrown solution that defies drying convention. Recycled lumber holds up a double layer of greenhouse plastic. A small blower ensures an insulating layer of air between the sheets of poly. Vertical wooden racks support the drying herbs laid across stapled fiberglass screening three feet in width. The five levels of racks average eighteen inches of reach between. Herbs get shifted several times a day, eventually making their way to the upper racks when they are about 75 percent dry. Field-moist herbs cannot be placed directly in the intensity of

*Text continues on page 202.*

# OUR SOLAR DRYING TUNNEL

**W**E CREATED an effective space for drying our herbs in a growing tunnel measuring 14 × 24 feet. A double layer of greenhouse plastic (UV-treated to slow degradation by sunlight) is kept inflated by a small blower fan available from horticultural supply houses. The air layer between helps stabilize the galvanized pipe frame of the tunnel and moderates temperature loss as twilight comes on. The end walls are a hodgepodge of framing lumber, fitted to bolt in on a curve with the end arches. Corrugated greenhouse plastic is the cover. Pressure-treated wood along the tunnel's bottom edges won't rot, so we agreed to its environmental karma. The drying frames are made of 1 × 4 pine with fiberglass screening stapled to the top edge, attached at a 16-inch spacing to salvaged 4 × 4 posts. The two side racks are 28 inches wide, three frames high. The middle rack stretches 36 inches across, five frames high. This leaves us 28-inch walkways between the frames, a good spac-

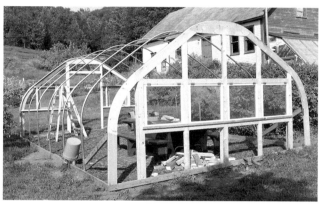

*The bones of a tunnel frame stand revealed for aspiring carpenters on other herb farms.*

ing for maneuvering with full herb baskets or a narrow wheelbarrow. A 65 percent shade cloth attached to the tunnel arches high up (with nylon clip ties) protects the upper frames in the middle from intense noonday sun, as well as moderating the overall temperature. Salvaged windows on both tunnel ends can be propped open when the temperature exceeds 100°F. High-velocity fans atop one of the side drying frames keep air moving at all times.

The frames are 9 feet long, with two attached in series in each aisle. This leaves room for a garbling table in one front corner and a backup heat source in the other. Scrap wood fires in an Ashley sheet-metal stove warm the space quickly on overcast days and at night. We placed the 6-inch-diameter stovepipe within an 8-inch-diameter outer pipe to shield the plastic from potential meltdown. Even so, a hand-held water mister to spray nearby surfaces is a reasonable precaution. The air space between the pipes is left exposed where the 6-inch stovepipe extends on out to the sky, thus allowing outside air to cool the exit framing.

This arrangement cost us just over $1,200, aside from the salvaged parts. Here's a breakdown of what we spent, so you can figure what to improvise:

| | |
|---|---|
| Galvanized pipe frame | $266 |
| Greenhouse plastic | 110 |
| Blower fan | 43 |
| Wiring supplies | 48 |
| Flexible corrugated plastic | 65 |
| Pressure-treated lumber | 104 |
| Spruce framing lumber | 90 |
| Fiberglass screening | 122 |
| Air-dried pine, 1 × 4 | 156 |
| Shade cloth and nylon ties | 83 |
| Stovepipe and wall thimble | 88 |
| Misc. bolts, screws, staples | 35 |
| Black bristle wallpaper brushes | 10 |
| (great for sweeping off the racks!) | |

The tunnel works well despite the vagaries of the weather. Going solar implies an ongoing commitment to micromanaging your drying space and planning harvest loading accordingly. We sweat happily with the good herb, mon.

the sun, as they will scald. If heat is forced too quickly over the outer cells of a leaf, those cells harden before moisture from deeper within can escape. Thus herbs brought into the greenhouse go on the lower racks, with arrival timed in the late afternoon to coincide with peak solar gain and the coming of the dark night. Maintaining the desired temperature at 100°F to 110°F (the thermometers are at eye level) requires a backup source of heat for cool nights and rainy days. Woodstoves work well, but Matthias recently switched to a self-feeding burner with a fuel source (corn kernels) that needs to be topped off only once a day. Air flows across and beneath each rack, thanks to strategically placed fans. Minimizing the drying time is key, with most herb leaf ready to be garbled and stored within 24 to 48 hours. Root drying times are doubled accordingly, with a follow-up spell after shredding to ensure that mold does not occur in storage.

Solar drying requires moving the herb through quickly. Given enough exposure, sunlight can cause many herbs to turn brown or black. The longer times specified for drying in the dark reflect this need to play it safe. Leaves from comfrey, coltsfoot, plantain, and mullein have high water content. These need to stay longer in the lower levels of the drying room where temperatures aren't quite as high. A slower pace results in less browning. Keeping the white side up on coltsfoot helps. Plants with readily volatilized essential oil content are best not dried in the sun at all: Angelica seed and root, valerian root, and blessed thistle come to mind. Temperatures pushed beyond 100°F will lessen these volatiles as well. Experience has taught us to use the dark attic on the end of our farmhouse for herbs

that dry down better there than in the solar tunnel. Lemon balm retains that divine lemony scent much better when dried in dark heat. Its volatile essential oil has sedative, antispasmodic (relieving spasms), and antibacterial effects. What smells good, treats good.

Growers in other regions need to take into account the intensity of a higher noonday sun. Later in the season at Desert Woman Botanicals, a 65 percent shade cloth covers the hoop-style greenhouse where Monica Rude grows both herbs and vegetables in early spring to sell as bedding plants. Cross-use of facilities on a small farm happens until we can someday contrive to afford the whole hog. Seedlings like moisture; herbs drying do not. A complete transition of the entire space needs to be made, or a plastic wall can be constructed to divide the greenhouse while the bedding plant season overlaps the earliest medicinal harvest. End-wall vents to the outside—which absolutely need to be closed as the sun sets to keep out moist night air—have large fans that keep the air circulating and help reduce heat buildup. Most leaf crops dry in two to three days, without supplemental heat, as desert rains are few and far between. Mugwort, chaparral leaf, and ashwagandha root dry well here. Monica eventually doubles up the shade cloth on what had been the spring end of the greenhouse to dry holy basil, wide leaf plantain, and calendula atop the bedding plant racks.

## Mechanical Drying

Other herb growers create curing rooms or chambers where drying heat is provided by fossil fuel or electricity. Minding the caveat to avoid direct sun provides more flexibility in achieving a high-quality product. The initial cost for a space of equal capacity to a solar structure will be greater, primarily due to the investment in a furnace/blower system. Being able to monitor the temperature precisely allows these growers to ease into the drying process at 85° to 90°F, and thus ensure a steady release of moisture from interior plant cells. The heat can easily be turned up, going as high as 120°F for roots and barks. Volatile oils are better preserved when the temperature does not exceed the century mark. Air flow from down under is directed up through the racks of herbs and out the top. Some systems employ dehumidifiers to keep the relative humidity below 30 percent. Be fire-sensitive: Drying rooms that go up in smoke within storage and apothecary facilities make for a huge infrastructure loss on any scale farm.

Renne Soberg in Minnesota put his drying room inside a former dairy barn. The 14 × 24-foot space is well insulated, which reduces how long the electric heater needs to run. An exhaust fan creates negative pressure in the room, thus keeping high-humidity conditions outside. Richard Wiswall at Cate Farm made use of another existing farm resource: a hot air furnace/heat exchanger used to heat the planting beds in the seeding greenhouse in springtime. A quick redirection of the ductwork funnels 90°F air (adjusted upward for root crops) outside through an 8 × 8 × 8-foot plywood box with four layers of sliding screen racks beneath a corrugated sheet metal cover. All combustion gases are exhausted through the furnace chimney, not through the herbs. This high-air-flow dryer can handle up to 450 pounds of fresh material without any space lost to walkways for turning over the herb. Loose sheets of screening atop each rack can be shaken out readily and thus cleaned to receive the next herb fresh from the field. Only one type of herb at a time is dried on either stack to prevent crumpled leaf or blossom petal from mixing.

### Homescale Drying

Innovation rules the day for drying medicinal herbs. Scale appropriately takes us from a bare minimum $3,000 investment in furnace hardware to a 60-watt lightbulb on the home front. Hand-crafted cabinets can be adapted at home to dry herbs for family needs using that lightbulb for both heat and air flow. Air intake at the bottom follows the rising heat out through vents in the top of such a cabinet. Spare hall closets can be set up with drying shelves, rigged with either a miniature vent fan to go with a heat source below or a dehumidifier. The pilot flame in our gas oven works well to dry small harvests of basil and parsley.[17] Screen racks lightly filled with calendula blossoms dry in a bedroom loft. Our attic served for years as our only drying area. Nighttime humidity above living quarters rises far less compared to an open-air shed or the haylofts of the barn. We still put aromatic herbs and everlasting flowers up in the attic despite the steep climb. We want calendula petals as bright orange as the day of harvest, so after one day in the greenhouse, these flowers are piled loosely in baskets on the floor of the attic for another week. Bunches of herbs can be dried from the kitchen rafters, with two caveats worth noting: Overly thick bunches will mold on the inside, and herbs that eventually gather dust have long since lost medicinal effect.

We once were given a drying rig built by Benedictine monks. It seemed to address both the solar gain of the day and the safe

*Text continues on page 206.*

# Matthias and Andrea Reisen

Matthias and Andrea Reisen embrace the primary tenets of successful farming: *Work hard and enjoy it.* Growing, wildcrafting, and drying each of more than sixty herbs is a phenomenal job that requires constant attention to detail. The season simply doesn't let up, except for an occasional teaching weekend, and these come with the opportunity to market the vibrant harvest of Healing Spirits Herb Farm.

Bartering and neighborly banter suit this agriculture. A nearby dairy farmer provides fresh milk in trade for prostate tincture. A Turkish friend bangs nails with Matthias on construction projects around the farm. Later, Andrea works on his back. An elderly lady, who comes by for goldenseal to relieve a respiratory condition, promises to have money next month when her check comes in. Trust is exchanged for care.

"Just compare that to a big herb company," Matthias points out. Several months can go by before payment for a substantial contract order is received back at the farm. Healing Spirits does one billing at the time of shipment but lacks a computerized invoice system to follow through with monthly reminders. Farm-

ers who honor their end of an agreement naturally expect the same courtesy in return. "You get too big," says this man of principle, "and you lose the personal connection."

Herbalists who know good herb order from the Reisens precisely because of the ardent connection Matthias and Andrea have with the plants. "To do well, you have to have a caring for the plants, an understanding of the energy of the plants," Matthias stresses. "This is what carries over into the final product and heals the person." The best niche crops for a small-scale herb grower tend to be hand intensive. Quality medicinals that can't be obtained by mechanized harvest can be offered on a more intimate scale. Red clover blossoms and milky oats are at the top of this list. Calendula requires picking every two days to keep abreast of virgin blooms. Alfalfa holds its green after drying only if it is picked just before the deep purple flowers open. Crampbark is gathered from highbush cranberry between late fall and early spring. Four- to six-year-old shoots are clipped off at the base of the shrub, the bark is slit open and removed, then cut

again into narrow strips that lie flat (rather than curl) to dry. Even common catnip maintains its quality when crafted by hand: its leaves dry much faster than the stalk, and can be hand stripped sooner to preserve more of the green.

*To do well, you have to have a caring for the plants, an understanding of the energy of the plants.*

—Matthias Reisen

Andrea gives a straightforward message to the herbs growing at Healing Spirits: "This is where we are. This is where you need to grow. It's the same for me." Avoca, New York, probably never had a more honest promoter. Down by the sweat lodge, shaded in the tree line along the property's edge, goldenseal leaves quake in awed consent.

Their gambrel-roofed barn has seen many modifications since its glory days, when it housed a herd of milking cows. Lines of posts and altered roof lines attest to the unassuming practicality of a farmer with a bold plan. Matthias has jumped right in to play with this giant Lego set. He created a solar drying greenhouse on one end, and another poly-sheeted space, dedicated to transplanting, beneath former shed rafters. Where once good hay went in to produce income, now it comes out. The herb leaf and roots dried here as a medicinal cash crop defy the conventional wisdom to avoid light in the drying process. All the words that describe good hay—green, vibrant, smelling like a summer day—are aptly applied to any order of herbs from Healing Spirits.

"We were dairy farmers," Matthias explains about questioning the axiom to dry herbs in the dark. "How do you make the best alfalfa hay? You take away all the water with conditions of low humidity and good air flow and dry it quickly. The greenhouse is the only way to do this in our region. The most important thing is moving the herbs through very quickly. If they sit too long, they wither and don't have any energy left in them. I also believe the powerful energy of the sun gets incorporated into the herbs during drying. Ideally, our herbs are dried within 24 to 48 hours."

"In the heat of the summer," Andrea explains, "we wait to put just-harvested herbs into the greenhouse until late afternoon. The herbs lose a lot of their wetness overnight." The high heat of the solar day carries well into the dark of the night, meaning significant drying does occur without light. Ceiling fans keep air circulating over the racks, and a corn-

fueled burner helps compensate for less-than-sunny weather. "We put our herbs up in the top of the barn in the beginning, just like the books said to, but quit that after a few weeks. There was no quality. The herbs weren't vibrant and green at all, but moldy. Here in the Northeast, we dry by a different set of rules.

"What we are doing may not work in California or even in Pennsylvania. Other growers should read as much as they can, talk to as many people as they can, and then use their own intuition and common sense in determining the best way to dry for their operation. If we were going to grow herbs in the Southwest, we would use a shade

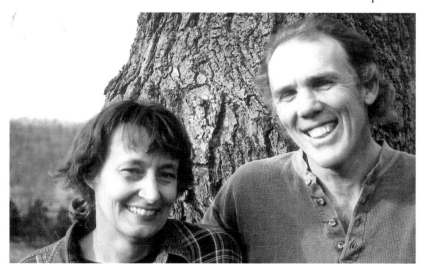

cloth. Here it gets hot, but we can ventilate and control the temperature. There are a few herbs that dry a little bit better in the shade, but they still need the heat, so we start them out on the bottom shelves with a sheet up top.

"Our favorite plants change. You can tell what we like because we often have an overabundance of them," says Andrea. "We have a lot of elecampane, because I really like 'Ellie.' The same goes for borage and blue vervain. When we started with ashwagandha, Matt got ten seeds and we really liked the plants. So the next year we started three thousand . . . without a marketing plan or even enough room to grow them!" Matthias laughs, acknowledging where his attachments lie: "We could probably grow all lemon balm here, and niche-market a whole line of lemon balm products. And then there are herbs that we would like to grow but haven't had the time. I'm drawn to par-

tridgeberry. I won't wildcraft it because there isn't enough of it, yet I think we could grow it. Or pipsissewa or uva ursi."

Most plants harvested for roots get clipped of tops out in the field. The one exception is ashwagandha, whose tough stalk gets machete treatment on the chopping table. Roots get a quick hose rinse to remove the clunkier soil, and then, in a move sure to warm the heart of any Amish farm wife, are dumped straight into a wringer/washer. The agitator on these old-fashioned machines can stand up to the rigors of a rooted load. Five precious minutes are spent on other tasks, usually stirring through leafy herbs on the drying screens, while the root laundry gets agitated. Then it's on to plastic trays to drip-dry before being spread across the solar drying racks of the greenhouse for two to four days. A Sears 6.5-horse-power chipper/shredder chops the dried roots. Matthias has come to prefer this tool over the more costly hammermill. The root pieces get dried for another day after grinding, "just to be sure," and then stored in plastic 5-gallon buckets until incoming orders direct the wares of Healing Spirits to their medicinal destiny.

"The plants are telling me they don't like rows," says Matthias, "yet my farm sense of how to do things knows only rows." The idea of diversified beds, where similarly lived herbs are planted together, has his attention: Lemon balm with echinacea, both of which would be in the field three growing seasons, creates a leaf/root crop dynamic. Such an interplanting comes one step closer to emulating the diverse plant communities found in Nature. "Maybe after you've had rye [to prepare a field for planting], you broadcast valerian, blue vervain, elecampane, and some boneset. Then you see what the relationship is. Throw in a little angelica. I don't know . . . we will experiment more with this."

Sharing hard-won knowledge about growing and drying herbs gives other wannabe farmers a jump-start on their experience. Matthias responds with a genuine smile to this notion of helping the competition: "Most people never follow through once they hear how hard we work." This journey with many different plants—from seed to medicine—toward a full-time living can be rather daunting. Listening to good teachers like Matthias and Andrea is easy. Making that experience work for you depends on dogged resolve. ✂

darkness of the night. The front side of this hefty cabinet was paned with sheets of overlapping glass, sloped to maximize solar gain. The glass was painted black. Screen-covered vent holes below and above ensured good solar air flow. No degrading light reached the plants drying on the slide-in racks. Drying conditions were excellent on a sunny day, but exceedingly poor when clouds hung low. The large size of this cabinet precluded moving such a beast into more hospitable shelter at night, and so evening humidity proved an additional problem. A small electric heating element and fan beneath the bottom rack could have solved the weak points of the first design. We never got that far. One day Michael backed the tiller right into the sloping glass. The idea of black solar in the hands of a surer-footed innovator has merit nevertheless.

## Storing Herbs

Herbs begin to reabsorb atmospheric moisture after temperatures drop below the 100°F average of the drying area. Therefore it's critical to get medicinal herbs properly stored once the drying is deemed complete, preferably during the hottest part of the day.

Many herbalists and apothecaries desire herb as whole as possible. Quality degrades much more rapidly after the herb has been processed into cut leaf or fine root powder. Thrashing leafy herb against half-inch mesh hardware screening (attached to a wooden frame) is a decent hand method of leaving pieces of plant stem behind before storing. The crisp leaves break apart somewhat in this garbling process and fall through the screen. Do wear a dust mask when working with herbs such as nettle and horsetail—sharp silica dust loosened from these plant surfaces can damage the respiratory tract. Nancy has an allergic reaction to yarrow, mask or no mask. Michael swears even a full body suit with oxygen supply isn't enough to garble wormwood. Contract growers get more involved with processing herb to suit customers looking for capsule-grade powders and bulk tea. Much commercial herb thus gets sold as a *cut and sift* grade, with the final screen pass determining the actual fineness of the cut. A hammermill makes these wholesale opportunities possible. This machine works by forcing the dried bulk leaf or root into a chamber where assorted cutting blades determine the shape and fineness of the cut. The plant material then passes through a series of screens to achieve a uniform sift. Echinacea and valerian root break down rapidly once milled, so it is best to store such herbs whole until the order comes through.

Dark glass is far and away the ideal container in which to keep freshly dried herb. Gallon jars lack the capacity to store much more than a pound or two at a time (depending on the herb of course), but they do hold in essential volatiles. Many growers utilize 5-gallon food-grade buckets with tight-fitting lids. Rigid plastic does not have the same contamination concern as do flexible poly bags. Garbage bags are definitely not kosher in contact with medicinal herbs. Nonaromatic herbs do well in paper or untreated cloth bags sealed within a large plastic bag or storage bin. The goal is to exclude light from the herb and seal out moisture.[18] It's advisable not to mix small lots of herbs in the same storage bin. Polypropylene bags are used by larger growers where bulk supply compels them to compromise on plastic contamination issues. Burlap bags aren't necessarily a benign alternative: Their fibers are often treated with fungicides to limit rot, and the weave does not seal out moisture on its own. *Fiber drums* kept in an underground storage room (which maintains the cool, dry, dark conditions herbs require for long-term storage) make for an Earth-friendly option in all respects. These paperboard barrels don't transmit occasional humidity to the herbs stored inside, as you might at first fear. Fiber does absorb strong fragrances, however, so designate the same drums for herbs such as peppermint and lemon balm every year.

Storage containers should be kept off the floor of the storage area. Simple wooden

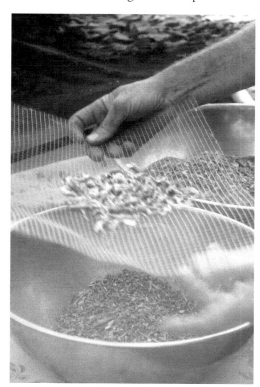

*Garbling herbs by hand against wire mesh works well for most leafy herbs.*

pallets spread across a concrete floor work well. Rodents are not appreciated, so choose a storage space where mice and rats can't come in. Think about where the herbs will go next. Bulk sales can be readily stockpiled. A mail-order herb business, however, requires more room to package and ship out orders. Most dried leaves and flowers will last a year in good condition. Many dried roots, stems, and barks will hold up even longer. A good record system, both on the containers and in a central notebook, is essential to ensure a proper stocking flow.

## HERBS FOR SALE

Building a reputation for quality makes for a sustainable living over the long haul. Direct sales beat the pants off the wholesale market for price, yet the benefits of a guaranteed contract are worth considering if you prefer to focus exclusively on growing. You want to sell your lovingly grown herb to buyers who fully appreciate quality. Someone used to buying run-of-the-mill commercial herbs can find just what they need on the open market. Medicine farmers, like premier vegetable and fruit growers, need to stick to their principles and set a price that fully covers production costs. The responsibility to set a price that makes a viable living possible belongs to us as producers, not the people buying our herbs. Be competitive within your quality niche, certainly, for price matters to even the most discerning customers at some point. Growing and processing an herb more efficiently isn't always possible—laying low with certain crop choices may be in order until the market comes to appreciate the nuances that make for quality. A gassed ethylene tomato will never be a homegrown tomato. The same is true of good plant medicine.

The people using the herbs we grow are the ultimate judges of the quality of our craft. Practicing herbalists look for and expect dried leafy herb as green as those last days out in the field. Greenness bespeaks medicinal value still intact. Not all herbs smell good, but they should always smell strong. Roots, whether fresh or preserved dry, need to be clean, smell of sweet earth, and be filled with the vigor of bustling fall days. The intimacy of the harvesting and cleaning effort leads to different degrees of quality. You market at prices that reflect the scale of your operation. Stem pieces in garbled St. John's wort, for instance, become indistinguishable upon pulverizing the works, or they can be tediously hand-picked out in order to leave the dried blossoms and upper leaves of the plant better intact. Charge accordingly for the work you do: High-end customers choose to pay for hand-crafted results precisely because such herb wows them.

Tincture makers generally prefer to work with fresh plant material, often specifying at what point in the growing cycle they prefer the appropriate plant part to be harvested. Offering consistently vibrant leaf and clean roots—shipped for next-day delivery if not carted just down the road—helps gain access to the fresh market. The difference in price generally favors fresh herb over dry. Fresh root of *Echinacea purpurea*, for instance, brings $8 to $12 a pound, whereas the whole root dried brings $18 to $30 a pound. Many roots dry down about four to five times by weight. The numbers show a definite advantage to selling fresh, on top of which the drying process gets skipped. Medicinal root crops can often be held over in the field when markets aren't forthcoming, whether for early spring harvest or another year of growth. Opting to dry the roots permits us to clean up remaining plantings in a block of ground, and allows us to venture for off-season cash flow despite the lack of a buyer at harvesttime.

Similar math carries over for aerial tops of medicinal herbs: Fresh catnip (*Nepeta cataria*) sells for $5 to $7 a pound, while dry brings anywhere from $2 to $14 a pound to the farmer. The stem of catnip has little medicinal value. Dry leaf can be stripped off by hand or with a belted thrasher, yet either way adds a processing cost. Discarding the stem nearly triples the weight of actual leaf remaining, however, and thus the wide range of price. Catnip is approximately 75 percent water, so a 4:1 fresh to dry ratio applies. Most people use dry catnip as a prime blending ingredient in a carminative or nervine infusion. The market for fresh leaf hinges on a narrower tincture market. Leaves stripped from newly cut stems will bruise considerably more than aerial tops left intact. Plan on harvesting leafy herb early in the morning for fresh shipment (much like salad greens) before the heat of the day builds up. This ensures the herb's arrival in prime shape the next day. Ice packs help forestall excessive wilting. Fresh orders need to be well coordinated on both ends of the sale.

Apothecaries need to decide between paying a higher price to get the utmost quality or toeing a more cost-conscious line. Machine harvesting of certain herbs can yield a satisfactory result in the hands of a caring grower. Rob Wooding of Southern Virginia Herbals grows several acres of red clover. A typical year's harvest amounts to 50 pounds dried of hand-picked blossoms. That amounts to a considerable 225 to 250 pounds of fresh red clover to pick (water

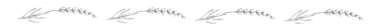

# HOME MEDICINE SHARE

W E'VE LONG HELD to the notion that a local farm can grow for local people. But some visions take a long time to become reality. Evolving a medicinal herb package can reach beyond the bounds of one's own community. Our version of community supported agriculture allows shareholders from anywhere to make a joint commitment to good Earth medicine. Sales start in spring; the promised harvest comes in early fall.

**A Very Shippable $50 Home Medicine Share**
These herbal preparations enhance a family's well-being. Our instructions will answer questions about how to best use the following herbs:
- One 4-ounce bottle of echinacea tincture (to enhance immunity)
- One pound of organic garlic (medicinal food at its best!)
- One 2-ounce jar of Nancy's healing salve (St. John's wort/comfrey/calendula)
- One 4-ounce bag of soothing relaxation tea
- One 4-ounce bottle of wild cherry bark cough syrup
- Free shipping anywhere in the continental United States
- Medicine shares are sent out "farm fresh" in September

content of these blooms totals 75 to 80 percent) to get the exquisite color only a meticulous effort can offer. The rest of his clover is machine cut and sells for a quarter the price of the hand-picked blooms. Leaf and stem of *Trifolium pratense* comes with blossoms ranging in age from developing bud to early maturity. This red clover—noticeably a different product from singly selected blooms—reflects the machine efficiency of the harvest in its price. Yet the scale of this Virginia farm does not go beyond caring craftsmanship: Perfectly timed blossoms still maintain a pinkish hue among the leafy mix coming out of Rob's drying trailers. The green of leaf and stem stands in contrast to the browned impropriety of megascale clover efforts.

Two sources exist for herbalists not involved with cultivating or wildcrafting their own medicinal plants. Direct connections can be made with a farmer/gatherer, or with industry brokers offering botanical wares in extensive catalogs. The range of quality from either can vary considerably. Good reputations are earned for solid reasons. The commendations of a colleague for a particular farmer or herb supplier are worth heeding, just as discontent with an herb purchase lacking in vital life force warns one to look elsewhere. Word-of-mouth praise takes time to build, but, once established, propels a farm effort toward many years of repeat customers and new demand. We heartily recommend asking other herbalists which growers and suppliers meet their expectations.

Marketing opportunities go the same two ways for the grower. Larger farms concentrate on wholesale contracts with herb brokers and manufacturers of herbal capsules and teas. The certainty of a guaranteed sale theoretically makes up for a lesser price per pound for a given herb. However, the quality achieved with mechanized harvest never approaches the handcrafted excellence garnered in harvesting and drying medicinal herbs on a more intimate scale. Capturing the direct sale remains the province of the small farmer. "The big herb companies don't necessarily pay higher prices for quality," points out Monica Rude, "so we look to sell no more than twenty-five pounds of any herb at a time directly to herbalists, small manufacturers of herbal products, and herb stores." Farms that go the mail-order route need a good selection of medicinal herbs to interest a broad customer base of home herbalists.

## Contract Growing

The buzz in agricultural advice these days says specialty crops are hot, with medicinal herbs at the head of the list. The drift of such sagacity keys on being able to get substantial contracts with larger herb companies. Be wary of great hopes: The herb industry can be capricious as bandwagon attention on the herb of the day continually shifts and more and more growers have crops to sell.

Renne Soberg bought his Minnesota farm just before the farm crisis hit in 1985. Here was a man from a dairy family anxious to find a new cropping direction. "I started out by doing a feasibility study with grant money provided by the Minnesota Department of Sustainable Agriculture. I identified about thirteen herbs that were either native here or showed a steady demand. I also selected on the basis that these be primarily an imported crop, as I didn't want to compete with other domestic growers. I was looking for large-volume herbs to grow that would fill a niche market, well-suited to my farm and well-suited to my personality. Catnip looked especially good."

The traditional method to overcome low labor costs overseas is to use technology. Renne retrofits old equipment to suit his herb crops. He has fabricated a header off a combine to cut his mints. His method of removing the stem from the dried catnip came about from previous experimenting with snap beans. His belt thrasher has two belts running at different speeds. When you feed the herb through, the top belt has a tendency to slow the material down, sometimes even stopping it. Meanwhile the lower belt thrashes the leaf off the stems. A series of rods carries the stems away, with the leaf falling between the rods. "Most of the leaf gets separated from the stem this way. I sift this to size, then for dust. I can do more in one day than I used to be able to do in a year by hand." Such innovation makes contract growing profitable, with dried catnip yields averaging 1,000 pounds to the acre.

Growers need to demonstrate an ability to deliver dependably quality herb before any company will offer an annual contract. Samples of your best stuff are what get buyers interested, along with an earnest desire to continue doing such good work. "You'll have to accept the going market price to get a start," says Renne. "And that might be lower than your cost of production, especially in the first year of a perennial crop. You haven't really established yourself as a high-quality producer yet, or as a consistent producer, to demand a higher price." Renne knows he could command a premium price in retail markets, but finds that selling lots of certified organic catnip at $3.75 a pound has established return commitment with his wholesale customers. Current research at Soberg Farms aims to achieve field capability for distilling essential oils and identifying Chinese herbs appropriate for regional markets. Good farmers continue tweaking even proven methods and crops choices. Renne has evolved a way that keeps his farm afloat. A developing herbal network in Minnesota between growers and practitioners might tie even the missing piece of his puzzle together in the end. "The one thing I miss as a contract grower is the chance to talk with the people using my herbs. The idea that keeps me going when I am tired and hot is that somewhere some child is being relieved by my catnip tea. That is what this herb business is all about."

Small growers understandably desire some preseason encouragement to augment future direct sales. Determining that a guaranteed influx of cash awaits after harvest—which might well be two or more years down the road in the case of perennial crops—helps when we're busting butt to build soil and have committed our time and resources to a full greenhouse. Yet not all contract agreements work out.

Grasshoppers plagued Monica Rude's 1999 cropping efforts, eating even her renowned hot peppers. She was glad to have prearranged a place to send the crop: "We started harvesting the cayenne weekly and shipping it fresh to a big herb company who had agreed to pay $2.50 a pound for 1,000 pounds. A good price for me, and shipping fresh meant I didn't have the labor and expense of drying it. This was all fine until I called them to ask when they were going to pay me for the initial shipment of 270 pounds." The company had put "60 Days Net" on the purchase order, which had never been discussed. Shipping costs had added to the urgency of Monica's cash flow. (Tip: Inquire about shipping labels so such costs are charged directly to the recipient.) Monica started calling the head of the company, who never returned her calls. "So I put Kyle on the case, and when he got off the phone, they knew they had been talked to! They agreed to send money. This victory lasted about an hour, then the buyer called and canceled the contract. It seems the company head had learned they were paying me $2.50 a pound plus shipping, which was too much. My calculations [based on their retail price for cayenne tincture] show they would have grossed over $230,000 on it after paying me for the full 1,000 pounds of cayenne." The modest payment for the hard-working farmer's end of this deal—with normal weight loss from shipping fresh deducted, to boot—finally came six months later.

Lot tracking is essential for contract sales, so assign a lot number to each shipment. Record which field the herb was harvested from, when it was harvested (which helps affirm constituent composition), and the specifications used for harvest. Blossom stage, part harvested, age of roots, and even the waxing moon satisfies this last set of criteria. Many companies provide a form listing all such requirements. Buyers will require a copy of the farm's organic certification, as only bureaucratic trust works in a distant relationship. Setting aside a representative sample of each lot shipped (use the same lot number) gives the contract grower some protection from a lawsuit claim that the herb was adulterated with another plant species.

## Healing Herbs for Your Community

"The medicinal herb market is a hard nut to crack," says Richard Wiswall. Cate Farm in Plainfield, Vermont, started growing herbs in a serious way five years ago. The initial focus was to find wholesale contracts with tea companies and bulk herb distributors. Fill-in sales to cottage-based tincture makers, brought about by crop failures elsewhere, came the farm's way on a hit-or-miss basis. "We didn't have any contracts then and we still don't. And that's unsettling when you're committing yourselves to four acres of medicinals. Now we're realizing that packaging sells." Quarter-pound bags of dried herb sell regularly at farmers' markets and at the Hunger Mountain Co-op. The farm's Web site, currently garnering an astounding seven hundred hits a week,[19] aims to bring in orders from herbalists for larger amounts. "Sally and I like providing a high-quality product to people who care, as opposed to selling a mediocre crop at rock-bottom prices."

Distinguishing a price break between retail and wholesale customers is a question of scale and emphasis. Quite simply, the costs per pound of herbs grown on a hand-intensive scale change little regardless of whether the quantity ordered is one or a hundred pounds. A contract grower, focusing on two or three main herb crops, and with equipment efficiency over a larger acreage, wholesales directly to herbal supply houses and tea companies that order in 500-pound lots or more. The two agricultures are entirely different, even when the crop is the same. Small-scale profit margins can't readily be lessened to accommodate a modest wholesale purchase. Growers need to decide right off the bat which market they can serve best, and it's essential to stick to prices that cover the costs and labor of doing an exquisite job.

Selling to community herbalists and neighborhood apothecaries can be made into an ongoing livelihood. An average order for five to ten pounds of assorted herbs is typical, but with the least expensive herb (say black walnut hull) selling at $8 a pound, and the most expensive (you try plucking enough red clover blossoms!) at $50 a pound, gross sales can add up quickly. A solid core of fifty to one hundred such customers providing repeat business, in addition to serious home herbalists, begins to make a year-round living possible. Looked at from the point of view of harvest, the average per pound price hovers just below $20 from small farms offering an extensive array of different medicinals. Each ton of assorted dried herb and roots theoretically amounts to a yearly gross of $40,000. Countless hours of work go into producing the quality that commands these prices, of course, but this mythical ton gives some idea of what it takes.

"You can look at what's happening in society and know what herbs to grow. We have a lot of stress, viruses, and infectious diseases. So we need nervines, antivirals, and immunity-enhancing herbs," says Matthias Reisen. This advice, to consider herb selection from the perspective of today's health needs, is invaluable. Invariably, sales of traditional herbs such as nettles and milky oats take off with the transition from fall to winter. Just as you begin wondering if your reserves of such herbs are going to sell, customers ask for the basics.

## Setting a Righteous Price

"We initially set our prices for medicinal herbs the usual way. Get ten different catalogs, both wholesale and retail, to see what everyone else charges," says Richard at Cate Farm. "Then we took the middle ground." What growers can eventually charge depends entirely on a good reputation earned over the years of selling to herbalists. A viable price needs to cover all the costs of growing and drying the crop, and to pay a respectable hourly wage. Then come marketing costs, the long-term investment in the farm itself, and that elusive term *profit* that accounts for our skill, dedication, and love. Spending half again as much time as in the field and drying shed to tend to the big picture of the farm shouldn't come as

TABLE 6-4. *Herb Price Ranges*

We surveyed price lists of several bioregional medicine farms and wildcrafters to get an idea of the going price per pound for high-quality herb sold directly to herbalists. Wholesale prices paid to the grower by large herb companies are often radically less. All the dried herbs listed here are either organically grown or ethically wildcrafted. Quality ultimately determines what a discerning market will bear.

| Common Name | Latin Name | Dollars per Pound |
| --- | --- | --- |
| Ashwagandha root | *Withania somnifera* | $16–22 |
| Borage leaf & flower | *Borage officinalis* | $14–20 |
| Boneset leaf & flower | *Eupatorium perfoliatum* | $12–24 |
| Burdock root | *Arctium lappa* | $10–14 |
| Calendula flower | *Calendula officinalis* | $24–36 |
| Wild Carrot (Queen Anne's Lace) seed | *Daucus carota* | $40 |
| Catnip leaf & flower | *Nepeta cataria* | $8–14 |
| Wild Cherry bark | *Prunus* spp. | $18–28 |
| Echinacea root | *Echinacea purpurea* | $20–30 |
| Goldenrod flower | *Solidago* spp. | $10–14 |
| Hawthorn berries | *Craetagus* spp. | $16–30 |
| Lemon Balm leaf | *Melissa officinalis* | $12–20 |
| Marsh Mallow root | *Althaea officinalis* | $10–16 |
| Motherwort leaf | *Leonurus cardiaca* | $12–18 |
| Mullein leaf | *Verbascum thapsus* | $12–16 |
| Nettle leaf | *Urtica dioica* | $16–24 |
| Oats, milky head | *Avena sativa* | $16–24 |
| Wild Raspberry leaf | *Rubus* spp. | $22–28 |
| Red Clover blossoms | *Trifolium pratense* | $26–50 |
| Skullcap leaf | *Scutellaria laterifolia* | $18–26 |
| Spilanthes leaf & flower | *Spilanthes* spp. | $24–32 |
| Valerian root | *Valerian officinalis* | $16–24 |
| Yarrow leaf & flower | *Achillea millefolium* | $12–18 |
| Yellow Dock root | *Rumex crispus* | $14–22 |

a surprise. Acknowledge those labor costs accordingly. A small grower on top of production reality can seemingly never set prices high enough.

"I think we should make a living in line with any other administrative position. Why shouldn't a farmer make the same amount of money that an executive managing a bank does? We do all the same management steps and take risks with our capital. Farmers just happen to do all the actual labor as well. Why shouldn't we expect the same return on our investments that large corporations expect to get?" asks Matthias Reisen, standing tall on the agrarian soapbox of parity. "Farmers manage the land, which is the backbone of everything. If a community doesn't have agriculture, it doesn't have anything. If the soil is not maintained, we don't have health in our nation. People don't seem to realize that."

Certainly the price of pharmaceuticals makes herbal medicine seem like a bargain-basement special. We entertain a strange cultural twist when we look at how much people are willing to spend on sustenance. Food is absurdly cheap. Much of what is sold in grocery stores would cost far less if we were to take into account nutritional worth. Small farms disappear daily because most human beings won't invest in optimal health by eating optimal food. Enter the medical system. Health insurance premiums are outrageous, but, in one way or another, people pay. The doctor prescribes a cure. People pay. The pharmaceutical industry provides a new wonder drug. People pay. Talk about getting what you pay for! The healing plants are giving us a chance to get back on track in many, many ways. That people might find a drug alternative in an herb is fine. Cultural thinking will readily accept a higher value for a medicinal plant than a food plant. We can work with that as farmers, paying our bills and earning a living wage, while our customers experience vast savings over pharmaceutical fare. Some-

thing deeper starts to click as people experience plants. Perhaps it's the healing, perhaps it's the exposure to holistic thinking. People who want to be well begin to realize that wholesome food is medicine. Nutrient-dense foods, of course, come from small local farms. One giant brain synapse later and we'll have a sustainable agriculture.

The value-added route holds promise for growers who might be inclined to run a cottage-based tincture business or to send out a mail-order catalog. Deb Soule and friends at Avena in Maine process much of the harvest of their one-acre herb garden to provide product for a thriving regional apothecary. This woman's circle draws a much vaster livelihood from the land by increasing the value of its crop resource. Paul Strauss of Equinox Botanicals in Ohio began his off-farm marketing with the Golden Salve he first concocted more than twenty years ago from woodland goldenseal to relieve the inevitable wounds that accompany farm life. Value-added approaches work best for small-scale enterprises that can plan in the time necessary for making products and all the marketing effort to ensue. You need a clear sense of goals and what you want to spend each day doing. Going around to herb fairs and stores is not the same as weeding under a hot sun. Packaging up mail orders and tallying inventory on the computer is not the same as harvesting an acre of roots. Team effort can be invaluable when wearing many hats.

Value-added becomes relevant as well when bulk pound prices are divided up into ounces. Four-ounce bags appeal to home herbalists who find a pound of dry herb daunting. A clear cellophane bag lets the depth of herb color resonate around a label identifying the homegrown plant medicine and the farm it came from. A markup of a third to a half gives the packaging effort justified value: Four ounces of motherwort leaf at a going price of $16 per pound tallies in at $4, which actually sells for $5 to $6 bagged. Medicinal use can be advertised to people verbally or by way of a poster board alongside a farmers' market display of herbs.

Every local grower's niche can extend beyond the expected herbs suitable for a particular bioregion. Freshness is a powerful marketing advantage that carries over to medicinal crops. Spilanthes in a growing tunnel may not be competitive, but it does produce some potent buds to tincture fresh. Or the leaves can be chewed fresh to ease a caffeine craving or put a summer respiratory infection at bay. "No herbs are going to be of any good to anybody unless they get used," says Richo Cech. "The fresher they are and more locally produced,

the better they're going to work. It may be more appropriate to grow *Bacopa monniera* in East India than in southern Oregon, but I'm able to improve local medicine by growing Brahmi here and distributing small amounts to people fresh." We're mighty appreciative of our faithful customers who are willing to drive out to the farm to purchase herbs and handcrafted medicines at a higher price than they might pay at a chain drugstore. Such friends acknowledge our hard work and respect for the land. Most important of all, these are people who know that fresh from the farm is better for them and their families.

The demand for good-quality herbs is on the rise. Seeing a thousand small farmers making a living on a few acres each rather than the corporate folk swinging fat on a hundred acres of a single herb rings true to the vision of local medicine.

## NOTES

1. The massive doses of antibiotics pumped into beef and dairy cattle in the last few decades are highly suspect in light of our current confrontations with this strain of *Escherichia coli* bacteria. Meat, lettuce and other field greens, and fresh fruit juice can be contaminated with this potentially deadly pathogen through contact with raw manure. Shipments of gotu kola grown in swamps in India have been rejected by herb companies because of *E. coli* contamination.

2. Austrian Rudolf Steiner gave a series of eight agricultural lectures in 1924, subsequently transcribed from stenographers' notes. Biodynamic agricultural practice is based on his teachings.

3. See Hugh Lovel, *A Biodynamic Farm* (Kansas City, Mo.: Acres USA, 1994), 105–13.

4. The positive influence of nettles on the oil content of aromatic herbs extends to valerian, marjoram, sage, and peppermint as well. See Steven Foster, *Herbal Renaissance* (Salt Lake City, Utah: Gibbs Smith, 1993), 154.

5. The sedative effect of fresh valerian root is attributed to isovaleric acid, which is also respon-

sible for the characteristic smell of the drug. The valepotriates—which develop when the dried root is processed—have a balancing, depressant effect on the autonomic nervous system. See Rudolf Fritz Weiss, M.D., *Herbal Medicine*, trans. (Beaconsfield, England: Beaconsfield, 1988), 281–84.

6. Lomatium is listed on United Plant Savers' At-Risk List. Concern stems from its fragile habitat on steep slopes, and the usual human greed to take until there is no more. Lomatium is a prime candidate for commercial exploitation because it is effective against serious viral infections of the respiratory tract. Wildcrafters in the Northwest see this member of the parsley family growing in rich abundance. The plants don't bear seed until they are ten years old or so. A forty-five-year-old root (weighing 12 pounds) with ninety crown buds offers a chance to harvest and replant.

7. BD 507 is a biodynamic compost preparation said to bring phosphorus into the organic process. Some biodynamic growers claim a foliar spray of 507 will protect fruit blossoms against late spring frosts (within four degrees of the freezing point). Interestingly, valerian demonstrates a stimulant effect medicinally in some instances as well.

8. Soil life forms an integrated community that our notions of seedbed preparation can throw asunder. Thus the customary recommendation to let ground set a week or two to allow elements, microbes, and fungi to reestablish essential balance. The introduction of oxygen (by tillage particularly) stimulates aerobic bacteria to consume organic matter ravenously. Root growth is inhibited in turn by induced nutrient imbalance. Probing the depths will always provide other viewpoints to take into consideration.

9. Cultivated raspberries are often spring-pruned of superfluous canes so those remaining bear larger berries. We harvest a similar proportion of wild canes knowing that the birds, animals, and the occasional browsing human will enjoy the berries on the canes we do not touch.

10. Oatstraw, machine cut at this same time, includes the milky heads along with the entire green oat stalk. The price accordingly runs about a third of that paid for the green seed heads alone.

11. Thanks go to Ryan Drum for tracking such intricacies for the rest of us.

12. Doug Elliot describes the fine art of "senging" quite eloquently in *Wild Roots* (Rochester, Vt.: Healing Arts Press, 1995), 117.

13. Our source for the mucilage content of marsh mallow is David Hoffmann's *Holistic Herbal*. In *King's American Dispensatory*, however, it's listed as being nearly 20 percent. Andrew Chevallier in the *Natural Health Encyclopedia of Herbal Medicine* reports the mucilage of marsh mallow is 11 percent. Go figure.

14. Garlic and lovage are the only other herbs that we know besides valerian for which floral pruning has merit in sizing the root crop.

15. Another danger for pipsissewa comes from being the "secret ingredient" in certain soft drinks. See Gregory Tilford, *From Earth to Herbalist* (Missoula, Mont.: Mountain Press, 1998), 6.

16. A seemingly workable plan until other wildcrafters get into the act, collectively moving the lower lomatium edge up the fragile slope unbeknownst to the others.

17. Admittedly, we don't worry about propane residues on our bread either. Just be sure to empty the oven of drying baskets whenever you do turn on the oven to bake. Ironically our kitchen filled with smoke the one evening a class arrived for a culinary herb cooking class.

18. Plastic bags allow the herb to breathe a little, as small oxygen molecules actually will pass through plastic. Moisture, however, is sealed out. Aromatic volatiles lessen in long-term storage whenever such breathing can occur.

19. An Internet hit by no means implies a sale. Cate Farm does not yet provide on-line ordering. Nor have Richard and Sally found a proprietary way of herbal networking on the World Wide Web. In this case, the aura of being a certified organic farm in Vermont carries the day.

# CHAPTER SEVEN

# Making Earth Medicines

CHAMOMILE
*Matricaria recutita*

*M*aking my first salve and, later, my first tincture were empowering events in my life. Not that either was so astounding in and of itself, being more like everyday cooking than rocket science. I loved the alchemy involved: experiencing these beloved herbs from my garden mix with the proper solvents and turn into medicine. I loved the connection to my ancestors; it was like reaching out and grasping the hands of a long lineage of medicine men and women. I loved the deep satisfaction of self-sufficiency. And, yes, a part of me relished thumbing my nose at corporate America. I caught an idealistic glimpse of never having to buy medicines or body care products again. I wouldn't need any drugstore again—I would provide for my family. ❧ I felt gratified giving my friends and relatives these preparations. It warmed my heart and stirred me on to hear that my salve was helping Uncle Hank's hemorrhoids and that another salve helped a friend's draft horse to heal after a bad leg wound. Honestly, making the salves was easy, but they were received with a bit of awe. That a mere mortal could produce a healing medicine in her own kitchen! "Don't you need to get approval from the doctor?" "What will the FDA say?" I was tasting blessed freedom and loving every minute of it. ❧ The pleasure of growing echinacea and harvesting in accord with the moon was not what made preparing that first tincture so special to me. Nor was it taking flower, leaf, and root into the kitchen to make them into a highly effective immune enhancer for my family. Nor would I say that the daily singing and offering of *healing prayers when shaking the extraction jar did it. Certainly all this was deeply satisfying. But the very best thing, deep down in my soul, was the feeling that, yes, I really was a medicine woman.* —N.P. ℘

THE AGE-OLD ART of making medicine is immensely empowering and great fun. Many of our medicines have been handed down through the ages because they are both simple to make and effective. The following guidelines for preparing herbal medicines are just that—guidelines. No two herbalists do everything exactly alike. Comparing different herb books will quickly reveal a wide range of opinion on everything from uses of herbs to the percentage of alcohol for a specific tincture. Indeed, the only thing all herbalists seem to agree upon is avoiding aluminum pans.

Use these suggestions, but experiment with your own preparations. Communicate with the plants you are using, talk to other herbalists, and read the suggested books from our herbal library (see page 88) to broaden your understanding of the apothecary's art. Keeping notes of how and when herbs are harvested and the proportion of ingredients will be invaluable in discerning what goes into a good remedy. Potency equates to mindfulness in this work.

Strive to be one with spirit as you co-create medicines that will help heal and strengthen lives. Many traditions believe you must ask the plant for permission to harvest it, or you will not get the full benefit of its medicine. Some people make offerings. Similar thinking applies to our focus in the medicine-making process. You can create rituals that resonate for you. Nancy dedicates the needed time solely to the making of medicine—whatever she may be brewing on a given day—rather than getting jumbled about doing too many things at once. Starting with an immaculate kitchen and having all ingredients and utensils handy sets the stage. We pause to offer a prayer of thankfulness and blessing. We may burn sage as well, especially when our work is intended to help a specific individual who really needs that extra energy. We build on this harmony with favorite healing songs. Medicine made without this spiritual alchemy will never be as good.

## COMMUNITY MEDICINE

Creating a neighborhood apothecary begins when friends start asking for those medicines we made first for our own families. Many herbalists soon find themselves happily engaged in offering more products to their communities. The ones who are especially adept at making good medicine can meet this ever present need by establishing a retail or mail-order business. Herbalists who choose to work more as practitioners can still use their medicine-making skills to formulate specific herbal remedies for their clients. The dispensary of a consulting herbalist and the apothecary of a more product-focused herbalist are really degrees of the same thing: places where people in the community can go to obtain safe and effective Earth medicines. Either way, intimacy and care underlies the quality of these herbal preparations.

Running a community herb store can be a bit overwhelming as well as quite exciting. What herbs do we need to have on hand? A minimum inventory is hard to predict, being different for every practice and every herb. The goal is to not let quantities get ahead of themselves. Bulk herbs keep best in the cool dark, so ideally the jars displayed on the shelf get refilled every month or so. Green vibrancy is quite obvious once you are tuned in to herb quality. A year's supply of each herb, obtained soon after harvest from reputable local growers, should run out just about the time summer's bounty calls again. Tinctures have a three-year shelf life (if not far more) and continue to be effective when a bulk supply runs to excess. Storing tinctures in large amber bottles, and only filling a few small dropper bottles ahead or on demand, encourages customers to return empty bottles to refill. Finding reasonable suppliers for the alcohol, bottles, and other required containers takes ongoing effort. Some herbal products may be better to buy at a wholesale price, allowing more energy for making those local medicines that are in high demand. Keeping a clean shop reflects a certain pride and assures our customers that attention to detail matters. Hygiene goes hand in hand with medicine making.

How one addresses fundamental business decisions establishes whether an herb store will thrive or not. Dashed hopes are avoided by being financially savvy from the start. Deciding how much to charge amounts to covering every cost of doing business. Questions about regulations and liability insurance have to be addressed. Time spent gathering herbs, making preparations, and tending store counts as much as the cost of supplies. Being generous to customers is important; being generous to yourself keeps the bills paid. We'll tackle the business mind a later in this chapter. Suffice it to say, herbal medicines are far more reasonable in price than allopathic options. People save considerably on health expenditures just by coming into an herb store. Providing the herbs and encouragement for families to make their own medicines saves them even more.

The Ozark herbalist Bob Liebert wears many hats. "We make fresh herb tinctures with an emphasis on herbs that are gathered by hand at the right time," explains Bob. "We make a few infused oils and salves as well. I feel that what makes us different is that many companies claim their wildcrafted herbs are so carefully gathered, and yet they deal with the same middlemen that buy from the locals around here who do not gather consciously at all. A big majority of echinacea and goldenseal are dug in June, for instance, exactly the wrong time for roots. And while they may say they are conscious of plant environments, these folks tear everything up. Our emphasis is in selling local herbs locally."

People will use herbs to the degree they are familiar with the presentation. Herb capsules are familiar to someone who has previously taken an allopathic prescription. A pill is synonymous with medicine for many folks. Tinctures fit into that same territory, but loose teas and fresh herbs require a bit more introduction. Our recommendations as herbal pharmacists need to reckon a client's comfort level with the form of the medicine.

"Capsules are for those who do not want to taste the herb and have no time in their life to deal with anything else," observes Melanie Osborne of Thyme to Heal Herbals in Lisbon, New Hampshire. "Tinctures are convenient, provide instant gratification, and are our best source for bitters. Tinctures can be put in water or teas, and can be taken just minutes before eating. Teas are for those needing nourishment of heart, body, and soul—those needing rituals and permission

*Just as the flowers grow from the earth, so the remedy grows in the hands of the physician. The remedy is nothing but a seed that must develop into that which it is destined to be.*

—PARACELSUS
(1493–1541)

to create, sit, and sip. Not that the others don't need this nurturing, but they are too busy to do this for themselves right now." Customers have a choice in this herbalist's shop. They can call ahead to request capsules (Melanie makes these only by arrangement) or come unannounced for loose teas and tinctures.

Many of the good associations we expect in a neighborhood food co-op hold just as aptly for the neighborhood herb store. Having herbs and tinctures in bulk saves on packaging. Basic family medicines such as echinacea shouldn't be sold in those tiny I-ounce bottles: That single day's megadose only begins to flex bodily immunity toward a persistent flu bug. Custom orders for capsules, suppositories, or formulated tinctures can be crafted on an individual basis. Specialty salves and body care products from other local producers can be included as well. The best herb stores we visited carried few national brands. Herbalists in these settings make time to chat and offer supporting advice. Workshops offered to home herbalists through the store build a community that understands how to use herbs responsibly.

Margi Flint of Earth Song Herbals in Massachusetts teaches her clients how to make their own herbal preparations. This herbal practitioner doesn't have a lot of spare time to make many products on top of a schedule filled with appointments. She offers herbs from an in-house dispensary and will make up a recommended formulation for a client the first time. After that, she prefers that people take responsibility for their own medicines. "They are putting their own energy into their healing," notes Margi. "What a wonderful way for clients to realize they are the ones in charge of their own health."

The knowledge and experience we bring to making herbal medicines in our communities is only as good as our integrity. We're convinced that a huge company with tremendously expensive lab equipment (used to confirm herb identity and constituent levels) cannot rival what skilled herbalists can do by transforming living plants into medicine. The multitude of tests that verify herb quality and identity are done for good reason. Frontier Herbs reports that 60 to 70 percent of pre-shipments (trial batches of herbs from commercial growers and wildcrafters) fail to meet the rigorous standards of their quality assurance lab. Herbs rejected there will inevitably be sold somewhere else. Problematic issues involve such things as high *E. coli* counts (not atypical with gotu kola grown in swamps in India, for example), off color, and rocks intertwined in goldenseal roots. Powdered herbs and essential oils that are misidentified—either mistakenly or willfully sold—can be checked for constituent levels using high-performance liquid chromatography (HPLC) testing.

Community herbalists know to what extremes they must go to clean a modest root harvest. They know their plants and the potent time to harvest. Herbs can't be tinctured any fresher than when the gatherer makes the medicine. Taste, smell, and appearance of dried whole herb alone confirms plant identity between a reputable grower and the apothecary. Such trust simply can't be assumed on a big-business scale.

Basic common sense is worth more than a triple stainless steel sink and other regulatory overloads. Anyone who has spent time in a commercial kitchen can confirm that having all the latest professional equipment is not what results in high-quality food arriving at the restaurant table. So it is with our medicines. Our right to make herbal preparations knowledgeably and lovingly in our communities should not be infringed on by overly strict regulations. We'll be reviewing the guidelines that any responsible herbalist does follow. Simply put, integrity will always be a prime ingredient in Earth medicines. Even if this sanitation-crazy culture rarely understands that neighborly efforts can be trusted far more than regulatory fiat.

## HERBAL PREPARATIONS

High-quality herbs are imperative for making plant medicines. Refer to chapter 6 for proper harvesting methods and guidelines. Know your sources well. Herbs that are full of vitality bring their life force to the medicine. The essence of the plant endures in the medicine when the plant is harvested in a respectful manner and processed soon after with healing intent.

Certain herbs are best dried before being processed. The changes in chemical composition effected by the drying process result in a better medicine. Cascara sagrada, for instance, actually has toxic qualities when used fresh. Fresh angelica root tends to be harsh on the digestive tract, but not the dried root. Practitioners get better results from an extract of freshly dried chickweed (*Stellaria media*) than from fresh chickweed.[1] The leafy stems just coming into flower need to have been dried very recently for this to be true, because chickweed does not retain its alkalinizing constituents for long.

The ultimate way to test for potency, used in big labs and small kitchens alike, is the *organoleptic method*. Sounds official, doesn't it? Nevertheless, herbalists have been using this test to determine the quality of herbs for eons. The perception of our senses discerns the quality of a particular herb. We

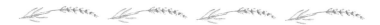

# THE MARSH CRONE

T HE BOOK CAME OUT of the blue, a tattered library copy from a part of Nancy's childhood long forgotten. The town librarian remembered a certain little girl enamored by this story of a marsh crone stirring a swampy concoction. No one had checked out *The Marsh Crone's Brew* (written and illustrated by Ib Spang Olsen) during the last twenty years. "Why not send this withdrawn book to Nancy?" thought Mrs. Gleue.

Talk about what a long, long trip it's been! And one so poignantly apt for a grown woman now enamored with herbs and making medicinal preparations of her own.

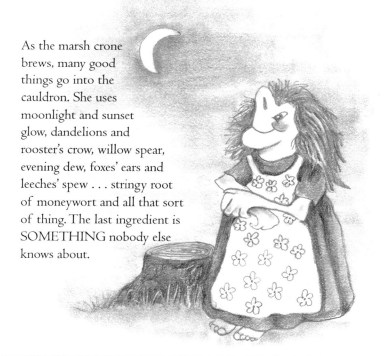

As the marsh crone brews, many good things go into the cauldron. She uses moonlight and sunset glow, dandelions and rooster's crow, willow spear, evening dew, foxes' ears and leeches' spew . . . stringy root of moneywort and all that sort of thing. The last ingredient is SOMETHING nobody else knows about.

use our eyes to observe the color and overall details of the plant material. A well-dried herb will retain the vibrant green of the fresh plant. Dried peppermint and other dark leafy green herbs should be bright and alive looking. Blossoms should be as bright and colorful as when the flowers were growing. Our dried calendula never fails to get an "Ahh!" when poured from a storage jar in the middle of winter: These bright orange blossoms just sing of summer. We use our noses to test an herb's smell. Many herbs will have a strong and unique scent. We always taste our herbs. Distinctive flavors indicate the expected constituent strength. Of course, be cautious when tasting low-dose, potentially toxic herbs. Taking a very small piece of such an herb to chew briefly before spitting it out tells us what we need to know.

What if you purchase herbs with which you are not familiar? Looking, smelling, and tasting only works when we know a plant already. Purchasing from a reputable source answers this dilemma, and then of course we can come to know the qualities of that herb. Community herbalists can and do obtain herbs from other sources and then pass these on to clients. Just remember: *Never offer medicine to someone else that you cannot clearly identify and have not experienced yourself*. If you haven't experienced the laxative effects of cascara sagrada, how are you to know the proper way to dose or formulate for its practically guaranteed "chittam" action?[2] If you have never put an eyewash in you own eye, don't formulate one to pass on to a mother for her baby's eye infection. Work with the herbs and become intimate with them before offering them to your community. Nancy allows one exception to this firm rule: Husbands are okay to practice on!

In addition to the scrutiny of the senses, herbs should be tested for their anticipated actions. Good-quality herbs are usually highly effective. If you are not obtaining the results expected with an herb, first question its quality. The nuance of harvest matters just as much as the age of the plant material and how it was stored. Other factors may be involved, of course. The herb chosen for a situation may not have been the right choice. Complex situations don't necessarily improve in the way we might expect. Or the herb may actually have been misidentified. Kate Gilday shared a good example of this. She had recommended preparations of Siberian ginseng (*Eleutherococcus senticosus*) to a variety of clients, with little effect. Kate found out later that another herb was being sold to her in place of it. Once she found a reputable source, the actual Siberian ginseng started making a big difference in her clients' well-being.

If you purchase herbs from bigger companies or abroad, be aware that many warehouses fumigate the herbs with phystoxin or ethyl bromide. Some companies also irradiate herbs, though this practice is yet to be approved by the FDA. Other companies use a $CO_2$ process to control storage pests. This is safe, but only effective for active infestations (the insect eggs are unaffected). Such information might not be available always, but do ask for it.

Once you harvest or obtain your dried herbs, keep them as whole as possible in containers in a dark place and at an even temperature. Always label the containers with the botanical name of the herb and the date on which it was purchased or harvested. Assigning a *harvest batch number* allows you to track other recorded information as well—where the herb came from and which products were made from it.

## A Few More Details Before We Start Making Medicines

Most of the equipment needed to make quality medicines is found in a well-stocked kitchen: accurate scales that measure ounces and grams; blender; coffee grinder; double boiler (glass, stainless-steel, or enamel); measuring spoons and cups; whisks; glass or plastic funnels in a variety of sizes; candy thermometer; mortar and pestle; sharp knives; large stainless steel strainers and colanders; muslin; cheesecloth; turkey baster; new cotton diapers; rubber gloves; stainless steel or glass pots and pans; rubber spatulas; and canning jars.

A few additional items can make the work more efficient: a tincture press; 100 ml measuring cylinder; 25 ml measuring cylinder in 1 ml gradations; turkey roaster; Vita-Mix; French-press coffeemaker; capsule filler; suppository molds. and percolator. You know you have gone off the herbal deep end when your loved ones ask what you want for your birthday and you request suppository molds and graduated cylinders!

When making tinctures for family use it is sufficient to strain the liquid through muslin and *squeeze, squeeze, squeeze* by hand every last drop you can get from the extracted herb. Other innovative home herbalists use a food mill or a potato ricer, and we've even heard of using a salad spinner. All are fine to a certain extent, but if you are making a lot of tinctures, a tincture press will soon pay for itself by recovering more of that precious menstruum. Presses consist of two parallel surfaces on a frame rigged with a hydraulic jack and a stainless-steel pan fitted with a drain hole and a hose. The extract is poured into a filter bag inside a stainless-steel bucket (perforated to allow free flow of the liquid) to get the sopping herb in place for squeezing. Each ounce of expensive tincture that can be garnered positively affects the profit margin. If you press around ten gallons of tincture a year, you will pay for a liter-sized tincture press in about a year's time. The math will please even a folklorist: A mere 10 percent gain

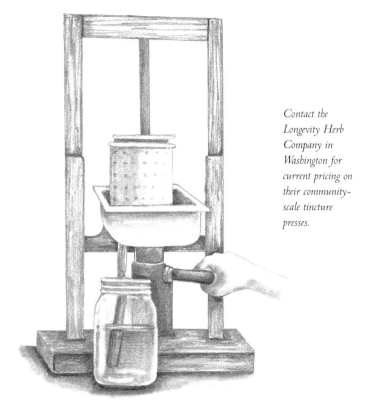

*Contact the Longevity Herb Company in Washington for current pricing on their community-scale tincture presses.*

from mechanical squeezing results in eight ounces or so of additional extract per gallon batch. Figuring a retail value of about $5 an ounce, more or less, this results in $400 of additional tincture from ten gallons of production. Then consider that *the last squeeze is the best*—the last drops out of the marc (herb solids under squeeze) are dense with constituents, which only ups the medicinal quality of a blended batch. Tincture presses for a small herb business run anywhere from $350 to $800. Wooden wine presses will be slightly more economical, but in the end you'll wish you'd gone the stainless-steel route.

The Vita-Mix is a food processor, juicer, blender, grain grinder, root chopper, and hammermill all rolled into one appliance. A well-made tool needs to justify a high price, and even at $450, this one does. A full 7-year warranty indicates quality. The Vita-Mix comes equipped with one polycarbonate container with wet blades, and a second with dry blades that handles pulverizing dried herb and roots alike. Realizing a degree of efficiency in processing herbs in preparation for medicine making on a community scale helps every herbalist make a sustainable living. We'll mention the other useful equipment for specific preparations just ahead.

---

## PRODUCTION RECORD

Preparation batch #  _____

Date prepared  _____

Date to press  _____

Common name(s)  _____

Botanical name(s)  _____

Harvest batch # of herb(s)  _____

Own quality assessment  _____

Total weight of herb used  _____

Total menstruum  _____

Volume of vodka  _____

Volume of 190-proof alcohol  _____

Volume of distilled water  _____

Volume of glycerin  _____

Volume of vinegar  _____

Notes on methods used, grinding, heat, and all other processing information  _____

Feedback from anyone using this extract  _____

---

Let's take a look at paperwork in the apothecary. By recording the weather conditions, time of year, and lunar phases of the herbs as we harvest, we learn over time which techniques and patterns give us the most potent herbs. For example, we may notice a higher quantity of mucilage when harvesting marsh mallow root in the spring or fall; or that we get a more resinous calendula by plucking blossoms in the middle of a hot sunny day rather than right after the morning dew evaporates. Just as nuance matters in the field, we observe over time which techniques and ratios in our herbal pharmacy result in better medicine for our clients. Community herbalists have a dream of a job when it comes to comprehending such nuance. A relationship with the plants that can be carried from the earth to the preparation table and then on to help people feel better is a complete one. We only learn the lessons, however, if we document the facts as we go.

Documentation is difficult for some of us. For years as a home herbalist, Nancy purposely did not label herb and spice jars in order to train her senses of sight and smell. This worked when we were dealing with thirty herbs we knew intimately, most of which we grew and harvested ourselves. Now we are dealing with a much larger number of herbs to serve our community, and some of them are purchased from elsewhere. Students use our herb pantry as well. Thorough labeling has become essential. Dried herbs are labeled with the common name, botanical name, when and where harvested, or when and where purchased.

Keeping a production record such as the one shown here for a tincture extraction is where the real learning kicks in. The details listed on this form will soon become self-explanatory. What counts is being able to repeat good formulas or trace any problems that arise. Production records allow us to recall the actual process used and know the story behind each herb involved (remember that harvest batch number mentioned earlier?). Developing such forms for each type of preparation allows herbalists to zero in on their own shades of nuance. Of course, we have to be diligent about doing the paperwork as we go.

## Water-Based Medicines

Nutritive, healing, and often comforting, water-based preparations are at the core of our tradition. Swallowing a pill is synonymous in this culture with taking medicine. Let's broaden that horizon: A cup of tea can be good for everyone! Once you and your clients have mastered the simple art of making medicinal teas, a whole range of ways to use herbs will follow. Herbal baths, eye washes, nasal washes, compresses, enemas, herbal steams, sitz baths, penis soaks, and douches all have a basis in the infusion/ decoction processes described below.

We like what some of the old doctors had to say about the wholesomeness of tea and other water-based preparations. The comments of John Scudder and L. E. Jones in *The American Eclectic Materia Medica and Therapeutics* written in 1863 ring just as true today:

> As far as success in practice is concerned, we have no doubt but infusion and decoction are the most eligible forms of administering such vegetable remedies as yield their properties to water. However much "tea practice" may be laughed at, we know that this practice has proven eminently successful in the hands of our old practitioners. In these forms, the remedy is readily absorbed; there need be no doubt of its purity, or that it is well prepared; and again, it is certain in this case, that the patient will receive sufficient [water], a matter that is of the first importance in the treatment of many diseases.

Many herbalists sell bulk herbs or prepackaged blends to make these water preparations. Otherwise, clients can be pointed in the right direction to obtain good herbs. Most of us do not actually make the tea itself for our clients. Therefore teaching people how to make these medicinal preparations correctly in their own homes is vital. We like to explain the preparations and even demonstrate the proper techniques with people at their first visit. Then we send them home with written instructions condensed from the following guidelines.

### Infusions

The art of making tea is healing in and of itself. We mix herbs with the elements of fire and water to behold a lovely cup of tasty, comforting tea. Use good-quality dried herbs or pick them fresh from the garden. Herbs help keep us healthy and wise provided we grasp the basics of a strong brew. The following measurements are for dried herbs, so if using fresh herbs use at least three times these amounts. For a *beverage tea,* add 1 teaspoon of dry herb to 1 cup of boiling water, cover, and let it steep five minutes. A pot of this tea is pleasant to share with friends after dinner or with an afternoon cookie. A lemon verbena tea or peppermint tea with honey is simply a delight for the palate.

A beverage tea can be healthful and relaxing, but it differs from a *medicinal-strength tea.* The choice of herbs used, the ratio of herbs to water, the length of time infused, and the amount and frequency that a tea is consumed distinguishes one from the other. Even how we speak of making each tea suggests a difference. We grow up familiar with *steeping* a pot of beverage tea and later learn to *infuse* our herbs to make medicinal tea.

Infusions can be potent medicines. These medicinal teas can be used in many acute situations such as cramps, indigestion, colds, and flus. But where infusions really excel is in building long-term health and healing chronic conditions—provided they are used consistently and over long periods of time. Leaves, flowers, aromatic seeds, and a few roots high in volatile oils (such as valerian, goldenseal, and osha) are best infused. The best way to make a good infusion is to put herbs in a quart canning jar or another container with a tight-fitting lid, then pour one quart of near boiling water over the herbs, cap, and steep at least twenty minutes. We let this brew sit overnight when a particularly strong infusion is desirable. A French-press coffeemaker that holds back the loose herbs when the tea is poured is well worth the $30 to $40 investment. Choose a glass pot designed to be held (and protected) by a metal frame, as these can be broken easily.

The standard amount of herb to water for infusions varies from 1 teaspoon to ½ ounce of herb per cup of water. We basically want a drinkable tea that is strong enough to deliver its healing virtue. (Of course, if we are making an infusion for something like a sitz bath it doesn't even have to be drinkable.) Experience brings a feel for the amount of herb to use for each situation. Consult the recommended books on medicine making or some of the old pharmacopoeias for recommended amounts of specific herbs for therapeutic doses. Consider the plant constituents being drawn into the water when making a medicinal tea.

Water-soluble plant constituents include starches, proteins, sugars, enzymes, mucilage, pectins, saponins, and polysaccharides. Some gums and tannins will be absorbed by water as well. Volatile oils evaporate quickly, and those that are slightly soluble in water (such as black peppermint) remain precisely because we never boil our infusions. Resins are completely insoluble in water.

*Cold-water infusions* are prepared by immersing herbs in cold water in a covered container for eight to twelve hours. This type of infusion is preferred when we want to extract mucilage or volatile oils, or when certain constituents such as tannic acid are not desired. Both marsh mallow and slippery elm are very mucilaginous and are easily extracted in cold water. Cold-water-infused peppermint tea retains more vitamin C and a brighter flavor than a hot infusion.

Solar infusions and lunar infusions are fun to experiment with. Each has its own special quality and flavor—and encompasses some of the healing powers of the sun and the moon. Simply place 1 cup of herbs in a 1-gallon glass jar, fill with cold water, cap, and set it in the sun for four to six hours for a *solar infusion*. Strain and enjoy as is or add honey and lemon.

A *lunar infusion* is best made when the moon is full or close to full. Certain plants seem to call out to us when we walk into the gardens for the herbs to prepare this infusion—angelica is one who expresses her charm when moonlight fills the air. Nancy and Gracie like to put the selected herbs in a special crystal bowl, left uncovered, and set out all night in the stone path garden. (Do use a bit of common sense here. One enthusiastic student of ours tried to make a lunar infusion during the Hunter's Moon on a cold fall night. The water froze and broke her bowl.) First thing in the morning we go out to sip this tea. Then we watch for those mysterious qualities during the next day or two that only fairy magic can bring.

## Decoctions

We use water to extract the properties of barks, roots, hulls, and some seeds. *Decoction* involves concentrating the flavors and constituents of the medicinal tea by boiling. Place herbs in an appropriate pot, pour in water, and slowly bring to a boil. Turn down the heat and simmer for at least twenty minutes. The decoction can be strained after it cools or left to steep overnight before straining and using.

Mixing roots and leaves in an herbal tea blend is not a good idea because the brewing process for each varies. The best way to brew these mixtures is to decoct the root portion first, turn off the heat, and then add the leaf herbs to infuse.

Dosage differs widely depending on the herbs used, the person, and the reason (ailment) that the tea has been chosen. A medicinal tea dosage is generally three cups a day for an adult and one-quarter cup to two cups a day for children, depending on their weight. Babies can benefit from herbal teas by drinking mother's milk fifteen to thirty minutes after Mom has consumed the tea. Small teaspoon-sized doses can be given to babies directly. Medicinal teas are best made up daily, but they will keep satisfactorily in the refrigerator for two days.

We're content to use our mountain springwater to make our teas. Chlorinated tap water from a municipal supply should never be used for medicinal remedies. City dwellers have the option of buying bottled water or installing a home water-purification system. Some medicine makers like to use distilled water in their preparations. Such "hungry water" will pull more of the medic-

inal properties of the plant into solution. You can distill your own or buy it in glass containers (preferable) or plastic jugs (more commonly available).

## Syrups

Delicious syrups result from knowing how to make infusions and decoctions. These work well for getting children to take their herbs. Great examples are wild cherry and coltsfoot for coughs, or a carminative herb mix with peppermint, catnip, and fennel for gassy tummies.

Making a syrup is actually a bit of a treat:

1. Use two ounces of dry herb mixture to one quart of water.
2. Simmer this down to one pint over low heat.
3. Strain the herbs from the liquid and compost the herbs. Return the liquid to the pot.
4. Add sweetener (honey, maple syrup, glycerin, or sugar can be used, but we like honey). Traditionally, to preserve it, two parts honey are added to one part of a strong tea. This is very sweet, so we prefer to add one cup honey to each pint of liquid and then refrigerate our syrups. These will last for two months or so kept refrigerated. If you want the syrup to be self-preserving at room temperature, the sugar content must be at least 60 percent by volume.
5. Bottle in sterilized jars, cap with sterilized lids. Label clearly.

The basic dosage of an herbal syrup is one tablespoon for adults taken up to five times a day. Children can have two teaspoons up to five times a day, depending on their weight. How soothing this can be on a sore throat!

# HEARTSONG FARM ELDERBERRY SYRUP

This delicious and healthful syrup can be used for cold and flu symptoms. Try filling a wine glass halfway with the syrup, add hot water, and lift a toast to your health when flu bogs you down. The color alone is enough to perk you up.

Simmer 1 gallon of fully ripened elderberries (stripped from their stalks) with ½ cup water in a large soup pot until soft. Strain the pulp out, compost it, and save the juice. Add ½ ounce grated ginger and a heaping teaspoon of whole cloves to the liquid and simmer uncovered until the liquid reduces to half the volume. Add 1 cup dried elderflowers to the hot juice, put the lid on and infuse for 20 minutes. Strain out the herbs and add one part raw honey to one part juice. Bottle and cap when cool.

This "low-sugar syrup" must be kept refrigerated and used within eight to twelve weeks. Whole berries can be frozen to make more syrup during the winter months when this anti-viral brew becomes essential medicine. Nancy's recipe yields approximately twelve 8-ounce bottles of elderberry syrup for our community.

### Dry Tea Powders

The dry tea method creates an herbal product that is alcohol-free and lasts a long time. These concentrated powders—sometimes called *solid extracts* (but not the solid extracts made in large laboratory settings involving vacuum distillation)—can easily be made at home or in the local apothecary. Dry teas are quite concentrated: ½ teaspoon is equal to 5 teaspoons of the dried herb. The finished powders can be added to smoothie drinks or juice or sprinkled on food. Using fresh herbs is ideal, but powders can be made with dry herbs as well.

Highly nutritional herbs such as nettles, dandelion, hawthorn, and alfalfa, and tonic herbs such as Siberian ginseng, codonopsis, and astragalus are good prepared this way. Depending on the herb, one teaspoon taken two or three times daily is a general dosage. Christopher Hobbs recommends preparing a dry tea powder this way:

1. Use chopped fresh herbs, cut and sifted dry leafy herbs, or freshly ground powdered roots.
2. Simmer herbs and water for two to four hours on very low heat. Use one part fresh herb to two parts water, or one part dry herb to five parts water.
3. Take half of the plant matter out at this time and press. Return any liquid to the pot and compost the marc.
4. Simmer the remains down to half the volume if you started with fresh herbs, or 20 percent of the original volume if you started with dry herbs.
5. Blend the remaining plant material and liquid to a creamy consistency. If this seems too thin, simmer longer.
6. Brush a thin coat of organic olive oil inside a glass baking pan. Spread the thick herbal paste on the pan, approximately ⅛ inch thick.
7. Put in a gas oven to dry for 18 to 38 hours, using only the gentle warmth generated by the pilot light. A food dehydrator set at 100°F to 120°F works equally well.
8. Remove from the pan and grind the hardened extract in a coffee grinder that

you've cleaned scrupulously, or one that's dedicated to grinding herbs.

9. This powder should keep in a glass airtight container for at least a year.

"We have made many of these powdered extracts over the past six years in our clinic and dispensed thousands of prescriptions containing them with awesome results," reports Christopher. "Reishi, nettles, ginseng and ginger, and American ginseng and ligustrum are some of my favorites. This process works very well with the tonic herbs to be taken for long periods. Alcoholic tinctures don't capture the vitamins, minerals, and large-molecular-weight polysaccharides that dried teas do. Tinctures are better for short-term use and for redirecting the energies of the body."

### Soups

Don't forget that age-old medicinal water preparation called soup. This time-honored way to get herbs and other nutrients into our systems has a place on the community medicine shelf. We add nutritional and immune-enhancing herbs to the cooking pot to make a fortified soup. Astragalus and burdock are regulars in the winter. Fresh or dry nettles, dandelion, and lots of garlic and onions are staples throughout the year.

The recipe for Deep Immune Tonic shown here is excellent for anyone, but it is especially appropriate for those convalescing or suffering from a weakened immune system. Our friend Kate Gilday from Woodland Essence based this tonic soup on a traditional Chinese Fu Zhang Tang formula. (This formulation, as well as most of the ingredients in this tonic, can be purchased from David Winston at Herbalist & Alchemist.) Even some herbalists who are primarily vegetarian recommend this heal-

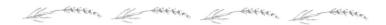

## DEEP IMMUNE TONIC

**10 to 12 cups water in nonaluminum pan**
**Several bones from an organically raised lamb or turkey**
**1 to 2 ounces astragalus roots**
**1 to 2 ounces codonopsis roots**
**3 to 4 ounces reishi mushrooms cut into small pieces**
**Good-sized handful each of shiitake mushrooms and turkey tails**
**Good-sized handful burdock root**
**Good-sized handful of atractylodes (bai zhu) rhizomes**

Place pan full of water and herbs on a very low flame. Simmer for three days, leaving the top slightly ajar, replacing water as it evaporates. At the end of the simmering time add two organic carrots and four stalks of organic celery chopped small. Simmer one more hour with cover on. Cool the entire contents. Strain the brew through cheesecloth. Place in ice cube trays. When frozen, pop out the cubes into freezer bags and store in freezer.

Dose is one "ice cube" of Deep Immune Tonic a day. Can be added to soups or water or taken alone once melted.

ing recipe: The bones, cartilage, and marrow make the soup extremely nutritious for people whose reserves and energy have in some way been compromised. Adding a little vinegar during cooking will help to draw minerals—particularly calcium, magnesium and potassium—into the broth.

### Spirit-Based Medicines

Many community herbalists base much of their business on making and selling tinctures. Tinctures have become very common in the past decade. We have heard many stories of people being introduced to using herbs simply because someone at work recommended using echinacea tincture for cold and flu symptoms. And it worked!

Generally speaking, spirit-based preparations are liquid preparations of herbs in a base of alcohol, vinegar, or glycerin. Rubbing alcohol serves as an appropriate base to make an herbal liniment for external use only. Water is a very good solvent, but it is not a good preservative. Spirit-based solvents do both. Some of the revered Eclectic medicine makers would roll over in their graves, but many modern herbalists have gotten a bit sloppy in referring to all spirit-based herb preparations as tinctures. Herbalists first need to distinguish between the terms *tincture* and *fluid extract* if we're to keep our dosage guidelines and methodologies straight.

Technically speaking, a *tincture* is a liquid preparation of an herb in which the solvent system used is an alcohol/water mixture and in which the volume of liquid exceeds the weight of herb extracted in it. Strength specifications for tinctures in pharmacopoeias and formularies are given as a ratio, such as 1:2 (fresh) or 1:5 (dry). The first number represents the weight of the herb and the second number is the volume of the combined solvents. We'll become more familiar with all this terminology soon. A *fluid extract*, on the other hand, is a liquid herbal preparation extracted in an alcohol/water mixture in which the proportion of herb matches the finished volume of liquid. The strength ratio now appears as 1:1, which in essence means the initial weight of crude drug equals the weight of remaining solvent. Making a fluid extract requires either the use of a percolator and calculated precision when starting out with equal parts of solvent to herb, or subsequent evaporation of a tincture to this desired concentration. The goal is to standardize dosage; however, the heat used to concentrate a fluid extract by evaporation destroys some of the constituents and therefore results in a less effective medicine.

Herbalists generally refer to the tincture-making process as *maceration*. The separate constituents in the herb(s) are released into solution by soaking in an appropriate menstruum. Tinctures are surprisingly easy to make, especially if using the *folkloric method* of maceration. The *measured method* of maceration involves straightforward math and an appreciation for constituent nuance. These variations share the same basic idea. Herbs are chopped or ground and mixed with the menstruum. The mixture is then allowed to soak (macerate) for at least two weeks before being pressed, filtered, and bottled. The spent herb, known as the *marc,* is then composted.

### Searching for Alkahest

Perhaps the hardest part of the whole maceration process is deciding on the appropri-

# BENEFITS OF TINCTURE EXTRACTS

1. Concentrate a wider range of constituents from the herb than water extraction alone.
2. Preserve fragile fresh constituents and activities that would be lost by drying herbs.
3. Easily assimilated by the body, much more so than capsules or tablets.
4. Retain potency much longer than bulk herbs. Properly made, most tinctures have a shelf life of three to five years stored at room temperature.
5. Tinctures are convenient to use in the home, on trips, or during emergencies. You don't need to wait for boiling water to steep tea.
6. Finally, from an herbal livelihood perspective, tinctures can be profitable at a fair market price.

ate menstruum or combinations of menstruums for each herb. A *menstruum* is the solvent used to pull the constituents of the plant into solution and thereby preserve its goodness. Alchemists once used combinations of alcohol, vinegar, and glycerin, and these continue to be our principal menstruums today. Still, medieval pharmacists liked the notion of narrowing down the choices for a good menstruum to one universal solvent. This hypothetical compound was named *alkahest* by Paracelsus (1493–1541) and was said to have been coined by him in imitation of the original Arabic words. Such a universal menstruum would have saved us from having to muse about solvent considerations. Alas! We'll just take a quick plunge now.

A decision to use alcohol correlates to the principal plant properties to be extracted. An *aqueous ethanol alcohol* combines the solvent abilities of both alcohol and water. Such a 40 to 70 percent alcohol menstruum dissolves the greatest amount of plant properties and becomes rapidly assimilated by the body. Salts, glycosides, sugars, vitamins, enzymes, bitters, alkaloids, and most tannins are pulled into solution by this deliberately calculated mix of alcohol and water. *Full-strength alcohol*[3] enables medicine makers to obtain waxes, resins, and essential oils from the plant material. Good herb books direct us to the herbs that traditionally make the best spirit-based extractions and the solvency range (percentage of alcohol) that might be used.

Distilled alcohols such as gin and brandy already contain a water portion. Every bottle label lists the percentage of alcohol contained as its *proof*—an 80-proof vodka, for instance, is 40 percent alcohol by volume. In other words, halving the numbered proof tells the percentage of alcohol in the liquor.

The folkloric method of tincture making naturally enough depends on these commonly available spirits. Commercial products generally do not exceed 100 proof, so herbalists need to mix full-strength alcohol with water for tincturing recommendations higher than 50 percent. The measured method of tincture making depends on using a close-to-pure alcohol. Grain alcohol tallies in at 190 proof. Just ahead, we will give directions for achieving the right ratio in a menstruum with such a potent spirit.

Grain alcohol is available right off the shelf in liquor stores in only a handful of states. A home medicine maker can either include Iowa, Louisiana, Oregon, and Texas on family trips to stock up, or try his or her hand at shuffling some forms. Here in New Hampshire we need to fill out paperwork to assure state authorities this straight alcohol is indeed destined for medicinal purposes before the liquor store clerks will place a special order. Grain alcohol retails under the brand names of Everclear and Clear Spring for about $16 a fifth (25 ounces) in our state. We've known some surreptitious herbalists who have managed to bring grain alcohol across the border from Mexico and Canada at a substantial savings. Our lips, however, are sealed.

Small herb businesses can purchase grain alcohol at wholesale prices direct from a company such as Aaper Alcohol. When first contacting them to order a 5-gallon drum, we were thrilled to hear that it was going to cost us $8.35 a gallon. This seemed an incredible bargain compared to $80 at the liquor store for a similar gallon's worth of grain alcohol. Over half the retail price for distilled liquors goes toward taxes, however, and the Aaper sales rep pointed out that this reality still applied. Federal excise taxes on wholesale grain alcohol amount to an additional $25.65 per gallon. Ouch! The clincher comes with shipping: Alcohol is categorized as a Class 3 flammable liquid and will be considerably more expensive to ship than another package of equal weight. Still, our wholesale savings amounted to almost 50 percent, and this gain improves for herbalists who live near city distribution centers and thus can forego shipping charges. One important note about ordering direct from these alcohol suppliers: Stress that you want alcohol fermented from grains, otherwise they may just ship a synthetic alternative made from petroleum. Alcohol apparently can be fermented from almost anything.

We are always asking ourselves, can't we grow and make all we need to create Earth medicines ourselves? We go to so much trouble to ensure the quality of our herbs, yet we add this distilled alcohol abounding in industrial karma to our herbal preparations. Homesteader guidelines direct that any homegrown effort should end up costing less and be of superior quality. Lord knows, we grow enough potatoes to make our own vodka. We even talked to a guy who would make us a still . . . Whoops! There are strict laws about moonshining. The legal requirement obviously needs to fit into our self-sufficiency equation when we talk about making hard alcohol.

Relatively small amounts of wine, beer, and cider are sanctioned for home production, but not brandy, vodka, and the other distilled liquors needed in the tincture process. Gene Logsdon discusses the legal situation at length in his book *Good Spirits: A New Look at Ol' Demon Alcohol.* The drift of this high-spirited farmer's perspective shows in his running commentary on the local injustice done by government to distilling entrepreneurs. Anybody can make spirits.

The whole chemistry rests on the singular fact that ethyl alcohol vaporizes at 173°F and water, of course, boils at 212°F. Heat properly applied can take a fermented mash all the way to grain alcohol by way of a multistep fractional distillation process.

We know when to pick our battles. When it comes to providing people with local herbs and the knowledge of how to use these plant medicines, consider us front-line warriors. So far we haven't felt that strongly about making our own vodka for extracting purposes, but Gene—well now he's got us thinking ever since we read his provocative little tome. Michael regularly makes hard cider from our organic apple cider. Nancy brews a bold nettle beer and an annual crock of dandelion wine.[4] But homemade alcohol in the legal category just doesn't have the intoxicating oomph to draw out plant constituents and subsequently preserve the extract. Cider's alcohol content runs around 5 to 8 percent, depending on the apple varieties pressed. Our elderberry wine approaches 12 percent. The alcohol used in tincturing fresh herbs, though, must be at least 40 percent pure alcohol (such as an 80-proof vodka), or it will not preserve the medicine effectively.[5]

We have heard discussions among herbalists advocating various types of alcohol as superior to others. Some say cane alcohol is better than grain alcohol, especially for people who are sensitive or allergic to wheat products. Other herbalists argue that the source of the neutral spirit is not important, since the result chemically is the same— nearly pure ethyl alcohol. Grain alcohol is chosen more for its lower price, as it is either a byproduct of what remains in the stills after the good whiskey has been bottled or a deliberate industrial distillation.

Oak barrel storage imparts good qualities in trace amounts to an aged brandy, according to Matthew Wood. "Grape alcohol [brandy] is penetrating, stimulates the circulation, and helps things go into the body," says Matthew, who is always on the lookout for energetic connection. "Corn alcohol [whiskey] has a fiery, overstimulating, violent quality. It was good for the wounded soldiers in the Civil War, but not everybody all the time. Rye alcohol [such as Belvedere vodka] is strengthening to the connective tissue."

Those folkloric herbalists who reach regularly for that vodka bottle probably don't realize this 80- to 100-proof spirit is actually a watered-down grain alcohol. The days of Russian peasant farmers fermenting their potatoes have mostly passed. Most gins and vodkas today are made from various grains and then distilled just like whiskey. These clear liquors, however, are not aged in wood barrels. The truth is, these folkloric staples are not aged at all. The better vodkas are distilled as many as four times, with scrupulous charcoal filtering accounting for the drink's mellowness. Juniper berries and other aromatics lend gin its distinctive flavor. The spring water added at bottling lowers the percentage of alcohol back to 40 to 50 percent. Herbalists pay top dollar for that water with every drop of vodka or gin they buy to use in medicine.

We know of one company in the United States that produces an organic vodka. Ancient Age Distilleries in Frankfort, Kentucky, makes their 80-proof "Rain" vodka just like the best Eastern European brands, except they start with organic grains. Organic alcohol runs about three times the cost of the cheapest nonorganic vodka. Should herbalists spring for the difference? The answer to that question lies in the eventual availability of an organic grain alcohol. Lending our support to an agriculture that's better for Earth always has impeccable value. Buying an expensive vodka, albeit organic, doesn't necessarily support the bottom line of an herbal apothecary. A neutral grain spirit is essentially pure alcohol after it has been filtered and purified, so we need not worry about pesticides in fully distilled products. The most cost-effective value clearly lies in using a 190-proof grain alcohol instead of any type of vodka for a starting point. Folkloric herbalists can dilute its alcohol content by half to achieve an equivalent-to-vodka menstruum for a tincture. Those preferring brandy, however, might want to take into consideration organic vineyard management; the grape alcohol process, by stopping far short of a complete distillation, does indeed carry residue ramifications into the brandy bottle itself.

Herbalists have one solvent that is toning and health-promoting in and of itself: organic apple cider vinegar. *Vinegar* serves as a passable solvent and a short-term preservative. We prefer vinegar for tonic remedies that will be used several times a day for lengths of time (these keep for several months if refrigerated), or when there is a religious or health reason to avoid an alcohol tincture. Being highly acidic, vinegar has the ability to extract calcium and other minerals. Regular use of apple cider vinegar tends to improve the assimilation of these minerals in the body as well. What Nancy calls her *high-calcium tonic* is actually a vinegar tincture of fresh oats, nettles, borage, and duck eggshells. Vinegar's solvency reach extends to sugars, tannins, glycosides, and bitter compounds as well.

Unpasteurized cider vinegar will sometimes look a bit cloudy due to a gelatinous mass of acetobacter commonly called the *mother of vinegar.* Good mother is akin to the sourdough starter passed down in a baking family. Its presence indicates that the vinegar is alive, a solvent fact that we certainly appreciate in our vinegar extracts as well. The vinegar offered for sale in the grocery store today is not real apple cider vinegar at all, but an apple-flavored, distilled grain vinegar that's been denatured. So-called white vinegar is not a wholesome food in any respect, though it does a respectable job of cleaning windows. These are not the vinegars with which to make healing remedies. We're blessed to have the right vinegar made right here on our farm. Those barrels of hard cider Michael always has brewing in our cellar provide all the impetus needed to make our own vinegar. An acetobacter mother basically converts the alcohol in the fermented cider in direct proportion to an acetic acid in the vinegar. Thus a 5 percent alcohol content in the hard cider produces a 5 percent acetic acid strength in the vinegar.[6] This age-old process places a vinegar menstruum very much in the camp of spirit-based preparation.

Vinegar tinctures can be made by the folkloric method described below. Nancy likes to heat the vinegar, to between 100°F to 120°F, in the belief that more flavor (and thus medicinal constituents) will be drawn into her tincture. Heat any higher than this, though, begins to destroy the health benefits of the living vinegar. The warm vinegar is poured over the chopped herbs and capped with a plastic lid. Vinegar will start to corrode a metal lid.

The sweet, soothing qualities of *glycerin* have become popular in recent years, especially as the preferred choice for making tinctures for children or people with sensitivities to alcohol. Glycerin may be taken by diabetics as well, as this solvent converts to glycogen, not glucose. Glycerin has preservative and solvent abilities about midway between alcohol and water. A glycerin menstruum works well for tannins and also will extract sugars, enzymes, glucosides, bitter compounds, and saponins to some extent. Glycerin does not work well for resinous herbs, or those containing a lot of alkaloids.

Glycerin tinctures, properly called *glycerites,* can be made with fresh or dried herbs. Be sure the herbs are exceptionally clean to avoid any bacteria growing in the product. Use one part fresh herb to two parts nondiluted glycerin, or one part dried herb to five parts menstruum (a 60 percent glycerin/distilled water combination). The absolute glycerin content in either must be at least 60 percent or there is a good chance of spoilage. Glycerites will last one to two years if stored in a cool, dark place. Vegetable glycerin from coconut oil has the highest quality. Herbalists choose to avoid the chemically synthesized glycerin and animal-derived glycerin.

*Combination menstruums* are useful for extracting certain types of constituents. For plants high in both tannins and volatile oils, like the bark of wild cherry (*Prunus virginiana*), we need to use some glycerin along with the alcohol to keep the tannins from precipitating out the volatile oils. Thus a 1:5 tincture of the dry bark is recommended to be made with 60 percent alcohol, 10 percent glycerin, and 30 percent water. Vinegar used in combination with alcohol assists in the extraction of alkaloidal (base) substances from certain herbs. The acid in the vinegar causes a chemical reaction whereby the alkaloids are turned into alkaloidal salts, which in turn become available in solution. Indian tobacco (*Lobelia inflata*) calls for just such an acetous tincture of the fresh herb at 1:5, with 75 percent alcohol and 25 percent apple cider vinegar.

As always, cross-checking several medicine-making references will often reveal such intriguing and pharmaceutically valuable information. Vinegar used for a longer-keeping extract is best heated to 160°F for two minutes to prevent the reestablishment of the acetobacter in the extract.

### Folkloric Method of Maceration

Folkloric herbalists generally use fresh plants to make tinctures. Some herbalists even go so far as to bring alcohol with them into the field when out on a wildcrafting expedition. These fresh tinctures are made without measuring—quite in contrast to the empirical calculations we'll soon be exploring. Plant alchemy works all the same.

Nancy learned the folkloric method years ago when she made her first tinctures. It's easy, and highly effective medicines can be made with many different herbs this way. Home herbalists need not be daunted. That empowerment alone gives the folkloric method a validity that more nuance-oriented herbalists shouldn't forget. People connect with the plants and receive healing virtues all the same making, these far simpler tinctures.

A 100-proof vodka extracts effectively a majority of the many plant constituents. This clear alcohol makes it easy to observe the color changes that a tincture goes through as more and more of the plant constituents dissolve into the menstruum. Vodka does not contain the flavorings of certain brandies or gin, all of which take up space in the menstruum. An extracting solution can hold only a finite amount of chemical constituents: Vodka allows the plant's goodness that much more space. Cost-conscious herbalists will want to remember that vodka is merely a 50/50 mix of grain alcohol and water.

The folkloric method of maceration is quite straightforward:

1. Harvest the herb in its prime, after asking its permission. Use the proper plant parts as identified in any good herbal (fully opened chamomile flowers, for example, not the entire leafy stem).

2. Chop the herbs as finely as possible to almost fill a glass jar. Pints, quarts, gallons—whatever amount of tincture you wish to make. Label this jar with the current date and name of the herb.

3. Fill the jar with vodka, stopping about an inch from the top of the jar. This allows space to slosh the extraction around easily. Add more vodka the following day if the plant material absorbs any solvent. The vodka absolutely must cover the herbs throughout the process.

4. Put the jar in a dark place at room temperature and shake it at least once daily. This is the time to put your good intentions into your medicine: sing healing songs and offer prayers. (Some of our dedicated students have taken this to an extreme and reported taking their tinctures on vacation with them, or leaving instructions for a friend to "tincture-sit" while they were away for a long weekend. Alas, we're not that faithful.) Keep the jar somewhere in sight, not forgotten in a cabinet.

5. After two to six weeks pour the whole contents of the jar through muslin or some other thin, clean cloth (new baby diapers work great). Ideally, let the contents macerate over the course of a whole lunar phase. Squeeze every drop possible out of the marc. Wringing the sopping herbs by hand works, as does using a food mill or potato ricer. This is where a wine press or a tincture press comes in handy.

# FOLKLORIC TINCTURE MAKING

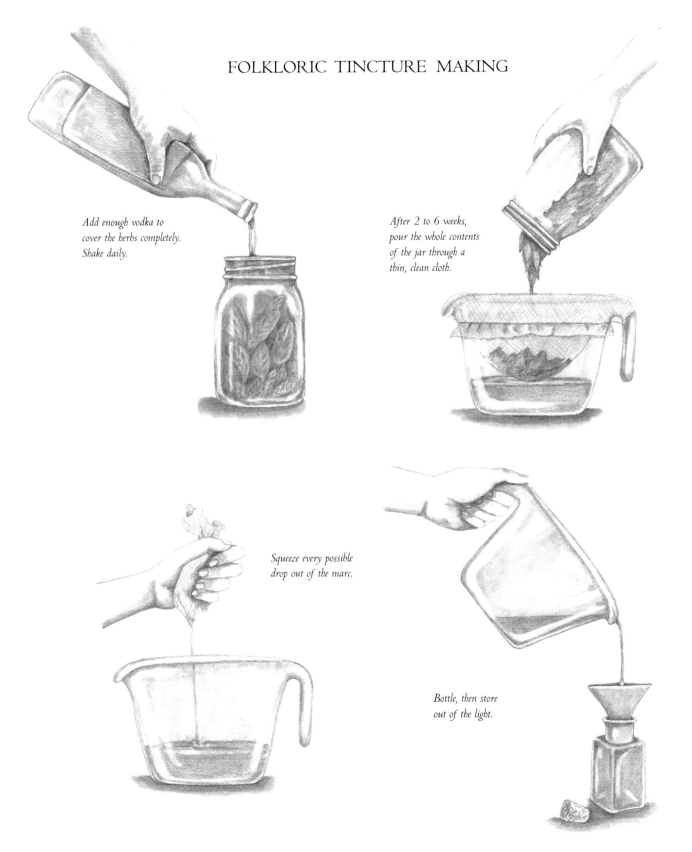

Add enough vodka to
cover the herbs completely.
Shake daily.

After 2 to 6 weeks,
pour the whole contents
of the jar through a
thin, clean cloth.

Squeeze every possible
drop out of the marc.

Bottle, then store
out of the light.

6. Store in a correctly labeled amber glass bottle out of the light.

Fresh herb tinctures made in this way use about one part fresh herb by weight to two parts menstruum by liquid measure. Such an approximation varies with how tightly packed the jar is with herb and how much water the herb being tinctured already contains. A plant's juices are mostly water, which decreases the 50 percent alcohol content of the menstruum by half (or so) in the actual tincture.

### Scientific or "Measured" Method of Maceration

Some people refer to the following as the standardized method of maceration. We prefer the term *measured method* to distinguish it from the dismantling and embellishing done to herbs in a large laboratory setting when standardizing levels of an isolated constituent. Some students hear the word *scientific* and automatically assume that this method is devoid of the mystery and spiritual connection embodied in the folkloric method. Not so. Herbalists can still ask the plant for permission to harvest and offer their thanks. It is just as easy to sing and say prayers while shaking our "measured tinctures." Even the math involved can add to our pleasure once we grasp how the valuable lessons learned by others about proportion can help our own medicine making. Could the time have come to unmask those secret aspirations to be more of a mad scientist than a marsh crone?

Getting out the beakers and graduated cylinders can be fun. Herbalists making large quantities of tinctures will save money by using grain alcohol and distilled water. Using the scientific/measured method makes it easier to repeat successful medicines. Dosage requirements become clearer, too, which is especially critical for low-dose herbs.

Unfortunately, somewhere in Nancy's past she acquired a mental block about math. Here's a village herbalist who has used the folkloric method for years with great success. As it turns out, many of the herbs we tincture for community use here at Heartsong Farm have a solubility range of around 50 percent. Echinacea, skullcap, and feverfew tincture quite nicely with a 100-proof vodka as the menstruum. Nancy deliberately avoided tincturing more resinous herbs such as myrrh, because she believed herself to be mathematically impaired. Constituent reality (as we've since come to understand it) matters if we wish to draw out the full action of a plant. The herb calendula offers a good example: Its bitter glycosides are extracted at 45 percent alcohol, but not the resins, which are only extracted at 90 percent.[7] Only a tincture made at the higher solvency possesses antifungal qualities.

Let's pause for a lesson in standard tincture ratios. These are the working formulas given in herbals for making tinctures of a given herb. For instance, look up St. John's wort and one sees "*Hypericum perforatum:* Tincture of dried flowering tips: 1:5 (70 percent alcohol)." The strength of the tincture (or a fluid extract) is indicated by the herb weight to menstruum volume ratio and the proportions of the various liquids used in the menstruum. The first number indicates herb weight in grams and the second number indicates menstruum volume in milliliters. A 1:5 strength means one part herb by weight was mixed with five parts fluid by volume, and so on. Strengths are typically specified either for fresh, recently dried, or dry plant material. The second ratio is commonly the percentage of alcohol used, but other ingredients in the menstruum such as vinegar can be listed as well.

TABLE 7-1. *Targeted Solvency for Twenty Herbs*

| LATIN NAME | COMMON NAME | PART USED | PREFERRED FORM | RECOMMENDED STRENGTH | PERCENT TARGETED SOLVENCY |
|---|---|---|---|---|---|
| *Achillea millefolium* | Yarrow | Flowering tops | Fresh or | 1:2 | 95 |
| | | | Dry | 1:5 | 70 |
| *Arctium lappa* | Burdock | First year roots | Dry | 1:5 | 60 |
| *Arctium lappa* | Burdock | Seeds | Dry | 1:4 | 60 |
| *Capsella bursa-pastoris* | Shepherd's purse | Aerial parts with seed | Fresh | 1:2 | 45 |
| *Cimicifuga racemosa* | Black cohosh | Roots | Dry | 1:5 | 80 |
| *Echinacea purpurea* | Purple coneflower | Aerial parts and roots | Fresh | 1:2 | 70 |
| *Equisetum arvense* | Horsetail | Leafy stems | Fresh | 1:2 | 40 |
| *Hypericum perforatum* | St. John's wort | Flowering tips | Fresh or | 1:2 | 95 |
| | | | Dry | 1:5 | 70 |
| *Juglans nigra* | Black walnut | Green hulls | Fresh | 1:2 | 40 |
| *Lactuca* spp. | Wild lettuce | Budding tops | Fresh | 1:2 | 95 |
| *Levisticum officinalis* | Lovage | Root | Dry | 1:5 | 50 |
| *Lobelia inflata* | Indian tobacco | Aerial parts with seeds | Fresh | 1:4 | 45 |
| *Melissa officinalis* | Lemon balm | Aerial parts in flower | Fresh or | 1:2 | 95 |
| | | | Dry | 1:5 | 70 |
| *Panax ginseng* | Asian ginseng | Roots | Dry | 1:5 | 70 |
| *Panax quinquefolius* | American ginseng | Roots | Fresh | 1:2 | 60 |
| *Salix alba* | White willow | Bark | Dry | 1:5 | 50 |
| *Sambucus* spp. | Elderberry | Flowers | Dry | 1:5 | 50 |
| *Scutellaria laterifolia* | Skullcap | Aerial parts in flower | Fresh | 1:2 | 60 |
| *Stellaria media* | Chickweed | Aerial parts | Recently dried | 1:5 | 45 |
| *Tanacetum parthenium* | Feverfew | Aerial parts in flower | Fresh or | 1:2 | 70 |
| | | | Dry | 1:5 | 50 |
| *Valeriana officinalis* | Valerian | Roots | Fresh | 1:2 | 95 |

For St. John's wort, the 70 percent portion of full strength alcohol given above assumes a 30 percent complement of distilled water in the combined menstruum. Some herbals will indicate this complete recommendation for solvency as (70A:30W).

Many Eclectic texts such as *King's American Dispensatory* and earlier versions of *The United States Pharmacopoeia* specify a solvency for making a liquid extract of each herb. The books we recommend on making herbal medicine offer extensive tincturing details as well. Combining all these opinions by contemporary herbalists and Eclectic doctors reveals a *solvent range* for extracting the active constituents in each herb. The standard tincture ratio for St. John's wort that we explained shows a typical spread of opinion from 55 to 75 percent for suggested solvency. The wider this range, the more the different constituent effects are drawn out. The chart on page 238 reflects the preferred form and recommended strength for making tincture extracts of twenty herbs. We've targeted a solvency that always falls within the accepted range and has been corroborated by other herbalists. This is the basis behind the math Nancy no longer seeks to avoid.

Don't be daunted by making tinctures with the measured method. Here are the basic steps for using dry herb:

1. Weigh the plant to be extracted. We recommend that herbalists learn to think in terms of grams and milliliters—modern-strength ratios are based on metrics—but conversion equivalents are available for those who insist on the confusion of English measurements.
2. Decide on the desired strength of the product.
3. Look up the percentage of alcohol recommended for the plant.
4. Calculate the amount of alcohol and water based on the strength ratio. For example, 200 grams of St. John's wort would require 1,000 ml of combined menstruum at 1:5.
5. Measure out the proper amounts of alcohol and water. Again, using the same example, 700 ml of alcohol plus 300 ml of distilled water reflects a 1,000-ml menstruum composed of 70 percent alcohol.
6. Combine the menstruum and herb. Put the mixture in a container with a tight-fitting lid. Store in a cool, dark place.
7. Shake daily until ready to press.
8. Press. Filter. Bottle and label.

Our example of a *Hypericum* tincture probably will not develop fully its character-

TABLE 7-2. *Measurement Equivalents*

*Solids:*

| | | | | |
|---|---|---|---|---|
| 1 ounce = | 28.4 grams | | | |
| 1 pound = | 453.6 grams | = | 16 | oz |
| | 1,000 grams | = | 35.2 | oz |

*Liquids:*

| | | | | |
|---|---|---|---|---|
| 1 ounce = | 29.57 ml | | | |
| 1 pint = | 473.3 ml | = | 16 | oz |
| 1 gallon = | 3,784.95 ml | = | 128 | oz |

istic blood-red color until four weeks have passed. One thing is certain, however: An empirically based tincture has been made successfully.

The measured method for working with fresh plant material differs only slightly from the steps outlined above for dry herb. The moisture contribution of the fresh plant needs to be determined as well. Drying a 100-gram sample of whatever herb allows you to determine its dry weight. Let's say 100g of fresh herb produces 30g dried. Therefore, the fresh plant consists of 30 percent solids and 70 percent plant moisture. The weight of the fresh herb from which an extraction will be made needs to be correspondingly lessened to account for its now known dry weight and moisture content. Thus 1,000g of fresh herb actually figures as 300g (30 percent worth) of solids and 700g (70 percent worth) of water in the plant itself. The recommended strength ratio for fresh St. John's wort stands at 1:2 at 95 percent alcohol, resulting in the need for a menstruum of 600ml of grain alcohol for the determined 300g of dry solids. A high-end solvency such as 95 percent cannot only be assumed to call for undiluted 190-proof grain spirits—it is the equivalent.[8] This measured maceration for fresh herb simplifies the more detailed examples found elsewhere when the alcohol content needs to be less than full strength. We hope you get the basic idea. Every herbalist is indeed capable of using the measured method.

### Standardized Extracts

We discussed standardized extracts at length in chapter I (see page 27). Here we want to add a bit to distinguish them from the maceration methods just described.

We establish a repeatable process for making tinctures when we apply a solvent ratio in the measured method of maceration. Experienced herbalists seek consistency as well in harvesting the correct herb at the optimal time from vibrant plants. In reality, however, no natural plant medicine comes completely standardized. The active constituents in a particular species can differ by as much as a factor of five.[9] Differences in soils, seasons, harvesttimes, and especially the differences in people who are taking herbal medicines, set an *unstandardized* pace. All we can do is strive to do our best and recognize that Mother Nature credits our good intentions by offering her best in return.

Some manufacturers "spike" their products by blending in additional concentrated or synthesized ingredients. Their goal is to achieve a standardized level of a single active constituent, usually the one currently being shown by research to have a strong medicinal effect. Thus determined, the percentage of isolated ingredient can be expressed on the label. This seemingly legitimate goal, however, often requires the aid of industrial solvents such as hexane and benzene, all of which are powerful toxins produced from petroleum. Healing virtue is thrown to the wind to create a marketing myth that standardized extracts somehow serve people better than whole-plant remedies.

Fair business practices are at stake here. Home herbalists and families have the right to know how herbal products are made and exactly what goes into them. We feel a good label will skip the standardization propaganda and tell people directly what menstruum was used and the weight/volume ratio of herb to menstruum. People should be able to know whether a product was made with fresh or dried herbs. An extract of a single flower in a vat of water would then stand revealed. Those standardized constituent levels with legitimate therapeutic worth don't lose validity when people understand the process involved (70 to 80 percent silymarin in a processed milk thistle extract used for severe liver disease, for instance).

### Percolation

The method where the menstruum slowly trickles through a column of the finely powdered herb is called *percolation*. This process allows every solid particle of the herb to be submitted to the solvent action of the menstruum as it flows down. Percolation must be done with dry herbs and specialized equipment. This method is valuable if you need a tincture or fluid extract relatively fast—these will be ready in two to three days. A maceration, in contrast, requires a minimum of two weeks. Properly absorbing the constituents of the dried herb into a menstruum so quickly requires meticulous attention to detail.

You can buy a standard percolator from an apothecary supplier. Innovative alchemists can make their own with a 2-liter wine bottle. Richard McDonald of Desert Bloom Herbs in New Mexico made us such a percolator. He used a tile saw with a continuous-rim-type blade on it to cut the bottle cleanly at the base. Then he smoothed the edges with a glass grinder. We supported this on a wooden shelf cut out to hold the upside-down bottle. A drip valve (that is, a screw-type cap) installed on the neck of the bottle allows us to control the rate of flow at so many drops per minute. Minimal warming of the menstruum coupled with a continuous pumping action through the herb (as opposed to a slow drip-drip-drip) reduces the extraction time to as little as six to eight hours and supposedly results in a 40 percent more potent tincture. Contact Dr. Earle Sweet at Sayfer Botanicals to learn more about the science of the percolation process.

Because we were steeped in the folkloric and wise woman tradition of herbalism, we had relatively no experience with the percolation technique of liquid extraction until we visited a variety of herb shops during our travels. Seeing herbalists such as Richard percolating herbal medicines in their labs made an impressive sight. At first glance, it didn't quite make sense that percolation could be as effective as maceration. Yet we saw how the slow dripping of an appropriate solvent through carefully packed powdered herbs at a controlled rate allowed enough concentrated time for the constituents to be drawn out. Nancy of course wanted a percolator of her own (assuming that Michael would do the math for her).

Percolation has merit. One place to find the working formula for each herb extraction is in an older edition of *The United States Pharmacopoeia*. Here's a summary of what you need to do:

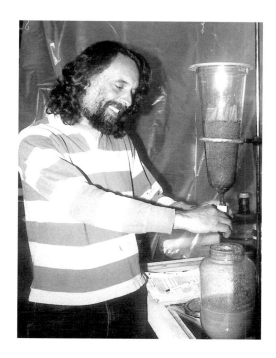

*Richard McDonald percolates a custom tincture in the back room pharmacy of Desert Bloom Herbs in Silver City, New Mexico.*

1. Measure the dry powdered herb or mixed herbs and place in a bowl. Be sure to measure the volume of dry herb as well, using a measuring cup, to determine how many fluid ounces of space it takes up.

2. Measure and mix the menstruum. Figure in an extra amount of menstruum to account for the liquid the herb will retain after the dripping process ends. On average, this amounts to an additional fluid ounce of space taken up by the dry herb.

3. Moisten the powdered herb in a bowl with a sufficient quantity of the menstruum to make it evenly damp. You want a "fine potting soil consistency" that can be squeezed into little clods that stick together. Leave the dampened herb in a closed container to "swell" for four hours.

4. Screw the cap loosely on the wine bottle, and then position the bottle (bottom up) on its stand over a half-gallon narrow-mouth canning jar. Allow enough room between the two containers to adjust easily the valve or cap on the neck of the percolator.

5. Dampen an unbleached coffee filter lightly with a small amount of menstruum so that it conforms to the inside of the bottle. Concentrate on forming a good seal that will prevent particles of herb from falling underneath the filter and clogging the flow rate valve.

6. Transfer the moistened herb carefully into the percolator, packing first along the top edge of the filter paper by pushing the moistened herb firmly against the paper using a wooden or plastic spoon. Holding the bottle in an almost horizontal position (once removed from its stand) helps with this circumferential packing. As you begin to fill the lower part of the filter (with the bottle now back in a vertical position), gently press the damp herb very lightly into place with a dowel rod. Place another filter paper atop the packed column of herb to prevent the menstruum from stirring up the works as it gets poured into the percolation cone.

7. Now partially open the bottom valve or cap to allow air to escape as the menstruum replaces the air within the percolation cone. This helps prevent stratification, caused by air trying to bubble up through the herb, instead of being pushed out of the bottom valve.

8. Pour as much menstruum as the cone will accommodate, leaving the valve open until the first drops come through. Close the valve, and cover the top of the percolator with a saucer (or plastic wrap held in place by a rubber band) and let the herb soak for at least twelve hours. An even longer time (up to two days with roots and barks) improves the strength of the extract considerably.

9. After this period, allow the percolation to proceed by gently unscrewing the cap part way until the menstruum drips out at the rate of approximately one drop every two seconds. An ounce of extract can be percolated every fifteen minutes or so at this rate. Add more menstruum to the top of the percolation cone as space allows, until the full volume measured out has dripped through the herb. Calculating the actual fluid retention rate of a particular herbal powder—and concentrating a last portion of the percolate by evaporation over a water bath if so desired—can yield very exacting results.

10. Bottle, label, and date the fluid extract or tincture.

The packing process is the hardest part to learn. If you pack the herb mass too tightly, it will be difficult for the menstruum to drip through. Packing it too loosely will cause it to separate, and then

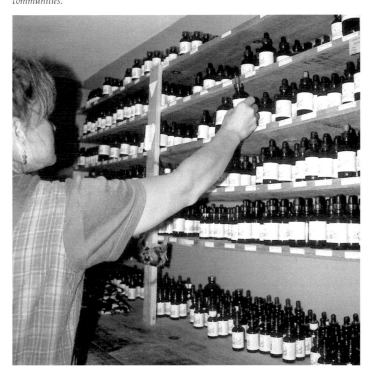

*The tincture racks at Avena Botanicals in Rockland, Maine, meet a multitude of healing needs for northern New England communities.*

you have to turn the whole thing into a maceration extraction. Watching someone else do a percolation helps. If you don't have a friend who is experienced in percolation techniques, but you have a VCR, you can watch Debra St. Claire's video *Herbal Preparations and Natural Therapies* (one of the best medicine-making videos available), which can be ordered from Morningstar Publications (see appendix five).

### Spirit-Based Dosages

We are reluctant to state general dosages for tinctures and fluid extracts because they vary widely. Dosage very much depends on the individual herb, the strength of the extract, and the size and condition of the person being treated. A general recommendation for an alcohol tincture of 1:2 strength might be for ¼ to ½ teaspoon of tincture three times a day for chronic conditions and ⅛ to ¼ teaspoon every hour or two for acute situations. Herbalists with a metric perspective will give the recommended dose in milliliters of a specified tincture. One teaspoon equals roughly five milliliters. Drop dosages, on the other hand, are not consistently accurate, as dropper size and air pressure affect the volume of each drop. Who wants to count all those drops anyway?

Tinctures can be administered directly under the tongue or diluted in water, tea, or juice. Alcohol is far less toxic than the industrial solvents (such as hexane or benzene) often used in standardized herbal preparations. Some people might be concerned about imbibing any spirits. Thirty to forty drops of tincture contain about the same amount of alcohol as one ripe banana. If desired, the alcohol can be evaporated partially, without impairing quality, by placing the recommended dose of extract in hot

## NAYSAYING HERBAL REMEDIES

EMBRACING HERBAL HEALING does not mean being naïve about using plant medicines. A good medicinal herb reference will point out known dangers and potentially adverse side effects. A clinical perspective considers contraindications of plant remedies used in conjunction with synthetic drug treatment as a matter of course. Prudence goes without saying. Clear warnings should always be given on the product label. But this line of reasonable concern can sometimes be crossed, to both confuse and outright dissuade those investigating plant remedies.

Two waves of thought pulse through our cultural blood in considering the rising tide of herbal medicine. Earth-centered herbalists hold great respect for both empirical tradition and rational understanding of whole-plant remedies. The medical-scientific crowd, gentlemen and ladies all, look for specific proofs that suit allopathic paradigms. Viewpoint must always be taken into account when evaluating the Herbs of Choice.

---

water (100°F to 105°F) for ten minutes. However, not all tinctures are heat-stable, and in those cases potency will be weakened.

### Herbal Liniments

Liniments are external preparations applied to the skin. Many are basically tinctures, although some liniments are oil based. Always remember to label liniments FOR EXTERNAL USE ONLY! We generally make our herbal liniments by the folkloric method, using vinegar or substituting rubbing alcohol or witch hazel for the vodka otherwise used as a menstruum. Liniments are used for varicose veins and for strained, sore, and tired muscles and joints. They also encourage healing for arthritis and bursitis inflammation. They can be used alone or can provide the moisture in herbal poultices, depending on the actions wanted. Witch hazel leaves soaked in witch hazel, for example is helpful with varicose veins. Use lobelia and cayenne for an antispasmodic liniment.

Kloss's liniment from the 1939 herb book *Back to Eden* is a classic. This excellent disinfectant can also be used on poison ivy and sore muscles. Simply combine two ounces of powdered myrrh, one ounce of powdered organically grown goldenseal, and ½ ounce of cayenne pepper with one quart of rubbing alcohol in a glass jar. Shake daily and decant after seven days.

## Oil-Based Medicines

Two types of oils are commonly used in herbal medicine: essential oils and fixed oils. Most of us do not produce either of these at home, but we do use oils by themselves and in combination with herbs for various therapies.

### Essential Oils

When we rub a sprig of lavender between our fingers, or pet the rosemary plant as we walk by, we are smelling essential oils. These are contained in tiny pockets, called glandular cells, in the plant. Most essential oils are extracted through steam distillation; some cannot be extracted this way and are currently processed with solvents including hexane, butane, methane, and propane, as well as the more toxic, even carcinogenic solvents benzene and acetone. Huge amounts of plant material are used to extract small amounts of oil. Thus, essential oils are expensive and somewhat wasteful of plant material. Plants that produce a relatively high percentage of essential oils, such as sage, thyme, and rosemary, take approximately 500 pounds of plant material to produce 32 ounces of essential oil.[10] Some plants, such as the rose, contain such a small amount that it takes one ton

of petals to produce just over 10 ounces of essential rose oil.

Be aware that there are poor-quality, highly diluted essential oils and synthetic "fragrance oils" on the market. If you see rose oil priced much lower than $250 per ¼-ounce bottle, the oil inside is not likely a pure essential oil. Adulteration and substitution are common, unfortunately. Lemon balm oil, for example, almost invariably turns out to be lemongrass oil. Sometimes it is difficult to get manufacturing details, so train your nose to be able to tell quality oils and buy from reputable sources. You actually can distill your own essential oils at home. Benzalco sells a home distillation unit and provides complete instructions— just plan on using a lot of herb!

Keeping in mind that essential oils are indeed precious, used sparingly, these can be invaluable in an herbal practice. Essential oils can be used in massage, body care products, steams, baths, disinfecting products, and salves, just to name a few uses. Learning the art of aromatherapy is a helpful adjunct to our work. Good books on aromatherapy include *Aromatherapy: A Complete Guide to the Healing Art* by Kathi Keville and Mindy Green and *The Practice of Aromatherapy: A Classic Compendium of Plant Medicines and Their Healing Properties* by Jean Valnet and Robert Tisserand. Study with an expert aromatherapist when the opportunity arises. Pay special attention to the safety precautions, as essential oils are extremely concentrated. Most of them are at least fifty times more potent than the herbs from which they are derived. Learn how to dilute and apply them properly, then befriend five or so oils. Get to know these well. We always have lavender, tea tree, peppermint, and eucalyptus oils on hand for treating many common ailments.

## Infused Oils

Infused oils are made by infusing herbs in a carrier or fixed oil such as olive, sesame, or sunflower. *Fixed oil* describes vegetable-derived oils made from crushing the plant material. Heat alters the quality of these oils. *Cold-pressed oils* are superior for cooking and herbal therapies. We prefer organic extra-virgin olive oil for most oil-based products, as this oil is highly nutritional and medicinal in and of itself. Unfortunately, vegetable oil is a good extractive medium for more than just certain soluble constituents of plants. Agricultural chemicals, including pesticides and herbicides, could lace any oil that is not certified as organically grown and produced.

Dina Falconi does a wonderful job explaining the different qualities of fixed oils in her book, *Earthly Bodies and Heavenly Hair*. She also includes numerous healing recipes for using essential, fixed, and infused oils.

Infused oils can be made in a variety of ways. The basic idea is to use the carrier oil to absorb the medicinal qualities of the herbs. Oil infusion is done slowly, with low heat. We have used the sun, a double boiler, and the pilot light on our stove, but the *slow-cooker method* is by far the best way to make larger quantities of infused oil. The ideal cooker is an electric turkey roaster or some other cooker with a temperature control device. The temperature of the oils should not exceed 125°F. The herbs lose medicinal value quickly if the temperature goes much higher. A Crock-Pot can be used, but the lowest setting on these is usually 125°F. Crock-Pots need to be turned on and off periodically so the oil does not get too hot. Oils should not go below 110°F, either. Although this will not decrease the quality of the infused oil it will prolong the process.

Herbal infused oils can be made with either fresh or dried herbs. Freshly dried herbs are the easiest to work with, as these present little chance of fermenting (because the water content of wilted herbs is accordingly reduced). The herbs we prefer to infuse fresh include elderflower, St. John's wort, and calendula. Nancy has never had an infused oil mold with either fresh or dried herbs when she used heat to prepare it. However, some real smelly ones resulted when she first started making oils and just set the jars in the pantry. Ugh!

The steps for making an herbal infused oil are:

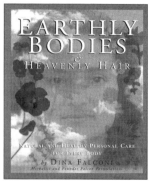

1. Place finely chopped herbs in a clean jar. Use approximately one part fresh herb to three parts oil. Increase this ratio to 1:4 for freshly dried herbs.
2. Pour the oil over the herbs, making sure to completely cover. The glass jar can then be set in the turkey roaster and water added to the roaster (not inside the jars) to help warm the oil. This strategy of separate jars allows two or more entirely different herbs to be infused at the same time. The herbs and oil can be placed directly in the turkey roaster for larger batches.
3. Heat the herbs and oil for at least ten days. Some herbalists heat them as long as four weeks. Keep the temperature between 110°F and 120°F. Stir daily. Leave the lid slightly ajar if using fresh herbs so any extra moisture can escape.
4. The oils will take on the color of the herb and some of the aroma. They should smell very herby, but not nearly as strong as an essential oil.
5. Pour the finished oil through several layers of cheesecloth into a clean glass jar. Squeeze out as much as you can, then compost the spent herbs.

*Dina Falconi believes that beauty involves working in partnership with Nature.* Earthly Bodies and Heavenly Hair *offers more than 450 original personal care formulas.*

6. Let the infused oil stand overnight so herb particles and moisture will settle to the bottom.
7. The next day you can decant the clear oil and leave the cloudy-looking stuff in the bottom of the jar. (You can compost this sludge. Nancy usually finds some creative way to use the oil residues within the next few days, such as slathering it all over herself when she gets out of the bathtub.)
8. Label your infused oils and store them in a cool dark place. Stored this way they will last at least a year.

We particularly like the infused St. John's wort oil for healing injuries that involve nerve pain, sciatica, and minor burns. Calendula oil is antiseptic and helps heal cuts, rashes, and scrapes. Arnica oil is good for bruises and sore muscles. Mullein flowers make an excellent oil for earache and ear infections.

### Salves

Infused oils are just one step away from becoming salves or balms. We simply add beeswax to solidify the oil. Many commercial salves are made from paraffin, but we don't like to put anything on our skin that we wouldn't eat. As paraffin is a petroleum product, beeswax makes a far superior ingredient.

Salves are effective for soothing and healing skin or sore muscles. They have a wide range of uses, from clearing up congestion and fungal infections to vaginal lubricants.[11] Infused oils and salves should not be used for inflammations: The oils tend to lock in the heat and exacerbate the swelling. Poultices are the herbal preparation to use for conditions that involve inflammation.

If you do not have the infused oils already prepared, you can make them quickly by heating the oil and herb over low heat in a double boiler until you get a rich, herby oil. The suggested oil-to-beeswax ratios for a salve range widely. The ratio chosen depends on the desired hardness of the finished salve. Lip balms (made exactly this same way) should be harder, especially if you are putting the balm in a push-up stick container. Many salve recipes typically call for using one part beeswax to four parts oil. For example, one cup oil would require ¼ cup beeswax. Nancy has found that melting the beeswax in advance and then letting it solidify in ice cube trays results in less clean up in the long run—each "ice cube" equals almost exactly ¼ cup by volume. These pre-measured cubes of beeswax can then be added to the heated oil.

A healing salve was the very first medicine—other than tea—that Nancy made. Here are her basic steps:

1. Prepare medicinal oil following instructions above. Strain.
2. Add ¼ cup beeswax to each cup of herbal oil. Heat these together gently over low heat in a double boiler until the beeswax is completely melted. Check the firmness by putting a tablespoon of oil in the freezer for a couple of minutes. Add more oil if it is too hard; add more beeswax if it is too soft.
3. Remove from the heat. If you are adding essential oils, do so now. Then immediately pour into containers.
4. While they are still hot, wipe out the pans and utensils with clean rags, newspapers, or paper towels, then wash them in hot, soapy water.
5. Let the salve cool and harden before putting on the container lids. Label.

Store in a cool dark place. These will keep for at least a year. Many last up to three years if stored properly.

Lip balms can be colored red by first dyeing the oil with dried alkanet root. The roots need to be strained out before adding the reddened oil to the beeswax. Dye the oil a much deeper red than you want it to appear on your lips, as the wax will somewhat lessen the alkanet sheen. A deep burgundy in the pot will show up as a rosy glow on the lips.

### Suppositories and Pessaries

Semisolid preparations made by adding dry herbs or tinctures to an oil base are called suppositories and pessaries. Cocoa butter is the most common base because it melts at body temperature.

*Suppositories* are used to introduce medicine to the rectum. They are often prescribed for local conditions such as anal fissures, constipation, hemorrhoids, inflammation of the lower bowel, and ulcerative colitis. They can also be used for acute conditions such as severe diarrhea and severe vomiting when the person cannot take medication orally. They are usually inserted after a bowel movement and before going to bed at night. Depending on the condition, they may be recommended two or more times a day.

*Pessaries* are similar to suppositories, but they are inserted into the vagina. They can be recommended for cervical cell dysplasia, labor induction, menopausal dryness, thrush, and vaginal infections. The pessary will melt and disperse its ingredients over a period of hours. It is a good idea to wear a pad to prevent staining of your underwear.

Reusable metal molds are available from pharmacy supply companies such as Apothecary Products. Molds can be fashioned as well from aluminum foil or thimbles fitted into a wire rack. Being creative works as long as the forms used are sanitary. Small cylinders can also be shaped by hand, if using a high herb-to-oil ratio. Roll these into long coils, first of approximately ¼-inch diameter and then cut into 1-inch-long chunks.

Depending on the condition and the density of the herbs used, the herb-to-oil ratio will vary. In general, use at least twice as much cocoa butter by weight than herb. These are the basic steps for making a suppository or pessary:

1. Lubricate the molds before you begin by brushing them with a little olive oil.
2. Grind herbs finely, then sift.
3. Melt cocoa butter in a double boiler or a Pyrex measuring cup placed in a water bath.
4. When the cocoa butter has melted, add the herbs and stir well.
5. Pour into molds directly from the measuring cup (provided it has a pouring spout) or use a turkey (bulb) baster.
6. Put the molds into the freezer to harden, then remove from the molds and store in an airtight container in the refrigerator. Don't forget to label each product.

The suppository recipe most in demand is the one for hemorrhoids. Use one ounce powdered white oak bark, ½ ounce powdered comfrey root, ¼ ounce powdered yarrow, ¼ ounce powdered calendula, and four ounces of cocoa butter for this preparation.

### Creams and Lotions

Keeping the skin soft and supple comes to mind when we reach for a cream or lotion. These oil-based preparations can be deeply healing as well when the ingredients

# ROSEMARY'S PERFECT CREAM

*Waters*

⅔ cup distilled water

⅓ cup aloe vera gel

1 to 2 drops of essential oil of choice

vitamins A and E as desired

*Oils*

¾ cup apricot, almond, or grape seed oil

⅓ cup coconut oil or cocoa butter

¼ teaspoon lanolin

½ to 1 ounce grated beeswax

Combine distilled water, aloe vera gel, essential oil, and vitamins A and E in a glass measuring cup. Set aside.

In a double boiler over low heat, combine remaining ingredients. Heat just enough to melt. Pour oils into a blender and let cool to room temperature. The mixture should become thick, creamy, semisolid, and cream colored.

Once the oils have cooled, turn the blender on its highest speed. In a slow thin drizzle, pour the water mixture into the center vortex. When most of the water mixture has been added to the oils, listen to the blender and watch the cream. When the blender coughs and chokes, and the cream looks thick and white like buttercream frosting, turn off the blender. Pour into cream or lotion jars; the recipe yields approximately eight 2-ounce containers. The cream will thicken a bit as it sets. Store in a cool place.

include herbs selected for an array of health conditions. The skin readily absorbs such medicine.

Body creams and lotions can sometimes be challenging to make: Oils and water don't like to mix. The best recipe we know of is Rosemary's Perfect Cream. This is one of many great recipes included in Rosemary Gladstar's *Herbs for Natural Beauty*. Master this basic recipe, and then you might choose

to substitute infused oils to embellish it. Oils of calendula and St. John's wort promote deep healing of skin. Tinctures can be added to the water portion for healing effect as well. The success of this cream hinges on having about the same proportion of waters to oils and having all the ingredients around the same temperature

### Dried Herb Preparations

Herb powders can be prepared in several ways. Herbs dried whole are ideal, with "cut-and-sift grade" the next best alternative. The more an herb has been broken down, the quicker it loses medicinal value. Herbs should be powdered as they are needed. Grind herbs in a mortar and pestle, or a coffee grinder, then carefully sift them through a fine mesh. Powders can be used in suppositories, capsules, herbal pastes, sinus snuffs, tooth powders, and made into pill balls. Spirulina, nettles, alfalfa, kelp, and rose hips make good nutritive tonics that can be sprinkled on food and into juices and smoothies. Herbal pastes are called *electuaries* and basically are just powdered herbs stirred into honey or vegetable glycerin. This is a particularly good way to give herbs to children or to make tonic preparations for adults.

### *Capsules*

Many people are used to the idea of taking aspirin and other medicines in pill form. Taking encapsulated herbs is comfortable for them. Capsules are convenient, especially for traveling. They are slower acting than tinctures or teas, since the capsule itself needs to be broken down by the stomach acids and the herbs assimilated through the digestive tract. People with poor digestion are not going to benefit as much from taking their medications in capsule form.

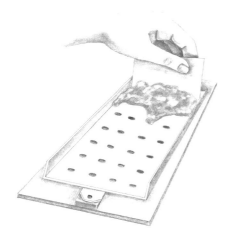

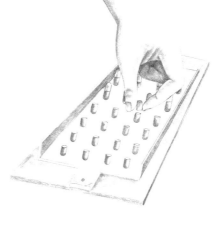

Capsules have no taste, which is an advantage for some situations, but they are definitely not suitable for bitters. Capsules do not keep a long time, as the finely powdered herb within has a limited shelf life of only two to four months. Don't make more than a month's supply at a time when assembling capsules for yourself or clients.

Capsules are easy but time consuming to make. You can buy gelatin or vegetable capsules. Gelatin is made from the hooves of animals; vegetable capsules are made from plant cellulose. These usually come in two sizes. The "00" capsules will hold roughly 0.5 gram of powdered herb. A single "0" capsule will hold roughly 0.35 gram of powdered herb. You can just scoop the powdered herbs from a bowl into the capsules by hand, which we don't recommend unless you have nothing better to do that day. Mail-order catalogs from sources such as Jean's Greens or many health foods stores sell small capping devices such as Cap'M'Quik for about $12. Professional capping machines are available from companies such as Apothecary Products.

Making capsules is easy.

1. Grind the herbs and sift to get a very fine powder.

2. Place the lower half of each capsule in the capsule filler. Spread the powder over the capsules and fill completely.
3. Top the capsules.
4. Place the capsules in sealed containers and clearly label.

Dosage will of course depend on the person, condition, and herbs being used. A common standard dose is two "00" capsules taken two to three times a day.

### Herbal Pills

You can make your own herbal pills by mixing the powdered herbs with equal parts of honey and water to form a paste. Balls of this paste should be rolled in carob powder to prevent them from sticking. Such pills can be made small enough to swallow or they can be a little larger and sucked on. The latter is especially good for sore throats, when you want the medicine to stay in the throat area a bit before going down. Pills will store longer if you dry them out overnight in the gas oven with only the pilot light on. Store in sealed containers.

Pill and capsule preparations more often than not diminish our herbs in the cultural quest for convenience and familiarity. Whole-plant remedies such as teas and tinctures are made from plants with their cell structures basically intact. Powders inevitably lose some of the essences, vitamins, trace minerals, and other goodness that the whole plants offer. The products found in Wal-Mart and other chain drugstores frequently contain fillers and herbs that have been processed with high heat. A community herbalist can deliver the unadulterated freshness that gives herbal pills and capsules medicinal integrity when the situation warrants.

### Poultices

Poultices are ground, chewed, or pulverized fresh or dried plant material that is moistened and applied directly to the skin or between a thin layer of gauze. The skin is the largest organ of the body and is able to absorb the healing qualities of plant medicines. Poultices can be used to help soothe irritations, heal bruises and wounds, break up congestion, and reduce muscle and joint inflammations. They withdraw pus, toxins, and embedded particles in the skin. Poultices can also help heal tumors, cysts, and cancers (both on the skin and within organ systems).

Here's the procedure for making a basic herb poultice:

1. Chop the herb or put it into a blender. Add moisture in the form of either vinegar or water. A bit of whole-grain flour helps to achieve the desired consistency. The blended herbs should be more like thick oatmeal than pea soup.
2. Pat this onto a cloth and place it, herb-side down, on the injury. Make sure open wounds are thoroughly cleaned and irrigated with an antiseptic first. Wrap the herb poultice in gauze before applying it to an open wound. This prevents any damage to the healing tissue when the poultice is removed.
3. Cover with plastic and wrap with an Ace bandage.
4. Leave in place for at least one hour. A poultice can be left on longer if no infection is present. Definitely change poultices every eight hours.

Common herbs and vegetables used for poultices include cabbage, onions, ginger, mustard, and lobelia. Choose the herb according to the action required. Be aware that some poultices, such as mustard, can irritate the skin, so check them frequently. The many beneficial healing properties of comfrey make it among our favorite herbs to poultice. We use both the leaves and the root at different times. Comfrey helps regenerate muscle, skin, and bone cells. It can be used for cysts, sprains, broken bones, and pulled or torn ligaments.

## PLANT ALCHEMY

The herbal pharmacist relies on a working knowledge of how to best draw the healing properties of each herb into useful medicine. Herbalists embrace varying degrees of detail to make those medicines as effective as possible. We'll be the first to admit, though, that the plants ultimately know more about these things than we might ever discern. We also acknowledge that folkloric tinctures have proved themselves again and again for our family. Plant alchemy based primarily on spiritual infusion indeed has healing virtue. Still, herbal medicine for many of us is that much more intriguing when we venture deeper into botanical nuance.

Years of scientific experimentation have pointed the way to the best methods for processing and extracting each crude herb. The heyday of Eclectic medicine determined much of what we understand today about optimal harvest timing, using fresh or dried herb, and the ideal ratio of menstruum solvents. John Uri Lloyd, the eminent late nineteenth-/early twentieth-century pharmacist, strove for strength in his medicines as well as quality. He achieved both with his sure-fire conviction that no one constituent could adequately represent the crude herb as a whole. His understanding of colloidal chemistry, reagents (such as the alkaloid adsorbent he named Alcrestain), and specialized equipment (have a look at the Lloyd cold extractor in the Smithsonian Museum sometime) allowed him to refine continually his medicinal plant products. The drug strength of Lloyd's Specific Medicines were generally considered to be about eight times that of tinctures. Inert and toxic solutes had been removed to achieve this concentration.

While many community herbalists are not likely to venture into such highly refined processing, our collective understanding of plant medicines benefits from those who contemplate the finer points of nuance. The essential minerals in a plant that are not soluble in alcohol, for instance, do not need to be lost in the tincturing process. David Winston of Herbalist & Alchemist has found that by calcining the plant residues (essentially burning the marc to white ash), these minerals can be rejoined with the liquid extract. "Most tinctures have zero minerals," David points out. "If you are taking a tincture like alfalfa, nettles, horsetail, or raspberry leaf—and you are taking them primarily because these herbs have mineral-rich qualities—you are not getting them in the tincture." We've already discussed the value of vinegar as a decent

solvent for pulling out some minerals as well. Understanding the qualities of the herb and the desired use points the way to a specific preparation process.

"We have not just a formula for each herb but a biospecific recipe," says David. "Some herbs need to first be acidified with vinegar. Others get hydrolyzed, meaning that herb is in water for eight hours before we add the alcohol. Certain roots and barks are best cooked in an overnight decoction. Take astragalus. If you grind up these roots, tincture it in alcohol and water for a couple of weeks, and then press it—you have garbage. You have to cook astragalus first in water for a substantial period of time, and, once it cools down, then add the alcohol. Or look at slippery elm. This herb works because of its polysaccharides. When you make a tincture of slippery elm, there are no polysaccharides absorbed. You can figure this out from learning about the chemical constituents, or you can just put some slippery elm in your mouth and chew it a bit. Feels slimy, right? But put the tincture in your mouth and there's no slime."

This herbalist's take on what works and what doesn't in medicine making derives from more than thirty years of attention to detail. All herbalists absorb the good bits of nuance with time. We're like a tincture in this respect. With our best possible plant preparations in hand, let's proceed to understanding how such medicines can be chosen for a specific healing purpose.

### The Art of Formulation

Seeing a master formulator in action inspires every new herb student. Experienced herbalists know which herbs are compatible and which ones possess a vital synergistic affinity

*Text continues on page 254.*

# Jean Argus

I WAS ON THE VERGE of tears with my job [customer service rep for Quaker State Oil] and having just gone through a divorce," Jean Argus recalls, when she joined her brother for a four-day sweat lodge at Sage Mountain in Vermont. That experience led her to Rosemary Gladstar's apprenticeship course in 1989, which "changed my life forever." This was a case where the early riser made the tea: "I loved blending the herbs on Rosemary's shelves to make the morning tea." And so was born the inkling of an idea.

The original conception of Jean's Greens keyed on Jean's knack for searching out good deals. Apprentices at Sage Mountain needed supplies to make medicines, and Jars From Jean offered the small quantities needed. This grew into a supply flyer distributed at herb conferences. "My brother, Phil, got my first big contract to supply a clinic with a detoxifying blend of tea herbs. We created a new formula which was better-tasting, more effective, and cheaper to use. Soon I was making up individual tea bags for patients, and today we sell our Z-Z-Z Tox tea to over fifty clinics," says Jean.

Demand grew as the business developed. Jean shocked everybody when she quit her job to pursue an herbal livelihood full-time. Jean's Greens started in a dining room, expanded to a larger house, and now has settled vibrantly on an abandoned dairy farm south of the Adirondacks. Whether happily directing her "Green Team" of women employees, tending to chickens run amok in a vast organic garden, or creating a new herbal formulation, this is a woman fulfilled.

Jean's business showed a profit in its third year. "We filled a need. You can't create a need on the marketplace, the need has to be there." The herb inventory is utilized for customer sales and to make products. "Herbs don't sit on the shelf long here," she explains. Purchasing from an herbalist who inherently knows such quality considerations is the best assurance going. Jean reports that demand has reached a plateau of sorts after ten years, for which she's glad: "You need to be able to run a business without it ruining your life. I've learned my limitations and to delegate more laborious aspects to others. Younger people want to grab a piece of everything, and once their business starts moving, they get greedy."

Sales for Jean's Greens hinge on her extensive mail-order catalog. "I had the idea on the beach in Belize of lightly imprinting a botanical image behind the product listings on each page." Artist friends offered their services, and soon each page was underlaid with a subtle green drawing and the botanical description and traditional uses of the plant pictured. The 10,000 catalogs printed for the year 2000 cost one dollar each to print and mail. Postage on mailing half these catalogs to the current customer list amounts to

*You can't create a need on the marketplace, the need has to be there.*

—JEAN ARGUS

$2,700; the other 5,000 catalogs go out by request in the year ahead. "We date when orders are received as a means of tracking who needs a new catalog. These only go out to people who've ordered in the past 18 months," says Jean, ever conscious of the high cost of a mail-order business. Customers from years past can always call when they notice their expected catalog missing, thus saving a precious paper resource from one-time whims. Catalogs are mailed in early November, and a spring newsletter keeps customers informed of new products and upcoming herbal events in upstate New York.

The retail shop component of Jean's Greens has increased considerably since the move to Norway, New York, and currently runs at about 20 percent of the business gross. "We see twelve to fifteen customers in here on an average Saturday, which is a lot for a rural area. I enjoy the retail part," says Jean, "but only because this is not

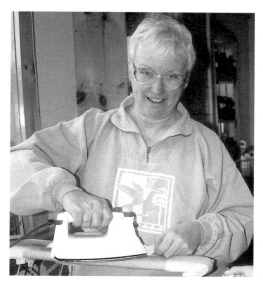

a shop where I sit around and wait for customers to come." A vibrant mail-order business needs such a day for Jean to keep up with the many details of good recordkeeping and planning. "And when I need to get away, all of the ladies on the 'Green Team' are willing to help out."

Herbs are kept in glass gallon jars, 5-gallon buckets, and 15-gallon plastic drums. Bulk purchases are received in an unheated storeroom for distribution according to need:

mixing teas, bagging herb orders, or maintaining reserves of the most requested herbs. An alphabetized listing of herbs in each size category keeps inventory dated and in proper rotation. Jean's greens come from an array of sources: "Trinity, Trout Lake, and Nature's Cathedral have been good, and locally I like Healing Spirits. Once my prices are locked in the catalog, however, I have to shop around when a regular supplier's price goes up." Jean learned a pricing lesson from a unique arrangement with a family of six home-schooled kids down the road. Each child brought in a basket full of corn silk, properly trimmed back to green wispy hairs, for the delivered promise of $2 an ounce in payment. Jean laughs, "Only later, once I dried the silks [a process in which weight goes considerably down], did I realize I'd be losing money selling at $3 an ounce in the catalog."

"I prefer to call our processing area the Lab. It was designed with the FDA in mind . . . they would not be happy if we called it a 'home kitchen' or 'kitchen.' There should be no food cooked or consumed in an area where preparations are made. We make all our custom products here," says Jean, as our eyes adjust to the glare of stainless steel. Tinctures made on

the premises can meet the most rigorous inspection standards. "We double macerate our echinacea tincture by adding the roots to the flowering tops already tinctured at the height of summer. I like to think that with two infusions I guarantee the customer maximum medicinal value. We get a delightful orange color with California poppy by doing this same thing.

"Here's where we make our own bug repellent, a sweet dream balm, even Jean's Green Shampoo with Irish Moss." Salves handcrafted by Gretchen Gould of Herb Hill in Rensselaerville offer an extensive catalog array to go with the home lab's one olive oil infusion of fresh plantain, comfrey, St. John's wort, and calendula. "Our Blue Chamomile Face Cream is quite popular. The recipe came from an old book given to me by a relative. I had learned the basics of making cream in Rosemary's course, added a few creative additions, and Blue Chamomile *happened.* We use an electric hand blender to mix the oils in a water base. Once the cream starts cooling, we work fast to get it in the jars to prevent layering."

*Jean has since sold her business with full intentions of enjoying her herbal retirement. The business carries on in capable hands, as you will find in our herbal resources section. The challenges and pleasures of meeting home herbalist needs with a mail order business are still one and the same.* ❧

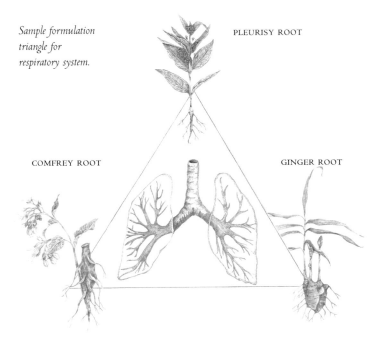

*Sample formulation triangle for respiratory system.*

PLEURISY ROOT

COMFREY ROOT

GINGER ROOT

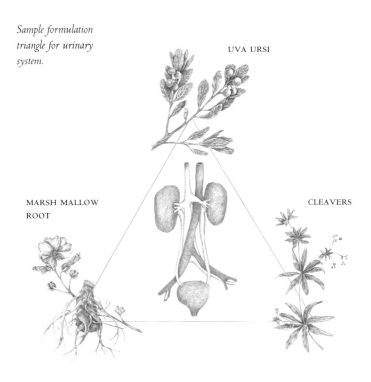

*Sample formulation triangle for urinary system.*

UVA URSI

MARSH MALLOW ROOT

CLEAVERS

for each other. These folks will step into their herb rooms and come out minutes later with a good-tasting and effective medicinal tea for a urinary infection; or herbal pill balls tasty enough for a five-year-old with a sore throat; or a compounded tincture extract that addresses one immediate symptom and the underlying constitutional imbalance.

Knowing an ever increasing repertoire of herbs well is integral to making sense of the art of formulating. We've seen the confused look in many an herb student's eye when formulation is being taught. Nancy thought at one point that teaching formulation to beginning students wasn't a good idea. Understanding the actions of enough herbs comes first. But now we understand the wisdom of introducing formulation early on in our classes. Students add to their materia medicas that much faster by experiencing how the known qualities of different herbs can be combined for healing purposes.

Some herbalists prefer to work with one herb at a time. Certainly this works well in some situations, such as ginger for nausea. However, this is not always the most advantageous way to use herbs. Some plants have a very strong medicinal effect and need to be buffered with other herbs. Senna, for example, is a powerful cathartic used for constipation, but it can cause painful gripping if used alone. Its action can be buffered with the addition of soothing slippery elm and carminitive herbs such as ginger and fennel.

The alchemy involved in combining herbs lies in the end result being greater than the sum of its parts. It's a kind of synergy whereby each herb in the formulation enhances the action of the other herbs. The combined herbs offer greater effectiveness and potency. Three major factors comprise the thinking behind a good formula. First, we choose herbs that address the primary area of concern. Second, we also want to include herbs that tone, build, and fortify the entire body. *Never waver from building overall health in an herbal practice!* Last, we need to stimulate and activate both the body organs and the herbs in the formula for healing purpose.

A master formulator starts out with a mission statement. A simple expression of the goal helps one focus on what needs to be accomplished with the formula. Here's a concise example: "I want to create a formula for a respiratory infection. It will help clear up symptoms of congestion, liquid in the lungs, and painful coughing."

All this comes together in visualizing a triangular framework to guide our formulating. The three points of the triangle represent the three goals stated above. Rosemary Gladstar has introduced many herbalists to this approach in her writings and teachings. Nancy has become well versed in this method by using it personally and for teaching students. We're going to assign certain herbs to the three points of the triangle as seen in the diagram on page 254.

### Point One: Primary or Specific Herbs

The herbs aimed at addressing the specific problem comprise 70 to 80 percent of the formula. These are the army generals, the ones that go out and get the job done. This point can consist of either one or more herbs. Any herb can be in this position depending on the formula, but for the sake of teaching, let's choose some powerful ones to get the idea across. Pleurisy root would serve well for a respiratory infection formula. Uva ursi would be included for a urinary tract infection. Crampbark would be a point one herb in a formula for severe menstrual cramps.

### Point Two: The Supporters, Builders, and Nourishers

Herbs that are soothing, toning, and nourishing usually comprise 10 to 20 percent of the formula. These are reminiscent of nurses, assisting the general(s) on point one, by gently going in and supporting body systems and specific organs. These herbs nourish the body as a whole and help restore vital life force. A nurse for pleurisy root in the respiratory formula could be comfrey root, which is astringent and mucilaginous at the same time. A nurse for uva ursi to help support healing of a urinary tract infection could be marsh mallow root. Chamomile would be soothing and supportive in the point two position for menstrual cramps.

### Point Three: The Activators and Catalysts

These herbs serve to activate both the specific body organs and to catalyze the action of the other herbs in the formula. These can perk up the organs, provide heat, break up congestion, and help the body eliminate. Herbal action groups that often get used here are stimulants, laxatives, diuretics, diaphoretics, and expectorants. Point three herbs comprise 10 to 20 percent of the formula. Ginger could be an activator for a respiratory infection formulation. It would bring warmth and movement. Cleavers, with its strong diuretic properties could be a mover in the urinary formula. Pennyroyal and ginger could be the activators in the menstrual cramp example. Pennyroyal can help bring on bleeding and ginger helps with nausea, so it would depend on the symptoms.

A few basic tenets go into choosing the herbs that occupy the three points of the formulation triangle. Do not get carried away by adding too many herbs into the formula just because all are apt for a certain situation. A few herbs wisely selected will be more effective than every herb under the sun haphazardly heaped together. Don't mix roots and leaves together in a medicinal tea formula, as these require different methods of preparation. Recommended proportions between the points can be shifted to meet the needs of the situation at hand. Good formulations evolve by adjusting the herbs according to what actually works, not by being rigid about rules. All the herbs used must not only harmonize among themselves, but be directed toward the specific intent of the formula.

Formulating is definitely both an art and a science. We use our intuition and our knowledge of plant actions, energetics, and constituents. We not only need to understand the plants but also the body. All of this is a plateful. Start simple. Be open to guidance and others' ideas. The nuances behind using our medicines become clear only with practice—lots and lots of practice!

### A Word about Dosages

Recommending effective dosages is the last step in bringing our preparation and formulation skills together. To do this, we have to have a good knowledge of the herbs, the strength of the preparations we are using, and the workings of the body. A wise approach is to start with a smaller dose and increase it if necessary. When recommending herbs to someone outside your home, follow up with a phone call after a couple of days to hear how your client is reacting.

Herbs are generally grouped as nourishing, tonifying, specifically medicinal, and potentially toxic. The nourishing herbs are the safest and rarely exhibit side effects, although just as with any food, they can cause an idiosyncratic response. Exact amounts of nourishing herbs are not so crucial, although again, like food, you certainly can overdo a good thing. Tonics are often used for long periods of time, and the specific medicinal herbs for shorter lengths. Dosages with these two groups are more critical to positive outcomes. Toxic herbs are really in a category all by themselves: Use only calculated low doses for very short periods of time.

Bodies come in all shapes and sizes, conditions and temperaments. Who we are affects the way Earth medicines are going to work. Large, robust individuals as a general rule require larger doses than small and frail folk. Conditions such as pregnancy, high blood pressure, and chronic kidney or liver imbalance all have to be taken into account. Many dosages are given for the hypothetical 150-pound adult male. Clark's Rule allows us to extrapolate from there: *Divide the weight in pounds by 150 to give the approximate fractional dose.* A 50-pound child, for example, would receive one-third of the recommended dose.

Herbalists have many different approaches to dosages. Some use only one drop of a tincture (not to mention those who don't even use leaves, flowers, or roots, but simply evoke the plant spirit), while other people use megadoses of standardized extracts. These huge variations always stem from one's underlying philosophies. Perhaps in the long and winding trail of our tradition, here is the one other place—besides avoiding those dang aluminum pans—we can come to some agreement. It's not about the actual dosages themselves, but about respecting why we indeed differ. The wisdom each herbalist holds of plant alchemy

# SIMPLES, FORMULAS, OR BOTH?

Herbs can be formulated and blended on the spot for each unique person. This medicinal combination of herbs can readily be adjusted as the person's symptoms change. What one person may need for a migraine headache or irritable bowel syndrome might not be what a generic remedy includes.

We leave the majority of our dried herbs in single bulk containers until needed. Then the person's tastes, health situation, symptoms, and constitution can all be taken into consideration when formulating the herbs. Grind whole herbs into powders right before they are needed, because most powdered herbs lose their potency more quickly than when they are left whole. Having a few broad-serving teas and capsules available in a community apothecary is helpful if the only person fluent in herbal formulating is unavailable to do custom blending. Herbal tea blends labeled as Respiratory Tonic or Fever Breaker become a godsend in those situations. The one marketing advantage of blending dried herbs in tea or capsule form ahead of time is the appeal that these remedies have for people buying herbs without a consultation.

Tinctures have additional advantages and disadvantages as either single (*simple*) or compound (*formula*) extracts. The herbs chosen for a specific tincture formulation often are not ready to be harvested at the same time. Nor is the recommended solvency for such an assortment of fresh herbs usually one and the same. Nancy's relaxation formula with skullcap, oats, hops, spearmint, and valerian, for example, features herbs that aren't necessarily at their peak vibrancy at the same moment. We make extracts of these herbs separately, each at its own determined solvency, and only later proportionally combine these simples to create the compound extract. On other occasions we deliberately blend a few fresh herbs (when possible from the point of view of harvest and solvency) with the belief that synergy during the macerating process adds to that formula's potency. But mostly we leave the majority of our tinctures as simples, so we can then individually tailor a formula for specific needs.

Most herbalists will agree that a combination of herbs in the body often works more effectively than one single herb alone. A good formula and bed rest can be all that's needed for an acute imbalance. Any botanical subtleties lost in a combination of herbs are offset by synergistic effects. Choosing to keep a variety of useful formulas on hand to cover the majority of a community's health situations might indeed be appropriate elsewhere. Each herbalist ultimately needs to decide which approach works best to serve his or her own people.

---

most definitely reflects those beliefs we hold so near and dear.

## HERBAL MARKETING PROSPECTUS

How wonderful it is to dream that one can make a viable livelihood by sharing genuine healing preparations within one's own community. Being able to supply a keen demand has always been integral to business success. And certainly interest in the healing herbs continues to grow every day. Natural approaches to common ailments work, as more and more people (and their doctors!) are discovering. The intense need for deeper healing by so many just about takes our breath away.

The availability of local plants, plus apothecary integrity, plus ever increasing demand is indeed a formula with great entrepreneurial promise. Flexing of the green—both in the generous nature of plants and the more prosaic dollar sense— gets the marketing blood raring to go. Herbs now make the Top Ten list of businesses on the rise. Yet before we bestow our blessings on any herbal venture, and possibly get caught up in dizzying finances, let's affirm the fundamental gift the plants themselves offer us human beings. *The plants freely give to help make us well.* Certainly we are entitled to make a good living at our craft. Yet the marketing precepts of the growth economy for profit's sake alone should not be allowed to alter our precious connection to what healing is all about. Next we're going to talk about community-based businesses that serve people with love, integrity, and respect. We're not going to trip into the lights fantastic of Wall Street and unfettered capitalism.

## Money Matters

Startup capital for any sound business idea is a must. Small beginnings can be humble and often serve as a good transition time to figure out marketing strategies and a reasonable production process. Yet supplies, labels, and brochures of even the simplest nature require an investment of hard-earned cash, preferably your own. A bootstrap operation requires a good, practical product with a quick turnaround in order to get a homegrown business up and running. Starting slow and steady gives a business time to grow sustainable roots and find appreciative markets.

Putting a price on each product that recoups all expenses and earns a livelihood is the crux of the matter. Prices for similar herbal products sold elsewhere somewhat determine the range within which we each must work. A market that values quality and

community connection will pay more for a local product only up to a point. However, underselling yourself ensures reaching that burnout point of no return. A fair price needs to be fair to the people your products can help and fair to you.

Distinguishing between wholesale and retail prices reflects the costs of being in two entirely different businesses. A *maker* covers the time and costs that go into creating a product. A *seller* ups that wholesale price to cover the time and costs of bringing those products to market. One all-too-common mistake on the home business front, for entrepreneurs who pursue wholesale marketing as well as sell their wares directly to local people, arises from not keeping these two aspects of their business separate. The wholesale price needs to work in the markets deemed ideal for the products being offered. Retail outlets have pricing formulas that range anywhere from a markup of 50 percent (typical in many grocery stores) to 100 or 200 percent in the community natural foods store, to as high as 300 or 400 percent in some high-end gift shops and glossy mail-order operations. Many companies offer a *suggested retail price* for each product. In reality, the maker has no control over the actual retail price his or her products will sell for. And once you accept the marketplace on its own terms— you really have little choice—it becomes easier to entertain your own retail prospects. As a seller, you essentially need to purchase your own products at the same wholesale price offered to any other business. You may choose to undersell your suggested retail price, thereby gaining a slight advantage for direct sales at the farmers' market or in the community apothecary over other stores carrying your local products at full price. You may establish tiers of retail pricing:

Sales that come knocking at the door incur less selling expense than mail-generated orders. A sensibly high retail price allows you to offer the occasional special without sacrificing profits on the margin over the entire year. Whatever the pricing choices you make as a seller, that fundamental rule of covering all costs remains.

Determining the costs of making a product requires good record keeping and a good sense of how to account for labor and overhead. *Pricing equations* provide an initial sense of where to begin. One simple approach to wholesale pricing is to double the cost of ingredients and then tack on a reasonable hourly wage based on the time it takes to make a product. If this ballpark figure sounds reasonably competitive, start with that price until you can get a firmer handle on your business as a whole. Others might decide to quadruple the cost of all the direct inputs (including packaging, as well as what actually goes into the herbal preparation) and forego trying to figure out the labor involved. Tracking hours allows you to determine if your time is worth $2 an hour or $20. Don't be discouraged in the beginning months or even in the first few years of a business, however, because a time investment goes hand in hand with capital investment to get a business established. What ultimately counts is having enough to live on and satisfying the goals you set for yourself.

If, in following these formulas, a price results that is much too high to be competitive, that's a clue you need to make some changes in production. Becoming more efficient could be as simple as investing in a tincture press. Conversely, maybe you are doing the best you can without sacrificing the virtues of healing plants and those lofty goals that launched your business. Grass-

roots marketing often involves educating your clientele that good quality and conscientious care indeed justify a higher price.

Stores generally rely on a *percentage markup* that results in a profitable bottom line when the financial tallies for the year are done. Different types of markets have their own markups that reflect the cost of doing business. A community herb store, for instance, might decide that marking up products from outside vendors at 100 percent (doubling the purchase price) and keeping a slightly lower markup on in-house products (based on an accurate in-house wholesale price) makes the hours put into retailing worthwhile. Play around with what works so that it all balances in the end. "Our markup varies," reports Shatoiya de la Tour of Dry Creek Herb Farm. "If we find a high-quality product that would really serve our customers, but it's pricey, we may choose to make less money on it, just to encourage sales."

Despite all those good healing intentions, a home-based business venture might not be suitable for everybody. Perhaps you will find success beyond your wildest dreams. Perhaps all that dedicated work just doesn't pay in the end. Either way, we need to adjust to make the business fit our lives. Finding balance and being happy ultimately count the most. Unexpected doors often lead to the vital answers we seek. Whatever happens, don't lose that precious connection to the plants and the joy of being of service.

## Marketing Mix

Some herbalists choose to specialize in a particular type of product line. A wide selection of healing salves, say, or cosmetics and body care products. Other community entrepreneurs with direct sales in mind entertain the challenge of offering it all: bulk teas,

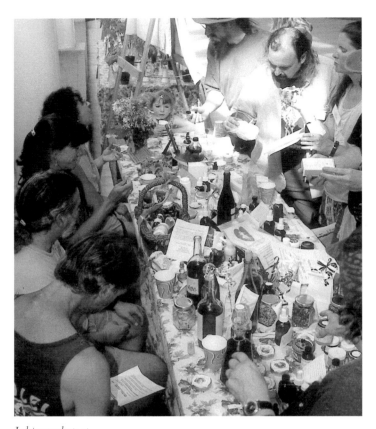

medicinal tinctures, select infused oils, an acclaimed syrup, a potent love potion, ceremonial smudge sticks, and soaps to boot.

We start off with our best products and expand from there. Filling a niche begins with a limited product line that can grow naturally. Offering a unique product can provide a vital foot in the door at regional markets, thereby ensuring a cash flow while venturing toward more commonly available products. Almost every community has healing needs that are not being met locally. Researching the production realities behind these possibilities can be as easy as touching base with other community herbalists. Networking through a regional or statewide association is the best way to learn where to get supplies, what regulations are inescapable, and about marketing approaches that work. Community medicine need not be so

competitive that we can't help each other meet the needs of local people everywhere.

Joyce Wardwell has found that purchasing essential oils helps support her more locally based medicines. "I do love a good whiff of rose attar," says Joyce. "I sell these little oil blends—holiday spice, tranquility, lavender—all made with essential oils. Those are my bread and butter; the oils pay for the other stuff I do. People smell them and buy them up. I can bring out good-quality herbs and tinctures [at gatherings and talks], and I am lucky if I sell $100 worth. But people buy the oils every time."

7Song sells his tinctures at the local co-op in Ithaca, New York. Other local products are emphasized in this food store as well. The support for local economy shows in the display. "Our products are right in your face," says 7Song, "and the other national brands are above and below. Ours sell the best. Echinacea is one of the only over-touted herbs that consistently works. I sell more of it than anything else." Once people discover that such a tried-and-true local product works effectively, their willingness to try similar local products grows.

The adage that *the customer is always right* might not necessarily be true, but we're best advised to treat our customers as though it were. Good service amounts to standing behind our product through both the good and the mistaken times. Being a good listener with a smile shows you care what customers think. People who are comfortable with us often help build our business in ways the big corporations can only envy.

And that thought brings us to advertising. Word-of-mouth praise from existing customers is the best bet by far. A printed brochure and business cards to hand out help make those mysterious connections that seem to come out of the blue months later. We'll explore brochure basics more thoroughly when we discuss word-of-mouth success in chapter 8 (see page 275). Building a mailing list from the moment that first customer walks through the door is crucial. Flyers, newsletters, and special product promotions follow from there. Community exposure helps spread the word about any local business. Giving free herb walks, presenting school programs, and talking to garden clubs are proven ways to let people know what you have to offer as a community herbalist. Many times a good press release—about such free events or your latest business venture—reaches many more readers of the local newspaper than money spent on display advertising. Regional ads work best in newsletters and quarterlies specifically aimed at interested herbalists.

## Supply-Side Economics

No matter how hard we try, we've yet to produce a New Hampshire coconut oil or a blown glass tincture bottle on our farm. Finding quality supplies at a reasonable price is a business necessity. The persistent effort that goes into comparing prices and assessing all the options available in packaging and additional product lines pays off every time.

*The Herbal Green Pages* put together by Maureen Rogers of the Herb Growing and Marketing Network (see appendix six) is by far the most complete source of herbal suppliers. Herbalists are well advised to get their own services and offerings listed here as well. Members receive as many words as needed to detail their business, as well as a free listing on the network's Web site; nonmembers are limited to a 45-word byline in the book version alone. This herbal resource guide sells for half the price of the $95 annual membership. Once in hand, you'll be able to find exactly the kind of connection you most need.

One way to make a positive difference in this throwaway society is to pack our good-Earth herbs using good-Earth common sense. Cellophane bags are much more environmentally friendly than plastic and equally good at protecting dry herbs from moisture. Unfortunately, cellophane is quite a bit more expensive and harder to track down. Glass jars are prettier by far than plastic, and often the more popular sizes come priced about the same. The best aspect of glass, and one of the things we like, is refilling bottles and jars for customers. Recycling the glass is the next best alternative. We've taken to offering those droppers that come with most tincture bottles separately for 75 cents apiece. People tend to save their droppers when they realize there's a direct cost otherwise.[12] We advise use of a measuring spoon for proper dosage anyway. All mail shipments can take advantage of recycled materials, from the box itself to reusable Styrofoam peanuts.

Bottling our medicines and applying labels adds to the labor cost of each product. The fastest (and thus the least expensive) way to fill tincture bottles is with a pump dispenser. Food-grade plastic containers with a 1-ounce pump dispenser are available from SKS Bottle and Packaging. Each press of the pump releases an ounce of tincture. We try to encourage the purchase of 2- and 4-ounce bottles of tinctures, which simply require additional pumps of the dispenser. Labeling remains a labor of love until the business gets big enough to afford a label-applying machine. Such machines do exist, but, because of their high cost no community herbalist will be setting one up at home anytime soon.

# THE REALITY OF THE FDA

THE ESTABLISHMENT of the Food and Drug Administration in 1938 led to federal oversight of the production and marketing of any drug, natural or synthetic, in the United States. New legislation in 1962 required drugs to be proved both safe and effective. The ensuing regulations set a financially successful course only for those medicines that could justify the investment cost of meeting those regulations. Unpatentable phytomedicines (those good precious herbs available to everyone on Earth) could not offset the costs required in the drug regulatory process precisely because the return on that investment could not be pro-

tected. Botanical medicines literally drifted out of the pharmacies and into health foods stores, where they are now regulated as dietary supplements under the Dietary Supplement Health and Education Act (DSHEA) of 1994. A current proposal in these days of so-called free trade to reclassify herbs and supplements as over-the-counter drugs will surely change the community-level leeway now available to herbalists.

Let's talk about regulatory reality as it exists today. Common sense and healing integrity need to go hand in hand with the making of plant medicines regardless of FDA oversight. The bureaucracy's problem is in not being able to

trust anybody. Regulations aimed at blatant disregard in the preparation process typically address the worst possible scenario. As herbs are considered to be foods, then food sanitation laws come into effect. These laws insist on such things as having a bathroom available that does not open into the preparation area, sealed walls and floors, and a triple stainless-steel sink.

Herbalists have every reason to applaud a clean environment in which to prepare healing herbs. The investment to modify a home or establish a commercial processing facility to meet legal requirements, however, could dash community-level hopes from the start. Enter

---

### Growing a Business

Extending your outreach beyond community boundaries may be key to establishing a viable trade. You'll need plenty of market savvy to launch a mail-based business. Wholesale connections require travel time and salesmanship of a different sort.

Sandy Maine of the Sun Feather Natural Soap Company shares her business odyssey in *Creating an Herbal Bodycare Business*. The stories behind several other successful herbal ventures are included in her book as well. She presents the ups and downs of marketing products, and gives a practical sense of what a business really costs to start—not only in money but also in time and effort.

Sandy reminds herbal entrepreneurs that planting a dream involves a lot of consideration. Lee Sturdivant offers up equally telling insights in her portion of *Medicinal Herbs in the Garden, Field and Marketplace.*

Good visions are worth pursuing. If you've got the gumption, know that the plants are willing and waiting partners in supporting an Earth-centered livelihood.

### A RIGHTEOUS LABEL

"We are safe in predicting that no patient will object to neatness and elegance in the dispensing of medicines; and that few there will be who do not rebel, mentally at least, when slovenly served," said Dr. Harvey Felthe human factor. Both state and federal inspectors have been known to overlook good faith efforts toward a "legal kitchen" that exhibit plain ol' common sense. Quite a few regional medicine makers we visited didn't have the infamous triple sink. Regulators have a big enough job just keeping up with larger food processors and commercial kitchens.

Avoiding antagonizing these folks makes a world of difference. Read about labeling concerns at the end of this chapter. Use only ingredients that are generally recognized as safe (such GRAS lists are available through the Federal Register). Keep your customers happy, as complaints usually trigger more formal investigations. Avoid alienating competitors. Manufac-

turers previously busted for a bogus label claim tend to want to point out a similar disregard to regulatory agencies. All in all, make your herbal preparations as clean, unadulterated, effective, and reasonably priced as humanly possible. Be proud of what you do.

And also remain wary. The current effort under way in the FDA to implement good manufacturing practices (GMP) guidelines will impose burdensome regulations on small-scale producers of herbal products. Requirements to submit samples of all herbs for testing and "laboratory-type conditions" for manufacturing facilities steps beyond the kitchen basics just described. The Codex Alimentarius Commission (of free-trade fame) has been charged

with harmonizing standards and laws of different countries, to create one single, uniform standard for the pharmaceutical industry. Most commission members are representatives of pharmaceutical companies. These are their recommendations: *No vitamin, mineral, herb, etc., can be sold for preventative or therapeutic use. None sold as food can exceed potency (dosage) levels set by the commission. Codex regulations for dietary supplements would become binding. All new dietary supplements would automatically be banned unless they go through the Codex approval process.*

The FDA has stated freely that it intends to implement the recommendations of the Codex Commission into its policies. We, the people, might wish to set a different agenda.

---

ter, speaking of the early days of Eclectic medicine, when physicians needed to be pharmacists as well.[13]

Community herbalists often provide tinctures and bulk herbs as indicated in a client's consultation. Commonsense instructions for use are given verbally and on a separate written sheet. A simple envelope label works to list the herb name and the date on a resealable plastic bag for tea mix or a bottled tincture. Nothing fancy, just fast and essentially cheap. Such basic medicine of the people comes without fanfare and is backed solely by experienced intent. You can certainly share a bit of herbal artistry, whether that means flower stickers used to embellish plain paper

stock sealed behind clear tape, or a hand-drawn design that celebrates your herbal energy. We wrote in tincture and salve ingredients for many years on 2 × 3-inch white label stock preprinted with a sketch of our farm and name/address in black ink.[14] Home-based labels serve the purpose well when no marketing plans exist to expand beyond day-to-day interactions within the community.

Which brings us to a second, slightly more commercial approach to label investment. Simplicity can still rule, but now we consider marketing tangibles that reach beyond the circle of our immediate neighborhoods. Once you find yourself offering a line of medicinal products in one or more venues, either directly at the local farmers' market or wholesaling to several natural foods stores, hand-writing labels gets tedious. The homey look may not falter beside the successful graphic art of established herb companies, but *you* most certainly will if you begin spending as much time on labeling as you do on growing the herbs and making the medicines.

Startup labels can be printed with space left to fill in the details for many different herbal products. That is, the logo, business address, and an information framework (*Ingredients:* or *Traditional dosage of __ ml per day,* for instance) are put onto full sheets of peel-off label stock at the printer. Richard McDonald in Silver City, New Mexico, uses a desktop publishing program on a computer to type in the product name and ingredients list on such blank labels as needed in his herb store. The herbalists down the street at Bear Creek Herbs fill in the blanks by hand with assorted colored pens to make a master label sheet for each product and then they run these through a color copier. Snip, snip—the labels are cut and then applied with slightly wider clear tape to protect them from damage. Labels for bags of bulk herbs, multiple-size tincture bottles, and salve jars can be printed.

Label size commits you to a certain bottle or jar size. Putting a small label on bigger containers works too, of course, but this option somehow always looks chintzy. The ability to utilize a personal computer to produce labels from start to finish on a color printer means you can adjust sizes, switch ingredient lists, even alter an initial logo whenever and in whatever quantity. But computers are a substantial investment too, and you might not want to come out of your gardens or medicine shop to learn computer skills. Bartering with someone in your neighborhood—family medicine and organic vegetables for revisable labels, say— might be the best startup bet of all.

The day that you can justify the expense of having labels printed in substantial quantities for each and every product will certainly signal a milestone in terms of your successful business savvy. Offset printing beats any computer-generated label we've seen for reproducing glorious logos. That glossy label stock designed to wear through wet and time does indeed catch the potential customer's eye. The temptation to go for the Cadillac model is best held in check by good business sense until your grassroots efforts have launched a humble enterprise to the regional level.

The specifics of what actually needs to be on any label comes down to four straightforward requirements. The *identity of the product* is its common name with which everyone is familiar, such as "herbal tea" or "skin care cream." Most labels highlight a creative product name prominently above the more prosaic identifying name. Smooth Move on a box of Traditional Medicinals tea speaks for itself; "herbal stimulant laxative" just below that clearly identifies the product. Many herbal product manufacturers have wisely stopped calling their spirit-

*A proper product label clearly exhibits the four FDA requirements.*

The identity of the product

Declaration of quantity

List of ingredients

Declaration of responsibility

## Immune Booster Caps

Herbal Dietary Supplement
*100 - 500 mg capsules.*

*New Improved formula containing Reishi and Shiitake mushrooms and Astragalus extract powders. Easily digested, will build vital energy and "calm the spirit", a Qi tonic.*

*Sugg: 1-2 caps 2-3 times per day as part of an overall wellness program. (Formula information available)*

*Jean's Greens Herbal Tea Works!*
*119 Sulphur Springs Rd. Norway, NY (315) 845-6500*

based preparations "tinctures" and instead opt for more innocuous words such as "compounded extract" or "concentrate." The T-word comes direct from the formularies and pharmacopoeias of the past, thereby designating a process once deemed as the manufacture of a drug. Do remember that avoiding such words will always please your local FDA inspector.

A *declaration of quantity* states the weight or measure of the product inside the packaging. This accurate net weight must appear on the front lower third of the label. It can be stated in whole units (pounds or quarts) or fractional units (ounces or fluid ounces). The metric conversion follows immediately behind in parentheses. The *declaration of responsibility* is what those of us outside of bureaucracy call the name, address, and zip code of our business. The company or farm name more often than not proudly gets included in an artistic logo design. Last comes a complete *list of ingredients* in decreasing order of weight or volume. A batch number should be located on the packaging in case the need arises to track the processing details of a problematic product. We've already recommended that tincture makers share the strength ratio and percentage of alcohol used in each maceration so community members can determine extract quality for themselves.

Keep in mind that economy of speech within the current legal framework serves herbalists well. Aggressive promotion of healing attributes is far more likely to put a medicine-making effort under scrutiny. The official attitude holds that food supplements (read "herbs") and good nutrition (read "real food") have little to do with healing anyway. Herb companies that don't blatantly buck that trend fly beneath the regulatory radar screen. The best product

names indicate what a specific herbal preparation traditionally achieves without saying outright what that product may be intended to treat. Again, Smooth Move provides a classic example. If one devises a product name that can be interpreted to have an innocent meaning—a name that has a reasonable nonmedical interpretation without being ridiculous—then it will probably be deemed acceptable, despite having a medical implication. So have fun, don't copy someone else, and trust Spirit to guide your healing purpose.

One standard end-around play when it comes to restrictive regulations goes like this: *I tell customers the truth and I tell the FDA what it wants to hear.* Bureaucratic mandates do not deter the one-to-one level of neighborly concern. We can talk freely about what we know and do not know as caring individuals. Local herbalists have a great advantage here: Our direct contact with the people we serve transcends the usual retail marketing game. Gloss can be replaced with sincerity. Demand for herbs can be based on actual needs met by traditional wisdom. Many small herb companies provide information sheets about certain health or wellness conditions that refer to the herbs historically found to be useful. Keeping such information-sharing separate from the products themselves and bearing little resemblance to the product labels of that company generally satisfies the regulatory folks that you are not making direct health claims.

The American Herbal Products Association can be a good source of information for herb business clarification. Dues start at around $600, however, effectively precluding small companies in their early years from participating in much of this collective experience. State health boards and the FDA do provide the appropriate standards upon inquiry, but it is an effort to wade through their wordy publications. *Herbalgram,* a publication published by the American Botanical Council (see appendix five), serves up breaking news on the regulatory front. However, much of this kind of information simply isn't relevant to helping people feel better. The American Herb Association's quarterly newsletter, edited by Kathi Keville, highlights these issues best and offers additional marketplace insights as well.

Our vision for community herbalists is to restore medicine making into the healing circle, where the direct relationship between plant, patient, and herbalist is celebrated. The gist of what we need to communicate in our labels should meet the regulations, yes, but truly shine when it comes to accentuating local connection.

## NOTES

1. The preferred form of a plant for making medicine is the kind of great details Richo Cech shares in his latest book. See *Making Plant Medicine* (Williams, Oreg.: Horizon Herbs, 2000), 125.

2. Here's a case where the common name for an herb quite accurately describes the bodily results of taking that herb. Just substitute "sh" for the "c" in chittam and you'll know what to expect from taking cascara sagrada.

3. We say "full-strength alcohol" in referring to a 190- or 195-proof spirit knowing damn well that the other 2 to 5 percent of distilled volatiles and water doesn't hold any mathematical relevance for our purposes. Medicine-making manuals that list a targeted solvency of 100 percent are in truth simply rounding up the proof of a grain spirit to reflect its nearly pure alcohol content.

4. Federal law allots an annual production of 200 gallons of cider (or beer or wine) per household.

5. The water content of the fresh herbs then reduces the final alcohol content of the medicine to the 20 to 25 percent range required for spirit-based preservation.

6. The potential alcohol content of cider needs to first be determined by measuring the sugar content (and thus the specific gravity) of the unfermented juice with a hydrometer. Complete fermentation being the norm in a 5 to 8 percent natural fermentation, a cidermaker can then assume the actual alcohol content of the hard cider to be the same as its anticipated potential.

7. Gilian Painter, *A Herbalist's Medicine-Making Workbook* (Auckland, New Zealand: 1998), 28.

8. A 190-proof spirit translates as having a 95 percent alcohol content and a 5 percent water content.

9. Debra St. Claire, *The Herbal Medicine Cabinet* (Berkeley, Calif.: Celestial Arts, 1997), 51.

10. Kathi Keville and Mindy Green, *Aromatherapy: A Complete Guide to the Healing Art* (Freedom, Calif.: Crossing Press, 1995), 120–21.

11. Margi Flint formulates a popular salve for her clients she calls *Slide and Glide.*

12. Be aware that the rubber bulb on an old dropper eventually begins to erode in the alcohol, subsequently contaminating the tincture.

13. H. W. Felter, *The Eclectic Materia Medica, Pharmacology, and Therapeutics* (Cincinnati: John K. Scudder, 1922), 51.

14. These generic Heartsong Farm labels worked equally well on gift jars of dill pickles and boxed beeswax candles adorned with a sprig of everlasting.

# CHAPTER EIGHT
# Spreading the Word

GOLDENSEAL
*Hydrastis canadensis*

*M*y guidance counselor in high school tried to sway me into teaching. I was as adamant as any youth: No way! Both my mom and dad were teachers, so I was sure that I was not going to follow in my parents' footsteps, no matter how admirable. Years later, I have to say that being a teacher gives me the greatest pleasure. I have taught special education and second grade in our local school, filled in at Gracie's Montessori school, led herb classes here at our farm and at conferences, and assisted Rosemary with her apprentice groups at Sage Mountain. This variety of working with both children and adults keeps me fresh. You learn so much yourself—through extra reading, writing up class handouts, and preparing your presentation—because you need to understand something fully to be able to teach it well. A good teacher learns from her students, no matter how young or old they may be. Sharing flows naturally once I've immersed myself in my chosen topic. ❧ Teaching about herbs is truly a double passion because I am able to share what I love. Seeing people become more empowered to take charge of their health fills me with hope and inspiration. I have always loved the old proverb, "If you give a man a fish, he can eat for a day. If you teach a man to fish, he will never go hungry." A core job of every herbalist is to give people their own handle on healing tradition.   —N.P. ❧

PEOPLE ARE THIRSTY for herbal knowledge. One of our most important jobs as community herbalists is teaching others how to care for themselves and their families. Herbs will only be used appropriately if people gain good information. When we share with a mother or father how to use foods and herbs to build overall health—and to have a reverence for Earth and the Creator—then their children are likely to learn this path as well. Our Gracie is constantly at work creating her own flower essences or mixing up an herbal brew in her kitchen play. Five-year-olds who know to chew up plantain leaves to apply as a spit poultice on a bee sting before coming crying to Mom or Dad have made a conscious connection to plant magic. Such a heritage endures for a lifetime. Herbal wisdom will be passed along to their own children when that day comes. Talk about being able to make an enormous impact on the future! We can restore healing tradition in this country simply by giving the next generation a footing in Earth-centered wisdom through their parents.

Much of what needs to be taught is very practical. Sage is used to dry up a mother's milk. Plantain is an excellent drawing poultice. Nettles are high in calcium and iron. The list of plant gifts goes on and on. People need to learn how to make herbal preparations and use them appropriately. We engage the plants directly when we teach about growing herbs, proper plant identification, and wildcrafting techniques. We truly succeed as teachers when our students make that conscious connection of their body and their mind and their spirit to the body/mind/spirit of the natural world. Trust for the body's ability to heal and function in balance and harmony flows from there. Teaching about herbal medicine then goes beyond the practical to the transformational.

## ENCOURAGING HOME HERBALISTS

The adage that *we all need to start somewhere* certainly applies to a caring spouse wondering just where herbs will fit into the family health picture. Enthusiastic teachers can get the medical sufficiency ball rolling once again in every home. Encouraging home herbalists is where we have our biggest influence on the health of our communities.

A home herbalist is someone who has grown up in a household with an herbal tradition or has been "smitten with herbs" somewhere along the way. Maybe he started growing a few herbs in the vegetable or flower gardens and gradually fell in love with the herbs' inner vitality and usefulness. Or possibly she grew dissatisfied with allopathic medicine and began using a natural remedy to treat a particular ailment. Motherhood especially inspires this need to do what's best for our little ones. A dawning realization about what all herbs can provide triggers the desire to learn more. One or two books from the herbal bookshelf help, but they don't quite provide vital hands-on experience and confidence. Community herbalists are that missing link.

If you know something, you can teach. We all know this is true on some level, of course, but most of us really have to work hard to teach well. Those common fears and anxieties about teaching—*Who am I to be doing this anyway?*—need not keep us down. Our credibility lies in loving the plants and being able to take care of our own families. We know enough about our topic to offer the right bits of knowledge that will excite home herbalists to learn more. Some of us have an encyclopedic grasp of a hundred or more herbs, while others are really quite happy celebrating life with a handful of favorites. No beginning student can handle countless details anyway. Merit often lies in the simpler approach.

Teaching, like any skill, needs to be practiced. Good teachers are the ones who have learned how best to articulate ideas by having tried different approaches. Some work great and others do not. Only practice reveals which techniques will engage students. We all have personal takes on stage fright and the like. Ultimately, we just need to plan well and take the plunge. Nancy always says a little prayer before each class: "Calm me and help me to share what will be helpful to these people. Let the teachings of the Creator and the plants flow through me."

Some basic tenets apply to any level of teaching. Having fun yourself makes it more than likely your audience will have fun, too. We share what we know and love, leaving the rest for someone else. Never be afraid to admit what you don't know.

People love handouts that detail the major points of your talk. Include addresses for resources and bibliographies of exemplary books. Establishing an agenda provides the class with a coherent structure for the day and a guidepost for the teacher. Being flexible with the structure can open great dialogue within a group. But spend too much time off-topic and you can disappoint those who really wanted your class presentation in full. Apportioning class time by the half hour helps a teacher stay on task and finish on time. Far-roaming questions are best left for a question-and-answer period at the end if you have a lot of material to cover. Classes that are about an hour and a half long work well with a cross-sectional audience.

*Do not try to satisfy your vanity by teaching a great many things. Awaken people's curiosity. It is enough to open minds; do not overload them. Put there just a spark. If there is some good inflammable stuff, it will catch fire.*

—Anatole France (1844–1924)

Our stories are what make teaching come alive. Sharing personal experiences about plant encounters and herbal remedies makes the knowledge offered more relevant. "My latest story," says Julie Manchester of Woodsong Herbals in Vermont, "involves the use of lavender essential oil to heal some severe second-degree burns I received during an 'unfortunate camping incident' in which our campfire exploded all over my legs. After being told I would have extensive scarring, I went home and used lavender essential oil exclusively on my legs, and have minimal scarring."

Teaching to all the senses beats the droning-on-and-on approach hands down. A few good props allow students to see what's being discussed. Nancy often arranges a platter of herbs according to the subject matter of the day. A class on the nervous system, for example, would feature a tray of eight artistically arranged nervines: chamomile, valerian, hops, St. John's wort, milky oats, skullcap, lemon balm, and linden blossoms. Similarly, freshly harvested plants make a stunning summer bouquet that can be divided up and passed around the class while you teach about each herb. Walks in the summer garden or along a medicinal trail allow each student to see, taste, touch, and smell living plants. It is a Sage Mountain tradition to taste teas in class, but our friend Amy came up with the

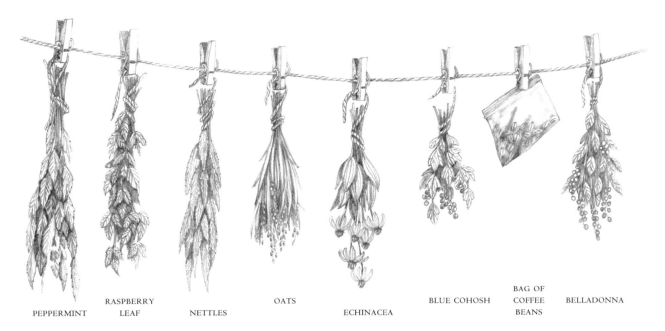

PEPPERMINT    RASPBERRY LEAF    NETTLES    OATS    ECHINACEA    BLUE COHOSH    BAG OF COFFEE BEANS    BELLADONNA

*We distinguish between nutritive, tonic, specific medicinals and low-dose herbs on the herbal clothesline. The line between the groups isn't always that clear. We should never view all herbs as gentle and nontoxic, nor should we view all herbs as relatively dangerous.*

smashing idea to put a Mason jar of herb tea outside by each plant being discussed. The introduction of each new plant friend then became an occasion to sip its sun-infused tea in dainty porcelain tea cups passed out at the start of the walk.

Students can play an active role. Learning about flower essences for the first time, for instance, can become quite personal. "As the essences go around the room," explains Linn Stilwell of Briarwood Farm Botanicals in New Hampshire, "I ask each person to describe the first thing that comes to their minds as they receive the bottle. Some giggle, some cry, some have heart-opening experiences. Pretty incredible reactions come from simply holding the essences." Making actual products—from formulated tinctures and soothing salves to a tasty tea blend and cayenne-ginger liniment—gets hands on the herbs. Students do it all: harvest the herbs, prepare the menstruum, heat the beeswax, label the bottles, judge the teas, and clean up the kitchen. An old Chinese proverb describes this type of learning quite aptly: *I hear, and I forget. I see, and I remember. I do, and I understand.*

Developing an effective repertoire of classes takes time. Offer an introduction to herbs at least twice a year at reduced cost to establish a core group of aspiring herbalists who will want to continue their studies. Other classes naturally follow from there. Nancy now has more than a dozen thoughtfully prepared "Home Herbalist Handouts" for various classes, designed on the computer, that she can print anew. Course offerings here at the farm include the art of herbal brewing, remedies for seasonal health, and the home medicine chest. Herbal body care always gets rave reviews, as everyone involved gives and receives a custom facial.

Class notes for the teacher correspond to the handouts passed out to students, serving to remind the instructor what to have on hand for a particular class. We all know how easy it can be to forget those visual props that make for an effective presentation. Nancy needs these materials when teaching the clothesline concept of categorizing herbs: clothespins, markers, plain paper, clothesline, and a selection of herbs to actually hang up. Two students are asked to hold the clothesline while others mark out the nourishing, tonic, specific medicinal, and low-dose herb categories. Then the fun begins as the students debate which herb goes where. Dry herb in clear bags as well as fresh plant tops can easily be clipped to the clothesline. Including a handful of coffee beans as one of the herbs makes for a stimulating quandary. Ideas such as this can be repeated next time around, provided you take time as a teacher to write down the organizational aspects of each class presentation. Materials (including books and color slides) for show and tell, a complete list of the handouts planned, and a detailed syllabus are all good. Next time you go to strain a freshly brewed tea, you will have a strainer on hand!

## TEACHING GARDENS

One of the best places to enter the teaching arena is through the garden. Gardens designed to showcase an array of cultivated herbs, and trails meandering through meadows and woodlands, offer a great introduction to healing plants. Jaunty signs identify each plant by common and Latin name and may even list some of the uses of each plant.

Developing teaching gardens and making them available for classes and open to the public at certain times helps bridge the gap between what people are hearing in the media and seeing on store shelves and actually beginning a healing relationship of their own.

The range of possibilities—from small backyard gardens to botanical sanctuaries— leaves no stone unturned. One traditional way of planting medicinal herbs in medieval monasteries was to feature beds of herbs according to specific ailments. Such infirmary gardens had beds of herbs for treating insomnia, digestion, colds, coughs, and so

forth. Similar plantings can be categorized according to the actions of the herbs: adaptogens, anti-inflammatories, demulcents, nervines, and so forth. Yet another approach has been to put the garden focus on herbs for the systems of the body.

### The Medicine Wheel

The circle is a classic design form for gardeners. Many herbalists organize a healing garden as a medicine wheel. The circle, symbolic of life, eternity, and our connection to all, gets divided into spokes, which can be marked by stones or narrow paths. The heart of the circle becomes the center of a healing mandala. A special plant, statue, or rock placed in the center focuses sacred intent into the garden. Each spoke section represents a body system. The herbs planted in each section tone, nourish, and correct imbalances for that particular body system. Such a garden can be small and meditative, with only a few plants, crystals, and stones representing the various healing energies involved. Larger circles can accommodate a full range of effective medicinal plants for each system. Overlap is good, for herbs often suit multiple therapeutic purpose. Seeing an herb such as garlic growing in the spokes for the respiratory system, the heart, and the immune system reinforces that teaching.

We made such a garden in 2000 with the help of the students taking our five-month course in Herbal Foundations. Nancy had to step back to let the group as a whole create the vision for the medicine wheel. The hands-on experience of digging in the dirt helped everyone bond. We chose a relatively small area about sixteen feet in diameter. We intended this as both a teaching garden and a ceremonial garden to hold beginning and closing circles. The space was marked out using a string line attached to a

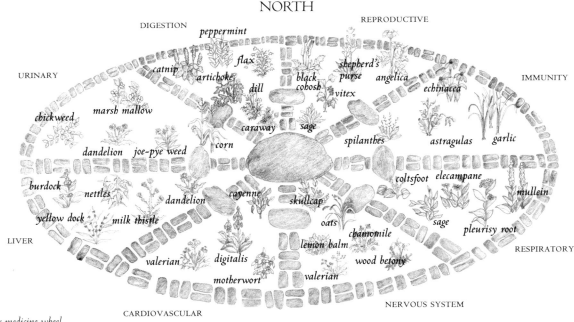

DIGESTION

REPRODUCTIVE

URINARY

IMMUNITY

*peppermint*

*flax*

*catnip*

*shepherd's purse*

*artichoke*

*angelica*

*black cohosh*

*echinacea*

*dill*

*vitex*

*marsh mallow*

*chickweed*

*caraway*

*sage*

*spilanthes*

*astragulas*

*garlic*

*corn*

*dandelion*

*joe-pye weed*

*coltsfoot*

*elecampane*

*burdock*

*nettles*

*dandelion*

*cayenne*

*skullcap*

*mullein*

*yellow dock*

*milk thistle*

*oats*

*sage*

*pleurisy root*

LIVER

*chamomile*

*lemon balm*

*valerian*

*digitalis*

*wood betony*

RESPIRATORY

*motherwort*

*valerian*

CARDIOVASCULAR

NERVOUS SYSTEM

SOUTH

*Our medicine wheel garden showcases healing plants for particular systems of the body.*

center stake to circumscribe a perfect circle. (Hint: Lay out a garden hose as you go to show where to commence digging the edge.) Eight sections were created within the circle, deliberately corresponding to the number of people in the group. We freed the circle of sod, leveled the ground, and marked the spokes of the wheel with a sprinkling of lime. Using a square-ended shovel, we scooped out the paths, throwing the extra soil on the garden sections and thereby creating raised beds. The resulting wedges were approximately three feet wide at the outer edge of the circle, with foot-wide pathways left between. Deciding which body systems to include in our medicine wheel made for insightful debate! We included the liver, knowing it isn't really a "body system" per se. Each student chose one section to research the plants to include.

We marked out the four directions by placing a small rock cairn to indicate the entrance to the medicine wheel in the East.

We consciously chose to position each body system near the direction we thought the most telling. Energy and rebirth are associated with the East, power and wisdom with the North, intuition and insight with the West, nurturing and peace with the South. Each student brought a flat "standing stone" to position halfway along each path toward the circle's center. Old bricks set in sand paved the remaining pathway, including the entire outer circumference of the wheel. We walk along this outer path in a clockwise direction (always upon entering in the East) to reach the eight pathways. An altar stone in the middle—rolled into place by concerted feminine mystique and one big guy— receives medicine pouches, crystals, and herb bundles placed for ceremonial intent.

Space in this intriguing plot of ground suddenly seemed to be in short supply, what with standing stones and brick walkways and central megaliths. The extensive list of botanical possibilities for each body system had to be whittled down, and we had to discuss if particular plants would really grow in a full sun garden in northern New Hampshire. Ginseng is good medicine, but it wants forest shade. A hawthorn tree would simply become too big for the space. We actually planted more than will comfortably fit once the plants are fully grown—the commonest of gardening mistakes—knowing that winter might temper our hopeful enthusiasm for less hardy species.

Our nervous system herbs include chamomile, skullcap, lemon balm, St. John's wort, wood betony, and oats; nervine standbys catnip and valerian got bumped elsewhere. Digestive system herbs are dill, peppermint, catnip, chamomile, fennel, and flax. The respiratory system herbs are coltsfoot, pleurisy, elecampane, sage, and mullein. Licorice, hyssop, lungwort, horehound, and red clover could just as well have been in the respiratory spoke—medicine wheel gardens are anything but rigid! Our liver herbs included nettles, red clover, burdock, yellow dock, and milk thistle. Good urinary system herbs are chickweed, corn, marsh mallow,

dandelion, parsley, and gravel root. Yarrow, mugwort, sage, black cohosh, and vitex (a summer resident at best) got the nod for the reproductive system. The circulatory system features motherwort, valerian, cayenne, digitalis, and lily of the valley; hawthorn is here in spirit. Finally, our immune system herbs include ashwagandha, astragalus, echinacea, spilanthes, and the practically all-purpose garlic. Annual and tender perennial herbs will need to be replanted each year.

## Medicinal Trails

Wildness should be celebrated in any teaching garden setting. Our sense of order falls short of Nature's design when it comes to mastering companion planting. Natural settings highlight the preferred environments that the plants themselves have chosen. Deep in the forest, the precious frailty of goldthread becomes apparent. Such medicinal plants can touch hearts without a single root being taken. Joe-pye weed in flower along a creek bank, elderberry clusters drooping down within reach, and fuzzy patches of boneset in late summer speak

*Get students involved with the plants with some hands-on garden time. Nancy had her Herbal Foundations class design, dig, and plant this medicine wheel garden one summer.*

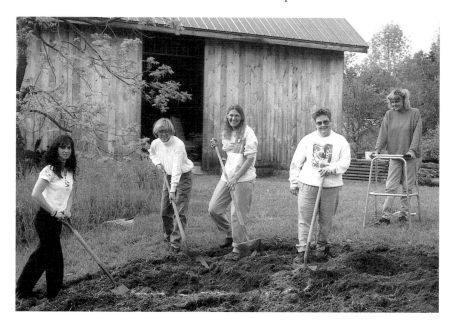

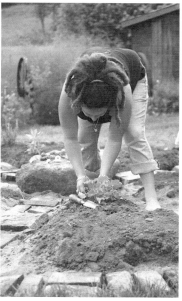

volumes for great gifts too easily over-looked. Students who help harvest a limited portion of any wild stand can grasp the ethics of wildcrafting. Abundance results from an abiding respect for diversity. A walk down any wild path leads to that irrefutable conclusion.

Medicinal trails can wind through a meadow, touch lightly along the edges of a bog, traverse a woodland stream, and lead ever upward to lonely vistas. However, such teaching trails can just as well head across town to find burdock in alleyways and black walnut in the park. The blazes for a medicinal trail are the plants themselves. Our job is simply to mark out these blazes for herb students to follow.

Crafting a medicinal trail does not need to be a monumental task. Twelve plant sightings give herb students twelve opportunities to learn about new plants and their medicinal uses. The field behind your house may be as far as you need to roam. More formal efforts may entail clearing brush, creating signs, and establishing a bulletin board at the trailhead for distributing a written guide to the plants to be found. Opening a trail to the general public encourages people to come out for the medicinal experience. Scheduling a guided tour gives people all the more reason to come. A medicinal trail in a town or state park furthers community awareness about local plants available for local healing.

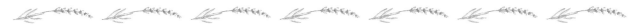

## THE SAGE MOUNTAIN MEDICINAL TRAIL

SAGE MOUNTAIN is a magical and powerful place that has become one of my homes away from home. Five hundred acres of forest and bog are set aside as a botanical sanctuary, thanks to cofounders Rosemary Gladstar and Karl Slick. I've learned much from Rosemary and the other wonderful herbalists who come to teach on the mountain. Yet the land and the plants in particular have been some of my best instructors.

My favorite medicinal garden is the winding mile-long trail through the woods. Medicinal plants are marked with bright orange flags with numbers that correspond to a written guide designed for self-guided tours. You can quiz yourself or a group of students before actually seeing the common name, Latin name, and traditional uses of each plant. All the plants are hardy in the Zone 3 climate found at higher elevations in northern Vermont, though some of them have been transplanted to establish certain species on this particular property. Black and blue cohosh, bloodroot, ginseng, and goldenseal are just five of the thirty-four species labeled and described. Trees such as slippery elm, balsam fir, and yellow birch are included as well. People are often surprised to find out that an ornamental tree like a white ash can be used for medicine. (White ash leaves are used as a spring tonic; they are known to be diuretic and slightly laxative, sometimes used to burn off winter fat and clear out the system.) Remembering which plant is which becomes easier when you can see it in the same spot again and again. Having that numbered cheat sheet along certainly helps.

The medicinal trail is open to the public on specific days for hiking and appreciating the woods. For more information, write Sage Mountain Herbal Retreat Center, P.O. Box 420, East Barre, VT 05649. —N.P.

## Production Gardens

We love hosting herb classes on a working herb farm. The intimacy of scale here allows students to experience the hard work and heartfelt joy that goes into every pound of dried herb. The vibes alone of so much healing energy in one place create a focused opportunity for learning about plant blessings.

Herb students walk down into the lower field to listen to Michael explain about the uncurling scapes of garlic. Growing energy can be directed entirely into the sizing garlic bulb by timely removal of this scape. (See page 172 for a full garlic exposé.) We reach down and scoop up some humus-rich earth. Contemplating that more microorganisms exist in each handful of that living soil than humans on the entire planet makes a lasting point about the importance of soil health. Nancy guides the group, plant by plant, across the farm. We are no longer teachers but students of these green seers ourselves.

Hands-on teaching about each herb builds self-reliance. Growing one or two plants worth of an herb looks manageable compared to five hundred anise hyssop plants calling for sweet attention. The secrets of successfully drying herbs become quite obvious in the drying tunnel on a warm day. The synchronized motion of gathering hands at work in the oat field impresses people. The milky oats, like any good food nurtured by skilled farmers, have shared a story that goes far beyond arguments about price. Time on a farm of any sort teaches lessons we all need to appreciate if we're to create a truly sustainable future.

## WORD-OF-MOUTH SUCCESS

Patience in the early years leads to eventual success in establishing an herbal teaching center. We learn how best to fill classes as we go, with a combination of brochures,

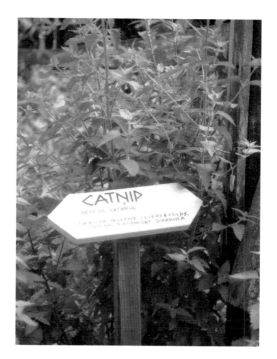

*Signs in the teaching garden help herb students to identify each plant, consider some of its traditional uses, and perhaps even absorb its Latin name.*

flyers, personalized invitations, and regional media attention. Ultimately, the satisfaction of past students will be the driving force behind any effort to make a viable living from herbal teaching .

Should you go for the gusto when it comes time to print your herbal brochures? We suggest a resounding yes to this investment aimed at getting your course offerings and herbal fare known in your community. Good art catches the eye. Establishing a logo—consisting of both name and graphic design—creates continuity for all subsequent publicity. Prominent words make it clear that this is the brochure for healing herb workshops in the area. Adding a second color won't be nearly as prohibitive in price as a full-color printing job. Our Heartsong Farm brochure utilizes purple and green ink on half of its eight pages. The front, back, and centerfold—as yet uncut and thus on one 11 × 17-inch sheet of paper—are run through the offset press a second time to imprint artwork and titles on those pages in a bold purple. An additional $75 toward 1,500 half-fold brochures provides this colorful flair. We have the order form printed as an insert page, front and back, bringing the total cost of each brochure to just under 30 cents.

A spring brochure announcing all classes and farm events scheduled through the summer and fall reaches those folks who tend to plan ahead. The Foundations of Herbal Healing course—offered one weekend a month for five months—needs to attract herb students early on. A seed gets planted for such an ongoing intensive that people will consider in future years. Brochures can be left at natural foods stores and with area health practitioners. Attaching several at a time on the community bulletin board at the grocery store (each time you go shopping) encourages interested people to take a brochure home. Single-page flyers need to be posted as a scheduled class draws nearer, ideally six to eight weeks in advance of each event. Classified ads can be useful if you have established a Web site where readers can find the full scoop on all your events.[1] Monthly publications advancing alternative health care and New Age consciousness in a region usually prove to be a far-reaching investment. Offering to write a small monthly column on herbal healing basics is a free way of getting your name in the public eye. Inviting a reporter to attend a class may well result in a profile story about all you do as an herbalist.

Promotion aimed at livelihood insists that modesty be put aside to some extent. Knowing you have important teaching to offer means putting yourself out there. Teachers with Earth-centered awareness are urgently needed to answer the call being put forth by traditional educational institutions. We journey to frontier territory teaching herbal medicine in schools, universities, and, especially, conventional medical schools. Three such herbal pioneers caught our attention in putting together this book.

Joyce Wardwell is teaching botany to thirteen- and fourteen-year-old girls at a charter school. "It took me a while to convince them to incorporate my ideas into their program. The school was concerned that I would push alternative healing as an herbalist," says Joyce. "I assured them that there was a lot more to botany than herbal medicine." She does have a chapter on herbs as part of the curriculum, and most certainly speaks for the plants and their gracious gifts whenever the opportunity arises. "We don't do any love potions, charms, and magic spells, however. I just want the kids to learn what a stamen and a pistil are. Yesterday they all made their own facial toner, and we are going to make birchbark baskets next." Joyce is developing a pilot program to create a similar class in a nearby public school.

Barbara Nardozzi had already been teaching horticulture at the University of Vermont (UVM) for ten years when she felt a really strong inner prompting to propose an herbalism class. She had to plug the idea for about a year and a half before the university business planners agreed to give it a try. "Introduction to Herbalism" has now been running for three years as a three-credit course. Barbara's class fills every time. "Then I proposed an intermediate class directed toward more medically oriented undergrads that started last fall. It has been a treat to be part of this huge web of interest among the students," says this herbalist cum professor. "Some want to go on to Naturopathy School and others get interested in ethnobotany. I also give guest lectures at the nursing school, and perhaps an herbalism course will soon be offered there as well."

A university course must fit certain professional parameters. Exams are necessary. Barbara gets to do far more field work with her apprentice groups at home. Delving into details about herbs for the various body systems and time for plant identification don't happen as much at UVM. Still, Barbara enjoys both settings. "Even now, when I stand up in front of my college class, I want to just pinch myself because I am so happy it is happening. Everyone seems happy. I like what I do, the students like the program, and the university is happy because the classes fill right up."

We talked earlier about Margi Flint's groundbreaking work at Tufts University School of Medicine in Boston (see page 134). "Part of my path has been to be a bridge," observes Margi. "I feel good about teaching at Tufts because the students will have one course where they will be loved and nurtured. They learn simple ways to survive and deal with their own colds and fatigue and their own brain overuse. They now have teas, salves, and oils that can assist them in a very brutal system." Herbs have a huge impact on the souls of these young doctors that will hopefully carry over into their future practice. Margi's own clinical experience with people on a weekly basis goes hand in hand with her ability to convey tenderness to her students. "If I didn't have clients," she notes, "I would not be able to teach from the heart."

## WORKSHOPS THAT INTRIGUE

Great fun awaits in determining course offerings with descriptive titles that resonate with herbal verve. The work lies in preparing yourself well and getting people as excited as you are about your herbal programs.

Stating the goals of a presentation makes clear what you intend to accomplish. Teach-ers can too easily overlook this important step of considering a workshop through the eyes of prospective students. Do send people home with at least one new practical skill to use right away. Balancing theory with practicality makes us effective as teachers. People need enough background information to think for themselves, certainly, but they also need that nudging how-to lesson that empowers them to *do* for themselves.

Presenting basic concepts of herbalism in beginning level classes is a must. Just how basic that can be is revealed rather quickly. *You mean you can use fresh herbs to make tea?* shows a deeply-ingrained Lipton consciousness. Intermediate students often benefit from a review of the basics but have come for a bit more profundity of thought. Advanced decorum implies no simpleton questions so the group as a whole maintains a high energy level. The same topic can be covered to different degrees of depth depending on who attends a presentation. Ideally, people sense that degree from our course write-ups before they register.

Most classes start with introductions. You tell about yourself as the teacher and what today's class will cover. Small groups lend themselves to having the students briefly tell about themselves and what they're looking for in the workshop. The job of gauging student expertise becomes relatively easy. We'll mention one last tidbit for the close of the session: Make a plug for your upcoming classes. Stir interest in the next step these students should ponder. Encourage people to add to a mailing list the names of friends who might be interested in your brochure. Offer books and herbs for sale in a low-key way. The captive audience before you represents a legitimate part of your livelihood as an herbal teacher.

*Text continues on page 279.*

# Jane Bothwell

Our search for the epitome of a community herbalist—excellent teacher, healer, community support person, and a lovely person to boot—led to Jane Bothwell in Kneeland, California. Being centered at home brings a different kind of distinction from that of being on the herbal lecture circuit. Here's a woman who had a pretty clear vision early on that her family life was vitally important. Jane has focused on raising her daughter and son, nurturing her marriage, and making time for friends in addition to immersing herself in the world of herbs. This college town of around 15,000 people has proved a good choice in her quest to fulfill a personal vision rooted in introducing others to the healing power of plants.

Dandelion Herbal Center is located in the coastal hills of northern California, an hour and a half from the Oregon border. The magnificence of surrounding redwoods, numerous mountain ranges, and the Pacific Ocean offers a vibrant setting. A former teacher and administrator at the California School of Herbal Studies in Sonoma County, Jane moved north to Humboldt County in 1988, bringing twenty years of experience with her.

"I wanted to be with live teachers and with the plants," says Jane, speaking of those hippie heydays in the early 1980s when many of today's well-known herbalists were stretching their collective wings at the California School of Herbal Studies. Rosemary Gladstar, who founded the school, remembers Jane taking some of the classes over and over again. "She was so dedicated to learning," recalls Rosemary. "She was a teacher beforehand, so she had good techniques for teaching. Jane began instructing some of the classes herself. She was completely committed and continued to add to her knowledge base. That is one of the things I really admire about her. She studied hypnotherapy and Bach Flower essences and really involved her life in them. So her work as an herbalist is really more expansive than mine on many levels."

"I am forever thankful to have had the opportunity to study with Rosemary," says Jane. "She continues to influence my life in profound ways. The study of herbalism is a way of life, a way of interacting, a spiritual awakening. Rosemary is an exceptionally inspiring teacher, a talented herbalist, a compassion-ate individual, and a gifted leader and visionary. She has a deep understanding of people and plants and an unending dedication to herbalism, our planet, and its occupants. My teachings are very much Rosemary's teachings, and I only hope to inspire and empower my students as she has me."

Being centered in one's community is a rich choice. Jane currently teaches an herbal apprentice course held one weekend a month from February through November. Her prerequisite course is a ten-class introductory series of eight evenings and two herb walks. The apprentice courses usually have around twenty-five students. A paid

*I realized what many people need is for someone to listen to what they are saying.*

—Jane Bothwell

assistant, Kathleen Nunley, does some of the teaching and preparation work, while work-study volunteers help with meals and setting up and breaking down for class. "The group takes turns bringing dishes like soup or cornbread, and we always make a wild greens salad," says Jane. "It works well, and is much nicer than everyone bringing their own lunch.

"I have thought of not calling my program an apprenticeship because it really isn't an appropriate use of the word. It is really an herbal study program." Jane carries the learning opportunities at Dandelion Herbal Center further with an advanced program of visiting teachers she calls a Festival of Herbs. "One weekend a month I have a visiting teacher: Rosemary, David Hoffmann, Richo Cech, Sunny Mavor, Cascade Anderson-Geller have all been here. I gear this for apprentice graduates or others who are already practicing herbalists, doctors, and acupuncturists: This is not the course to find out what a tincture is."

Jane serves her community as a health care practitioner as well, though she sees fewer clients these days since the arrival of her son, Forest. "I mostly see people that have been coming for years and need to come again, or people that I have an affinity to for some rea-

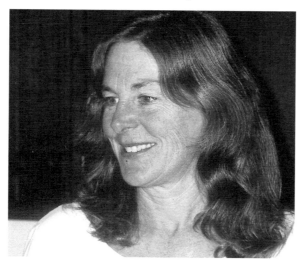

son and I think once or twice will help them. I do fill formulas for these clients, though I don't sell products otherwise.

"I also practice hypnotherapy. Generally people come for one or the other, but if they start coming regularly then they usually get mixed. I definitely use my hyp-

notherapy tools in my herbal consultations. People don't know that's what I'm doing, but that's why I took that training. I realized what many people need is for someone to listen to what they are saying."

Keeping family life and work in balance is difficult with herbalism because it is such a passion. Perspective helps in considering the day-to-day possibilities that await us. "I look at all the things I want to do, knowing I have a lifetime to do it all," says Jane. "Yet with my children there's this concentrated time, maybe eighteen years, which seems like a long time, but it really isn't. Our daughter, Jennifer, is already nine, and I think that special time with her is half gone. I chose to have children, and my children are really my priority. My passion with the plants is a priority as well, but how much time do I have? I can be a better parent and wife if I am more personally fulfilled.

"Herbalism fills me up and gives me energy and enthusiasm for life that is very valuable to share with my family." 🙵

---

We find interacting with people to be magical. Look directly into the eyes of individual students as you speak and let that warm connection empower you as you teach. You'll find class time can pass much too quickly.

## Herbal Class Themes

If you are not a seasoned teacher—and more than a bit hesitant—then start out with topics such as herbal cosmetics, designing the herb garden, culinary herbs, making herbal dream pillows, and herbed vinegars. A huge contingent of people are very hooked and enthusiastic about herbs that rarely touch on medicinal aspects.[2] Bertha Reppert, Adelma Simmons, and Phyllis Shaudys are queens of this genre. These amazing women have written books that are jam-packed full of ideas and recipes. Many of the topics they teach about appeal to a wide range of audiences, helping to make a bridge for people who go on to discover the brilliance of using herbs for health.

Teaching plant identification invariably kindles green magic. People on herb walks find themselves intrigued about possible uses of each plant. This introduction to the herbs as friends evokes the deeper interest that leads to the workshops we really want to teach.

No rhyme or reason exists to the way these classes evolve. We teach what we love and what we have incorporated into our own lives. Parenting sets us up to know about natural remedies for children. Being a woman makes us keenly aware of women's health issues—and vice versa for the menfolk. People like to come to talks that center on one topic such as winter health care. Our own experiences, perhaps working through a personal condition or someone else's in the family may point to a class on herbal approaches to hepatitis or high blood pressure. Other classes are designed specifically because people in our communities ask if we can teach on a certain topic.

Focusing on herbs for a particular body system can draw more interest simply by going beyond anatomy. People will identify more readily with "Herbs for Stress, Sleep, and Dreaming" than a workshop title such as "Herbs for the Nervous System." Just as "Herbs for Women's Health" sounds a bit more appealing than "Reproductive System Herbs." A good title and an irresistible course description can make all the difference in attendance. We emphasize that products will not only be made but taken home in our "Home Medicine Chest" workshop. We remind folks: *Bring a basket for your herbal goodies.* Be specific about tangible benefits. Offering a book as part of the class registra-

tion fee makes the deal more generous. Three plants to take home complements a class on "Ten Family Herbs" nicely.

Creating a series of workshops encourages people to commit upfront to a block of classes. Six evening sessions over a two-month period provides your students with a solid introduction to herbal medicine. Individuals can step in for one or two of the classes of any series as long as it doesn't seem to interfere with group continuity. Offering a discount on the whole package often encourages people to sign up for every class. A single class fee of $20, for instance, would result in a six-class fee of $120. Show basic marketing savvy by charging an even $100 for the entire course.

Our Herbal Foundations class meets one full weekend a month over the course of five months. Nancy loves having a continuous, enthusiastic group coming here to the farm on a regular basis. We start off at square one, so both beginning and intermediate herbalists can move ahead together. Nancy relies on Rosemary Gladstar's *Science and Art of Herbology* as the "text" for this course.[3] We do most of the hands-on projects here together on class days, with written assignments left to student initiative to hand in for review. Nancy finds having much of the written material already structured and organized allows more time on class days to have her students be with the plants. We open with song and blessings, lecture in a rocking chair circle in our post-and-beam barn, bounce out to the gardens for herb walks, share a lunch brought each time by two of the students, make herbal preparations in the kitchen, and teach some more. We often linger long after closing circle ends the formal class to work on the medicine wheel garden, share volunteer seedlings, and enjoy our newest herbal friends.

## Teaching Children

Children are born naturalists with an innate curiosity about life. Our call is to guide them in the ways of Earth wisdom. Showing that we too belong to Nature—as a humble *part*, not belligerently *apart*—makes the connectedness of all life clear.

The weaving in of stories and songs that celebrate these concepts has proved to be integral in teaching the next generation. A couple of current favorites that we draw upon regularly are *Song of the Seven Herbs* and Lesley Tierra's *A Kid's Herb Book*. The short stories in these books can be read and acted out with the children. When we ask who wants to be Kosi, the young boy who grows to be a wise medicine man, hands fly up, quick to volunteer. The other children are just as happy to be supporting characters such as the tribal chief and the eagle, or to sprout forth at the end as a powerful medicine plant. Lesley's herbal workbook just flows with fun ideas for getting kids involved with herbal magic. Swirling marshmallows in a cup of hot chocolate can be both tasty and healthy when we return to the root of this tradition, for instance. Using pieces of marsh mallow root (*Althaea officinalis*) at the center of this confectionery treat teaches children all about its virtues in a way they won't soon forget.

The best teaching tip we know for working with children is pretty common knowledge, but not always followed: Don't make them sit too long. Allow them to move, taste, smell, mix, get their hands in the earth, wiggle, and giggle! Their inner exuberance for life can be quite contagious.

The legacy of an Earth-centered lifestyle shows when our children respond to the values we project as herbalists. "My five-year-old was helping me mix an herbal concoction for somebody last week," says Aviva Romm. "She looked me right in the eyes and said, 'Mom, this is just what I want to do for the rest of my life. I want to help people with herbs.'"

Phyllis Light has five young ones in her herbal tow. "The kids like helping dig plants," notes this proud mother. "It brings me back to the times that I went out into the woods with my grandparents and parents when I was little. They are learning that if we don't feel well, the first thing we go to is the plants. They take their brews (see page 112) and let me know if it is a good batch or not as good as the last one. Making medicine is often a family affair."

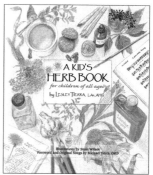

A Kid's Herb Book *by Lesley Tierra gets children caring about their health at an early age with all sorts of fun activities. Every family will find this magical herbal workbook just the ticket to rekindle home healing tradition.*

## Nature and Spirit Camp

One week each summer we have a day camp for girls and boys to enjoy the magic and mysteries of Nature. Each day quickly fills with hiking, singing, stories, Nature skits, making herbal wreaths, brewing herbal teas and potions, playing games, learning edible and wild medicinal plants, and much more.

Nancy's aim as a teacher is to celebrate the fun of being a kid:

> I want the girls and boys to share our peaceful spot here on Earth. I want them to run, laugh, sing, listen to the birds, breathe lots of fresh air, and wade in the brook. I want them to be introduced firsthand to herbs that grow almost anywhere and can be used for first aid. I want them to experience touching, smelling, feeling, harvesting, and using herbs. I want them to get their hands dirty in rich soil, while introducing them to concepts like making compost and growing crops organically. I want them to affirm the spiritual aspect of themselves, to know the light within is just as real as the physical. I want them to know that when

*Text continues on page 284.*

# PLANT ACTIVITIES FOR CHILDREN

THE FOLLOWING are tried-and-true plant activities with children that work well at our Nature and Spirit Camp, in classrooms, and with Gracie and her friends here at home. Most are applicable at different levels with older children and adults, too.

*Plant identification books.* Use small notebooks and clear contact paper sheets  the same size (cut in advance). Identify only a few herbs each day. Place a leaf and/or a flower on each page and write a few sentences about its medicinal use. Make it simple for younger children: "Chamomile is good for stomachaches." Older children can add more information. Cover with contact paper.

*Plant presses and herbariums.* A simple wooden herb press consists of two 10 × 12-inch pieces of plywood, four corner bolts, and four wing nuts. The herbs are pressed between interior layers of cardboard and blotting paper. Mounted samples kept in a binder can be labeled and described. Or the kids can craft cards and bookmarks with the pressed flowers and leaves.

*Meeting the herbs.* Choose only a few to focus on. Make tea ahead of time and have it in a capped jar right by the plant in the garden.

Kids taste the tea when being introduced to each herb.

*Make herbal sun tea.* This is almost too easy to write about! Let the kids put fresh herbs (steer them toward tasty choices) in a big clear glass jar, cover with water, and infuse all day in the sun. Strain and drink as is or add a little ice, honey, and lemon. Yum!

*Tea table.* Kids blend their own herbal tea to take home and share with their families. Use herbs such as peppermint, lemon balm, raspberry, spearmint, nettles, oats, calendula, roses, fennel, anise hyssop, and red clover. A pinch of stevia adds natural sweetness. These choices are pretty mild and tasty so everybody ends up with a delicious blend.

*Tummy potion.* Talk to the kids about which herbs are good for upset, gassy stomach problems. Let them pick fresh peppermint, chamomile, and catnip. Add fennel and ginger. Infuse, strain, and make a syrup. Assign a few kids to make labels while the others help bottle. We assure parents the medicine is effective and very safe by sending home a tummy potion write-up.

*Mini herb gardens to take home.* Greenhouse seedlings and divisions straight from the garden work well in creating a windowsill planter. Save seed-planting for longer-term projects. German thyme, parsley, garlic chives, peppermint, and a Thai hot pepper (for color and intrigue) are good choices.

*Impromptu plays.* Presenting complete rehearsed play can be quite time consuming. Assigning parts and reading a good story aloud can be just as much fun for kids. Nancy whispers the main lines to the actors so they can say their parts as they act it out spontaneously. This brings the stories to life and gets their bodies moving. *The Lorax* by Dr. Suess, *Keepers of the Earth* by Michael Caduto and Joseph Bruchac, and *The Herbalist of Yarrow* are particularly good. Other books are listed on page 89.

*Making herbal wreaths.* This is another all-time favorite with young and old alike. For the younger students, buy small wreath rings around eight inches in diameter, and cover with several dried sprigs of wormwood, silver king, mugwort, or sweet Annie. Attach this by spiraling floral wire to hold the chosen artemesia sprigs in place. The older students can do this part. The students then simply glue dried herbs and strawflowers all over the wreath.

Elmer's glue works fine. Each wreath turns out different and quite beautiful.

*Dyeing with herbs.* Dyeing is a colorful way to play with Nature. Plants that don't require a mordant (a reagent that fixes the dye to the textile) are the easiest to use. Use a food-grade alum as a mordant for those that do. Choose dye baths for children that can be made in one step. The decoction method is similar to making a big pot of tea. Onion skins produce a tannish-orange color. Dyer's chamomile, goldenrod, madder, and some types of lichens are also good. Cotton will not dye as easily as wool, but silk will dye in a one-step dye pot. Wool fleece and wool yarn can be dyed for puppet projects. Nancy likes to purchase silk so the children can make precious little silk pouches to keep their treasures.

*Sleep pillows.* Use a small square of fabric and tie together with a ribbon to make a "sleep bundle" or sew into little pillows. Fill with some or all of the following herbs: roses, lavender, hops, chamomile, rosemary, lamb's-ears, balsam fir needles.

*Natural snacks.* Happy children like to make snacks and they like to eat snacks. Here are some of our favorite recipes.

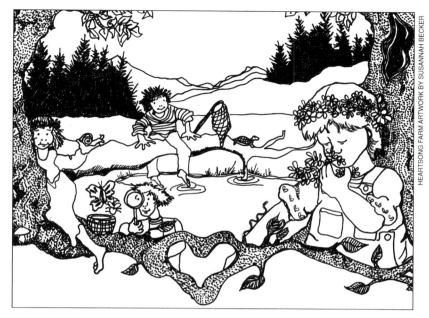

HEARTSONG FARM ARTWORK BY SUSANNAH BECKER

### Herb Cream Cheese Spread

Let cream cheese soften at room temperature, then chop finely any herbs the kids choose. Blend with a fork. A shot of lemon juice helps. Here is one yummy example: 1 clove garlic finely chopped; 1 tablespoon parsley; 1 teaspoon each sage, rosemary, and thyme. Add some calendula petals for color and subtle flavor. Now you can serve in a pretty bowl, or roll in chopped nuts for a cheese ball. Kids love squeezing this spread through a cake icing bag to top off veggie slices and crackers.

### Homemade "Good for Ya" Ginger Ale

Simmer 2 cups of chopped fresh ginger root in 1 quart of water for 30 minutes in a covered pot.

Strain and add ⅔ cup of raw honey and 4 tablespoons of lemon juice. Keep in refrigerator until ready to use. Add 3 to 6 tablespoons of this "ginger shrub" to an 8-ounce glass of sparkling water.

### Peppermint Cookies

Blend 1 cup of butter, 1 cup of honey, 3 eggs, and 1 teaspoon of vanilla in a mixing bowl until creamy. Mix in 1 teaspoon of cream of tartar and 1 cup of dried peppermint leaf. Gradually add 3 to 4 cups of flour until the dough is smooth and elastic. Form into a ball and chill for 30 minutes. Preheat oven to 350°F. Roll out to ¼ inch thick on a floured surface. Cut into shapes. Bake 7 to 10 minutes, or until edges are slightly brown.

we need something for our health—either food or medicine—we can often find what we need right around us.

Each morning we begin with a welcoming circle. We play percussion instruments and sing while one student walks around with a smudge bundle of sage. Then we have a moment of silence. Nancy usually leads a prayer of thankfulness and asks if anyone wants to add something. Some do, some don't. One boy, Dana, who was so shy he would hardly speak when he first came, offered to give the whole prayer the last day of camp. He stood up and gave thanks for the snakes, the brook, his mother, father, brother, and sister, the birds, the sky, and all that lived. All this love just poured out of that little boy's heart.

The real work of a kids' camp lies in organizing all the details ahead of time. Once the children arrive, we have just as much fun as they do. We choose a narrow age range, currently from five to eight, so the activities work for everyone involved. A teenage friend helps out as Nancy's assistant, in addition to a parent volunteer each day. We deliberately limit the size of the group to twelve to fifteen kids. Camp lasts from 9 A.M. to 2 P.M., with each child bringing his or her own lunch. We have a hands-on activity going on (that can easily be done with minimal direction) first thing because some children arrive earlier than others. Such activities include making leaf prints or adding an herb to their plant identification books. The schedule for each day is written out for all to see.

Children are much closer to the essence of life than most adults, but lose much of this spiritual perceptiveness over the years simply because it is not nurtured in our soci-

*Kids learn direct from the source— the plants themselves —at our Nature and Spirit Camp.*

ety. We incorporate activities during Nature Camp that enhance all the senses. We listen, touch, feel, smell, and taste many plants. We have periodic moments of silence, either as part of the morning circle or while out on a hike, to share what we experience. The trick is not to hold the silence too long, because children can't maintain it. Nancy carries a pretty-sounding bell that signals the beginning and ending of the silence. We talk about practicing being attuned to Nature just like we practice dribbling a soccer ball. The more we do it, the more acute our senses become. People long ago needed adeptness to survive, be they predator or prey. We pretend to be Native American hunters stalking deer in the forest, or cave people traveling through saber-toothed tiger country. This helps kids connect to their roots and remember forgotten skills.

On the last day of camp, Nancy takes the children to her sacred place, a comforting nook in the forest that we call "The

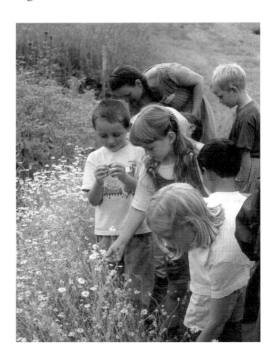

Sisters." This humble grove of red and white pine, spruce, and fir trees regularly draws us to sit and connect with Earth, ourselves, and the Creator. Nancy has the children whisper as we get close, then sit quietly for a few minutes once we arrive. She shares her feelings about coming here and then asks if anyone has a special place just to sit and be. Some already do. Giving credence to solitude and meditation helps children nurture their own relationship with Earth and Spirit.

## Advanced Classes

Herbal teaching centers need not only hold appeal for home herbalists. All of us have more to learn. Advanced herbal classes offer both a chance for detailed review and answers to deeper questions. Guest teachers offer our communities broader perspectives than ours alone. The interest in regional intensives is growing, as more herbalists come on the scene and other health care practitioners pursue this gentler medicine.

Some teachers may not feel ready or able to offer advanced classes. Inviting guest teachers is one way to learn more yourself. Local interest may be sufficient in an urban area, but often we need to attract herbalists throughout a region for such events. Traveling expenses can add greatly to the costs when a teacher comes from a distance away. Commitments often are made a year ahead when nationally prominent herbalists schedule conference appearances and try to coordinate some sanity into crowded calendars. Advance promotion for advanced classes is requisite. Don't be shy to let other herbal teachers know of your plans so they in turn can notify their students. The more we network with each other, the greater the possibilities.

# TEN INTRIGUING HERBAL WORKSHOPS

WE INVARIABLY FIND great workshop titles while going through other herbalists' brochures and conference flyers. Some imply pure inspiration, others offer a witty play on words. Some are appreciated for simply steering a right course and offering good teamwork. Here, not necessarily in order, are our favorites, with due credit given:

- "Fun Guys: Medicinal Mushrooms" with Christopher Hobbs
- "What's Science Got to Do with It?" with Susun Weed
- "The End of Antibiotics and the Herbal Medicines that Will Replace Them" with Stephen Buhner
- "Stepping Beyond Fear: Using Herbs in Our Practice" with Aviva Romm
- "Botanica Erotica and the Green Goddess" with Diana de Luca
- "Non-Medical Diagnosis for the Herbalist" with Matthew Wood
- "Nurturing Our Daughters with Herbs" with Tammi Hartung
- "The Roots and Spirit of Herbal Medicine" with David Winston and Donald Yance
- "Eat Your Weedies" with Gail Ulrich
- "Dirty Fingernails: A Grower's Intensive" with Andrea and Matthias Reisen

---

Many advanced classes focus on clinical practice, where diagnostic skills and actual practice working with clients is the emphasis. Clearly, taking this step from helping one's family to working with a wide array of conditions and all sorts of people requires more concerted teaching effort.

Kate Gilday and Don Babineau offer an intriguing advanced program at their teaching center in upstate New York. Three extended "Tending the Spirit" weekends focus on different aspects of being an herbal practitioner. "Tending Those in Need" looks at beginning a consulting practice, including diagnostic and intake skills. Kate delves in to why people heal by tuning in to the emotional and spiritual aspects of illness as well. "Tending the Spirit of the Plants" lets herbalists experience new environments and the subtle energies of the plants growing there. Finally, "Tending One's Own Spirit" offers introspective renewal in the sweet stillness of the forest for any healer, as well as an introduction to plant spirit medicine.

The Sage Mountain Advanced Program hosts a practicing guest herbalist once a month for seven months. The program is designed to provide advanced students of herbalism an opportunity to pursue their studies in a focused and systematic manner with some of the most respected herbal instructors in the country. Each guest teacher shares details about his or her own practice and expertise and perspective about herbs, health, and healing. The Friday afternoon session always keys on an actual intake with a client-volunteer from the local community. Each instructor focuses some of the weekend on a body system and the corresponding herbs and herbal therapies. Students find it sometimes overwhelming, frequently thought provoking, and always inspiring. Sometimes we learn the most from the teachers who "rattle our cages" and demand that we reevaluate our own beliefs. Other times, the ones who we can identify with the most have us saying in our hearts, "I want to learn what he knows, I want to help others as she does!"

Stirring the soup with diverse teachings strengthens one's herbal foundation. Each herbalist is different and has his or her own unique style of helping people. Frequently teachers contradict each other. One month we might hear a teacher say, "I don't bother to deal with the client's diet—the herbs themselves will provide the healing." Then our next herbal instructor adamantly asserts that digestion and diet are the only way to really effect long-term change. Idiosyncratic strengths and weaknesses provide the spark that someday will mark our own stirring of the pot.

One of the best experiences during the advanced program is observing the guest teacher conduct an actual case study. Other members of the local community come up the mountain for a free consultation as well. Students take turns doing an intake with each client, while the other students listen and later contribute suggestions toward a therapeutic course of action. Talk about nerve-racking! We venture our opinions on each matter in a fish bowl of herbal opinion. Getting feedback from one's peers as well as from experienced practitioners makes this an invaluable way to learn the practicing side of herbalism.

Developing an ongoing clinic in one's community gives advanced students the experience needed to start an herbal practice. Kathleen Maier at the Sacred Plant Traditions Center for Herbal Studies in Charlottesville, Virginia, combines years of insight as an herbalist with medical training as a physician's assistant to give her students grounding in both worlds of care. "We are not teaching the herbalists to be pseudo-allopaths," Kathleen explains, "but rather helping them with the language so they can be bridges for their clients. People coming to our herbal clinic are often standing on the bank of the allopathic tradition—they need herbalists who can translate the medical language for them so they know it is safe on both sides."

The Sacred Plant Traditions program includes several key ingredients that make it such an exemplary teaching model:

- A knowledgeable and dynamic herbalist as the director.
- A group of four students meets once a week for nine months.
- Prerequisites for students in herbal foundations as well as anatomy and physiology.
- The teaching day is split in half, with the mornings devoted to advanced lectures and the afternoons for seeing clients. Issues such as thyroid health and various protocols for hyperthyroid or hypothyroid imbalances are reviewed. Energetic models and medical terminology broaden the students' understanding of each health situation.
- Consultations are free to clients, but people are required to commit to coming at least three times, so students can learn from the follow-up consultations.
- Students observe for the first three months and gradually take over the role of practitioner with supervision. Second-year clinic students have more responsibility and autonomy. Apprentices see clients privately (or with other apprentices), complete all the casework, and research therapeutic protocols. They meet together with Kathleen to discuss all aspects of their case studies and receive supervision.

This clinic model benefits people who perhaps aren't in a position to afford such quality care. Fledgling herbalists acquire vital experience with a variety of health sit-

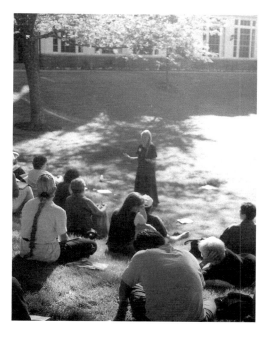

*Trishua teaching at the International Herb Symposium, held every other year at Wheaton College in Norton, Massachusetts.*

uations. Isn't it incredible how good answers meet everyone's needs?

## TRADITIONAL APPRENTICESHIPS

Learning the depths of any path hinges on intimacy. As teachers we know only too well that our brief time with students in a class setting can be too disjointed for complete learning to ever take place. Clinical insight can be explained in a workshop, but never conveyed fully. Students need more time to probe diagnostic techniques for themselves, time ideally spent in an ongoing relationship with a holistic practitioner. Nuance becomes one's own only when experienced, whether we're talking about plant harvesting, medicine making, or fine-tuning therapeutic recommendations. Practicing newfound skills under the tutelage of a good teacher over an extended period of time will make competent herbalists. The traditional apprenticeship marks the surest way to get there.

*Text continues on page 290.*

# Kate Gilday and Don Babineau

LIVING ON a dirt road where the stars shine in all their awesome glory helps define a good place to call home. In upstate New York, where the foothills rise to meet the Adirondacks, Kate Gilday and Don Babineau have conscientiously crafted a solar home and established an herbal livelihood centered on the forest. Their gardens, alternating with beds of echinacea and homegrown greens, incorporate those "best of *Mother Earth News*" ideas that every homesteader aims to accomplish. The true essence of this place, however, begins in the surrounding woods.

Kate and Don have a deep connection to Earth and the plants. Their relationship to Nature is just as close and real as their human relationships. "We're in a time," observes Don, "when people know so little about the hands-on aspects of living on this Earth. A big part of this for Kate and me is that incredible connection of Spirit and personal psychology on the level of our environment. How it shapes us and we correspondingly shape it." The gift of helping people get in touch with the spirit of the land integrates across the board at Woodland Essence. Other herbalists can teach about three hundred different herbs and make recommendations for untold medical conditions, but the healing focus here never deviates from this first and deeper truth.

"Sometimes we feel like midwives," says Kate. "We try to bring people back in touch with their birthright as part of Nature, not separate from it. And the transformation that happens can be amazing! When people remember and choose conscious connection to Nature, to self and community, deep and lasting healing can happen. We're honored to assist in this reawakening."

Kate began her herbal journey in 1975, becoming interested in herbs when her young daughters had ear infections. She was not happy with the choices she was offered by the conventional medical system. Using the two herb books she could find at the time (John Lust's *The Herb Book* and Jethro Kloss's *Back to Eden*), Kate began treating her girls with the recommended herbs. "They all worked! Which was especially amazing, considering what passed for marketable herbs in those days," recalls Kate. "The other parents that had children at day care started asking why our kids weren't getting sick as much or why were they getting over things so quickly. Then I would share the information with them. It all started very experientially, just sharing the little bits that I knew."

Herbal connections started to flow for this former nursing student. *Well Being* magazine introduced Kate to the writings of California herbalists including Rosemary Gladstar, Michael Tierra, and Kathi Keville. Then came a couple of long weekend

*We try to bring people back in touch with their birthright as part of Nature, not separate from it.*

—KATE GILDAY

programs with Susun Weed in 1985. "I am really glad I had the opportunity to study with Susun at that time. She put words to a lot of ideas that I had," says Kate, who is now an esteemed herbal teacher in her own right. "I really appreciated someone who was radical enough to challenge the present paradigm of health care."

Inspired in her herb garden

by comfrey, calendula, and echinacea, Kate began selling medicinal products in the local food co-op. "Whenever you put your name on a bottle and get it out there, your phone starts to ring. As the phone started to ring more, I got very excited. Whatever people would ask, I would spend long periods of time on the phone trying to answer. Then my family started to tell me, 'Mom, we never

would plan my life around them. Other people began to show up at the door. I was considered a community herbalist in their eyes, though just beginning to claim it for myself. We really step into this gently.

"People first came to me with coughs, scrapes, colds, and bruises. I was never overchallenged by the people coming to me. Then slowly but surely other things came along

Kate is very clear about personal priorities. She currently sees clients one day a week at Jean's Greens, the mail-order herb apothecary nearby. "Your business will grow exponentially as much as you want it to grow. You have to make sure that you are asking the universe for just what you want. The answer can only be as good as the question."

A unique line of Woodland Flower Essences—embracing tree spirits such as black birch and quaking aspen, and conserving at-risk species such as lady's slipper and blue cohosh—along with a full teaching schedule fills much of the rest of Kate's universe. "It would be hard to be a community herbalist without a support system. My family is great, and each one of them helps others in their own way. We are more like a community herbalist family than just me being the community herbalist." Together, Don and Kate make a gifted team of guides into the forest, leading groups to old-growth trees, identifying medicinal mushrooms, making ash bark baskets, and bringing forth the underlying spirit power in Nature. The apprenticeship programs at Woodland Essence run one weekend a month on the beginning and intermediate levels, with advanced three-day seminars focused on tending the spirit of those in need, the plants, and one's own. "The reality," says Kate, "is that no matter how great your program is, and

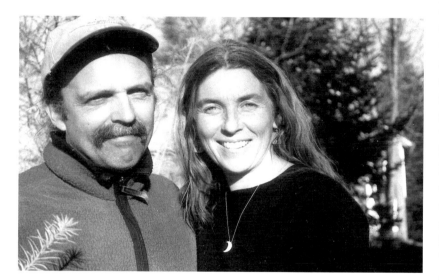

see you. We see you at meals and when you wake up, but then the rest of the time you are on the phone.'" Kate understood things needed to change.

It's a disservice to give quick, one-herb answers to people if constitutional issues lie at the root of their problems. Working with diet and lifestyle becomes the forte of any holistic herbalist. "Then I made the mistake of asking people when they could come over," continues Kate, "and I

—urinary tract infection, chronic coughs, trouble conceiving, broken bones that needed help healing. Now I'm working with people with cancer. There are definitely times when I feel stretched . . . if it's beyond something I can do, I'm the first to say, 'This is something I have never worked with. I can support you in these ways and then maybe you want to see this person over here.' I know my parameters and feel comfortable with what I know and with what I don't know."

no matter how open and bright your participants are, they can only take in so much in a day. What people need besides the studies is the time in between the learning: the smudging, the prayers, the songs, touching and feeling the herbs."

Don, ever a man to head to the hills when opportunity beckons, adds to the family income by gathering woodland medicinals. Don says, "I'll walk four to six miles up into the mountains to gather chaga," which is a shelflike fungus found on trees, and known for its immune-enhancing properties. Chaga dries down 60 percent by weight. White, yellow, and gray birch are the host trees. Don uses a 20-foot pole saw, leaving anything above that height. Harvesting the mature fungus doesn't affect chaga's return. The reproductive spores are found higher up still, among the leaves. "I harvest in the winter, when the shelves are easier to see on the tree trunks. Our son, Sean, has a real gift for spotting chaga. We hike in on snowshoes. A day's work yields about 100 pounds, carried out in backpacks, which dries down to forty pounds of marketable chaga." Don bought a chipper/ shredder at a roadside sale, thinking he'd use it for compost making. It wasn't that effective, but turned out to be great for grinding the chaga (broken up with an ax beforehand) and medicinal roots.

"The forest supports us personally in so many ways," says Don. "We consciously harvest plant medicines from the trees and forest floor to sell to other practitioners and herb compa-nies. Our herbal retreats intro-duce others to a renewed under-standing of the nature of the forest. Kate and I rest in the deep silence and ever present cycles of life, Earth, and rebirth held here."

We're compelled to point out one more talent in this fine fam-ily: Kate's singing carries across the opening circle at the Green Nations gathering in the Catskills each September. Voices come together in the enrapturing cradle of this herbal sister's song:

*May I walk in beauty on the*
> *Mother,*
*Like a river flowing over rocks.*
*May I walk in beauty on the*
> *Mother,*
*Like a river flowing over rocks.*
*May I walk, may I walk,*
*In beauty and balance on the*
> *Mother.*

"I have an apprenticeship that I think is barely an apprenticeship," points out 7Song of the Northeast School of Botan-ical Medicine. "This thing people call an apprenticeship—one weekend a month—that is just a class." 7Song picks his apprentices carefully, knowing the next six months to two years will be spent working side by side with this person for five full days a week, sometimes six. He requires that students do not take another job dur-ing this time. "We've allowed a discrep-ancy around the word *apprenticeship.* A stu-dent who apprentices with an experienced herbalist for a long time develops a per-sonal relationship with that teacher. We've bastardized a fairly good term."

The apprentice agreement at Desert Bloom Herbs in New Mexico seems very traditional, much like artisans have done throughout history. Herbalist Richard McDonald insists on a year's commit-ment: "It's just not worth my energy to have people work with me without learn-ing the basics of herbalism." Apprentices work alongside Richard in his store, mak-ing medicine and assisting customers. Apprentices attend all classes and field trips he offers in the Silver City commu-nity. They join in on wildcrafting expeditions and eventually get to sit in on consultations. Richard neither asks for money for this training, nor does he pay a living stipend. A retainer of $800—the kind of upfront commitment not readily forgotten—is set aside in a bank account, to be returned to the apprentice with interest at the end of the year. An apprentice either needs to have enough saved up to make it through this year, or take on odd jobs on days off from the store. Sharon (apprenticing at the time of our visit) found Richard to be a fun alternative to the costlier option of a certified program in herbalism.

Just as it takes a certain hankering for knowledge and experience in the herbal student, teachers need to embrace equally the give-and-take nature of this traditional arrangement. Mutually beneficial commitments between the student and the teacher are what make an apprenticeship bear fruit. The help we receive in our work should never be the sole reason behind taking someone into our fold. The gifts of the healing plants quite frankly need to be passed on. Part of our call as herbalists is to encourage the innate goodness in others who would share green medicine. Yet, just like any other human relationship, we need to choose our companions wisely.

Clarity from the onset about each other's expectations establishes where you are headed together. Apprentices should be told what they will learn and what you expect in exchange for your teaching energy and patience. A trial period of two to four weeks allows leeway for either party to back out of an incompatible situation.

Herbalists vary widely in how formal they wish to make this learning experience for long-term students. Sharing personal libraries and establishing certain times for questions sets a self-motivated pace that's reasonable to expect in a committed apprentice. Some teachers will give specific written assignments based on required reading. Still others will hone inner capabilities by cutting no slack. Basically, apprentices learn by observing humbly a knowledgeable person in action and then implementing the teaching for themselves.

Ryan Drum spent twelve years apprenticing off and on with Ella Birzneck at the Dominion Herbal College in British Columbia before she died. Some of this came as formal class time, other times he simply watched quietly as Ella treated a client. The day came when the torch of healing was passed into his hands with but one obligation. Ryan recalls this succinctly: "My teacher said, 'If you know, you must tell.'"

## NOTES

1. A Chelsea Green book we can recommend wholeheartedly to any herbalist considering a Web site—and business promotion in general—is *Grassroots Marketing* by Shel Horowitz. Getting noticed in a noisy world can be done with plenty of class.

2. The American Herbalists Association, by way of example, disavows any medical use for herbs.

3. Sage Mountain offers a bulk discount to herbal teachers who choose Rosemary's home study course as a reference. Other teachers have used an introductory book such as David Hoffmann's *Holistic Herbal*. Still others spend a phenomenal amount of time to create their own course materials.

# CHAPTER NINE
# Healing Visions for Today

BLACK PEPPERMINT
*Mentha piperita*

*F*riends and family members often come to me with their prepackaged tablets from the discount store, wondering if this is a good herb for a particular ailment. The plastic bottles all have fancy labels usually with "nature something" in the title. I feel kind of stuck, because I want to encourage people who are searching out a more natural way of healing. They want something that is safer and possibly more effective than pharmaceutical choices. I try to encourage them gently and lead them to wholesome choices—but I just can't advocate the "this herb for that ailment" approach. Taking a pill is so much easier than walking every day and cleaning up one's diet. Filling up on Cool Whip, Twinkies, and Coke makes it hard for even the best herbs to make a dent. Buying that quick fix is the tip of the iceberg when it comes to what herbalism is about. ℘ Using herbs as a way of countering symptoms will be beneficial to an extent, but the bigger picture of holistic thinking offers more. You have to be connected with the plants in some direct way to really know the essence of herbs. You don't have to grow and harvest every plant you'll ever use, but you need to make that connection on some level. Maybe you just grow some mint in a container and make your own tea. That small step gets you started on the right path. Living herbs connect us to Nature. Herbalism is about nourishment and connecting with the plants. It's about drinking in the healing qualities of a flower, or having a siesta while sitting under a big oak. Herbalism is about reveling in the beauty of Creation. This includes the healing herbs and our own magnificent bodies that spontaneously heal. —N.P. ℘

LOCAL HERBALISTS understanding how to use local plants help local people stay in good health. The medicine offered to us by the plants is health care at its finest, right up there with eating right, being joyful, and knowing meaning in life.

The push for reductionist science as the sole determinant of worth in herbal medicine does not puzzle us in the least. Everyday blessings become less accessible when *expertise* and *standardized process* are regulated into cultural reality. Layer upon layer of corporate and professional ingress burdens too much of our lives today. The plants bestow upon us countless earthly and spiritual graces. It's simply audacious to think people should not embrace homegrown cures and personal involvement in their well-being. Herbalists keep the medicine of the people alive by nurturing this embrace. We can and do integrate the fantastic findings that science reveals into traditional healing wisdom. Yet to say that this constituent here, this mighty phyto-silver bullet, is solely why a given plant medicine works, is to begin to shut the door on whole-plant remedies. The true source of healing magic that grows outside our door also awaits us inside our heart.

Our bodies are miracles we'll never fully comprehend. Holistic healers seek to understand the sum effects of mind and spirit on our dis-ease. We know that the good bacteria surrounding every square inch of us parry mightily against consistent pathological odds. Building immunity depends on healthy organs supported by eating and living sensibly. We artfully use differential diagnosis to determine the most efficacious herbal treatment that will assist the body's innate ability to heal. Medicine couldn't be more complex. A doctorate degree in med-

ical science only initiates a lifetime of humble study. Physicians with a desire to serve as healers know this well. Similarly, herbalists never stop learning from the plants and the people they serve. The notion that everyone finds a piece of the truth certainly applies. We need to celebrate each other's insights. We need to honor the wisdom of past generations. We need to look toward a future where herbalists, doctors, and all healers work side by side in our communities.

We've begun to be integrative in our view of medicine. Talk of conventional medicine and alternative medicine sidesteps this far more helpful perspective. The purpose of any healing modality is to help people be well. Those modalities with a track record of effectiveness—be it physical, emotional, or spiritual healing—have a rightful place in medical practice. The tradition of herbalism has been validated throughout the ages of history. Put in perspective, modern allopathic medicine, for all its purported orthodoxy, is rather a new kid on the block.

A united effort by doctors in the last century to monopolize and control the medical field pushed herbs and other healing traditions to the background. Now public consciousness has shifted. In 1997, Americans made an estimated 629 million visits to alternative practitioners offering long-standing therapies such as massage, acupuncture, and herbal remedies. Conventional doctors, on the other hand, received only 386 million visits. None of this takes into account the simple exchange of neighborly advice and motherly love. The demand and appreciation for so-called alternative medicine has brought herbs to the fore. Now, we face a critical choice. Those who argue for the use of herbs within a Western allopathic framework are simply substituting single plant

*So great was the enthusiasm for medical breakthroughs based upon the chemical analysis of drugs, systematic record keeping, surgical innovations, and scientific research, and so boundless the optimism in medicine's future progress, that the past seemed to hold no value either for doctors or for their patients. The consequences of this shift in medical mind-set are still with us today. Indeed, it is not uncommon for medical researchers and physicians to restrict their studies to the last five or ten years of medical progress. Of the history of medicine the average person is likely to know only the tall tales of supposedly nonsensical treatments such as phlebotomy, poultices, and purges. . . . Such flippant rejection of many millennia of accumulated knowledge has its price, as does the rejection of traditional medicines from foreign cultures. Ignorance of the past has never been a firm foundation for the present.*

—ROBERT AND MICHÈLE ROOT-BERNSTEIN,
*Honey, Mud, Maggots and Other Medical Marvels*

constituents for synthetic drugs. Encapsulated herbs are now available everywhere and are being purchased in record numbers. When prescribed to treat a symptom—be it through self-diagnosis or through a practitioner—the thinking behind the pill remains the same. Immersing yourself in the whole experience of a healing plant, on the other hand, literally changes lives.

Physicians are gradually opening up to the possibilities of herbal medicine and a holistic view of healing. While set minds may shift slowly, younger doctors with Hippocratic idealism intact often do choose broader perspectives. Conventional medical programs now offer elective courses in phytomedicinals, and attendance is growing. Knowledge of medicinal plant use, however much it gets cloaked in constituent garble, guides inquisitive minds to further discovery. Recently, Dr. George Lundberg, editor of the *Journal of the American Medical Association* (JAMA), was quoted as saying, "There's no such thing as alternative medicine. There is only medicine." Respect for one another as healers can only be a good thing. Integrative medicine leads us all to an inclusive vantage point. Healing, at its finest, is both an individual and a collective process.

The herbal movement itself is in need of healing. The herb industry, hepped up on consumer demand for tackling symptoms, has traveled far from the center of the natural world in offering an array of plant-derived medicines without a holistic interface. Constituent science provides the fuel behind the advertising of these standardized extracts and food supplements. Community herbalists continue on as ever, committed to the proofs of tradition and whole-plant use. Plant spirit medicine advocates find their harmony in direct communion with green consciousness.

"There is a split," acknowledges Rosemary Gladstar. "We all try not to admit that. There is a split between a linear/rational way of thinking and the folkloric/intuitive. People are structurally and mentally just very different from the day we're born. It's easiest for me to understand a folkloric approach, nor have I trained myself to think linearly. Each person is trying to make it seem that what we are each doing is right and acceptable. Some are trying so hard to make herbalism accessible to the American public, so that it integrates with the medical system. The American Herbalists Guild is struggling to do that. People outside of the organization basically view it as moving toward a more medical model. Yet within the group there is a desire to preserve folkloric tradition. I am still hopeful that there is a way of bridging this gap, but I think we have a long struggle to get there. We all just keep doing the very best we can."

The ultimate integration of medicine lies on a more personal level, which complementary therapies at their best encourage. Each person is his or her own healer. Health care practitioners can serve as vital partners available to assist along the way. Our unique healing paths encounter body, mind, and spirit to the degree we personally empower these manifestations of human existence. How we use this harmony in healing parallels how we live our everyday lives. People who view physical reality as the extent of existence act within a material cosmology. For them, a pharmaceutical or herbal medicine offers certain physical effects, hopefully applied to the good. Encountering the power of the mind brings belief and hope into what we do. Journeying into the vastness of the Great Mystery opens our hearts to the affirmations of divine love.

To deny spirit only lessens one's ability to tap into the miracle of being. Few of us achieve the stature of a bodhisattva,[1] just as few of us really see our wholeness as a right combination of chemical elements hanging out together to form a lifetime. We are a mix of what we believe and sense and experience. Our personal power flows from this mix. Equally important, Creation takes the form of what we perceive our mix to be. The plants can offer constituent relief, welcome assurance, and spirit guidance to the extent that we extend ourselves into wholeness. Conveying this with words reduces the fundamental essence of what might well be at the core of healing perception. Certainly herbal medicine is subject to the very same tidal pulls as any human tradition. Now, as we stumble toward what we hope is an integration of medical care and economic fairness, getting a grip on collective reality becomes all the more essential.

## COMMUNITY HEALTH

Health care begins with *people care* long before illness makes its presence known. The all-consuming pace of material living seems to insist we leave behind neighborly connection. Our current system of medicine too often seems in line with an alternative definition of that word—something that is unpleasant, but necessary or unavoidable[2]—than with a mutual embracing of the human condition.

Common purpose and interpersonal relationships help to make us happy. Friendship and happiness make for good health. Chronic loneliness, on the other hand, drains away every vestige of intimacy and connection. Far too many people are lonely today. We spend more time fearing each other than we do loving each other. This herbal discussion of an affordable health care system will step beyond fear. The values we urgently need to consider may not be profitable in a business sense. The risks we need to take in caring for one another might not be insurable. The hopes we need to express, however, will most definitely be realistic. The plant world reaches out with a shared vibrancy that offers more than we can ever repay. That spirit of generosity will be our guide.

### Truly Integrative Medicine

Modern allopathic medicine has been a blessing to the world in many ways.

Certainly we wouldn't want to be without it should anyone in our family ever have a serious accident. Yet conventional medicine is just one of the choices on the road to healing, and not necessarily always the best choice for every situation. Sadly, many of us have lost touch with our own intuitive wisdom about what is right or wrong for our bodies. We wait instead to hear what the doctor has to say. Many have given up control and just go to the physician and say, "Fix me."

Each of us has to discern which healing therapies are the best choice in each situation. One of the blessings of this age is having so many choices, from acupuncture and body work and psychotherapy to energy work and nutritional therapy and the herbs we love so well. Herbs can be used in combination with other healing paths to enhance their benefits. Herbs also can be an excellent secondary therapy to complement allopathic medicine. A person making the decision to undergo chemotherapy or radiation therapy for cancer, for example, can be supported with herbs to help rid the body of toxins and help soothe and nourish the body systems.

"The conventional system works to a certain point," says herb grower Matthias Reisen. "The hospitals have some great technology that we couldn't do without. I can't set bones, I can't take X-rays. But once they're X-rayed and set, I can help the bones mend a lot faster than they can in the hospital. Both of the systems need to come together, we need to integrate them."

Alternative and allopathic practitioners should be able to work together without worrying about offending each other. How utterly tantalizing it would be if *grand rounds* would consist of allopathic doctors, tradi-

tional healers, a massage therapist, and a nutritionist who would sit down together in mutual respect and plan a truly holistic recovery plan for hospitalized patients. All members of the team would have a voice, and then options that would benefit the patient would be offered. All would recognize the patient as the ultimate decision maker.

Similarly, open-practice clinics would replace the traditional doctor's office. People would see their primary care physician for a diagnosis and recommendations, and then check with an herbalist or naturopath for a second opinion. Additional care from an acupuncturist or massage therapist would be available at the clinic. A nutritionist on site could offer specific dietary information and even teach people how to prepare whole foods. A lending library of phenomenal breadth would encourage people to delve further into their health situations. Self-healing would be encouraged and abetted by the holistic care of skilled partners—the medical team—in each individual's therapeutic odyssey.

We visited one such clinic in Lyme, New Hampshire, to talk with Robert Rufsvold, the founding doctor-in-residence. The consulting team at the New England Center for Integrative Health consists of one M.D., a naturopathic doctor, a physician's assistant, an acupuncturist trained in Traditional Chinese Medicine, a chiropractor, a nutritionist, a massage therapist, a Reiki practitioner, and teachers of yoga and qi gong. Bridging these differing cultures in medicine places Bob in a rather unique position to discern the collective journey ahead. "We need to be able to rationally accept some of the good things of our Western, scientific, technical medicine *and* accept that there are other healing ways to explore as well.

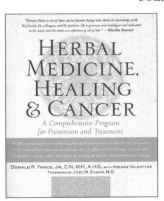

*Donald Yance provides us with compassionate understanding to using healing herbs and good foods in treating cancer.* Herbal Medicine, Healing & Cancer *is a holistic manual for the patient, the doctor, the herbalist, and the nutritionist.*

Shouldn't the common denominator," asks this good doctor, "be to find out what works? Let's try to use all avenues that are safe and that work with the body's own natural abilities to heal."

Integrating quite different systems of medicine will be an ongoing process. Herbalist Margi Flint began having office hours at a hospital near her Massachusetts home. An acupuncturist, massage therapist, and Reiki practitioner are available there as well. "The Healing Atrium at AtlantiCare has a really good vibration. But even with all of that, you still have the old model and the old model is pretty harsh. My feelings get hurt," says Margi. "I am fifty years old. I have to decide how much of that I want to put up with and where my devotion lies. One of the advantages of being associated with the hospital is that you see very sick people, and because you are affiliated with the hospital, they have more faith in your ability. I have had some pretty miraculous results with herbs. One man, a paraplegic, had horrible bedsores that were down to the bone. The doctors had just given up on him. It was so beautiful to see those bedsores heal up with herbs and to see this man get his hope again."

Two hospitals have asked herbalist Kate Gilday to do in-service training for physicians and nurses in upstate New York. Another area hospital is developing a cancer center. One room drawn on the architectural designs is labeled as an herbalist's office. "Isn't that amazing?" asks Kate. "The hospital wants to do it because the patients are asking for this." The medical powers-that-be are not going to invite herbalists to join such an integrated effort if they have only accomplished a mere six months of herb training. All those steps in between, from home herbalist to consultant, take time. Despite her considerable seasoning, Kate's first reaction to being asked was, "Can I do this?" But then she remembered that first rule: to do no harm. "Responsible herbalists definitely do no harm. We just support," acknowledges this gentle woman, "by offering nutritive herbs and trusting our own experience with the herbs that we have used ourselves."

Creating this new medical paradigm is not just a question of bringing all health care practitioners together in the same place at the same time. The most comprehensive healing available only gets off the ground when our culture drops the current adversarial model of medicine. The far more important connection lies in patient empowerment. Our bodies are genius. Their natural ability to heal lies at the heart of all this integrative promise. Alternative remedies and even prescribed medications are often necessary, but these merely assist in the healing process. Each one of us holds the reins for who we are and how we feel. Illness invites us to ask questions that go beyond the physical body. Do I need to make a change in the dynamics of a relationship? Are old belief patterns no longer serving? Am I stuck in a situation where a positive change of attitude alone could make an incredible difference? A healthier way to be makes room for more joy, creativity, and sense of purpose in life. A truly integrative medicine is about people integrating personal responsibility into the process of achieving lifelong wellness.

Obviously we need to orient ourselves toward health rather than disease, to emphasize prevention above treatment. Medicine that goes beyond heroics to the everyday will need to center on new values, not money, and not patriarchal control. Service, love, and fun need to be the driving goals behind this care. And to do that, medicine must be taken out of the business sector. Greed and selfishness, as Dr. Patch Adams constantly points out, have placed society and its health care system in great peril.[3] We need to create a sense of belonging and of community, where medicine is seen as a part of ourselves, a natural endowment, a true gift of sharing.

Perhaps this is where the community herbalist fits in best. We live within our

## REACHING THOSE WE LOVE

How do we educate our loved ones about alternatives to the assaultive, crisis-intervention medical treatments to which they've become accustomed? Our own health choices, rooted as they are in Earth consciousness, aren't necessarily viewed as on the up and up by the other generations in our families. The holistic framework from which we steer the course for our own health (and advise others in our communities) makes sense to us. We have a trust in the herbs based on direct experience and reverence.

Those same principles of personal integration apply equally to our children and elderly parents. People should feel confident in the healing path they undertake. Trying to convince others that herbal medicine is for them will not work unless it flows for them. Some people respond really well to other medicines, but not so well to herbal treatments. No one system works well for everybody. The best we can do is support people in their choices.

Education is key. We can tell a parent or child, *Do you know that people have used this? Here are some medical studies. This herb is not harmful to take with your medication—I checked for any contraindications. If you would like to take it, I can get it for you and send it to you.* If our loved ones say no to that, then we have to respect their choice. Offering the loan of a good book such as *An Elder's Herbal* by David Hoffmann can help clarify a health situation and lend credence to unfamiliar therapies. Sharing information from a place of concern differs greatly from being a holistic zealot intent on preaching herb-righteous sermons. Yet in time, casually given handouts on the caffeine habit or ill-advised margarine use may resonate. Herbal alternatives for stroke prevention sound pretty good when pharmaceutical side effects prove irksome. Cancer patients at the failed end of conventional treatment could be ready to consider alternatives. Still, regardless of the choices made, being supportive of those we love means the most.

"Some students tell me they want to put herbs in others' food," says Rosemary Gladstar. "I tell them that I would never want someone to come to my home and put medicine in my food! I would want them to educate me about that and allow me to make my choice and respect me for that. We need to have that same respect. My father was exposed to harmful chemicals in the war and now has cancer in his ear. All of his five children really wanted him to go to this Seventh-Day Adventist sanitarium where they treat people holistically. They use herbs and have medical specialists. We wanted him to go to this place because it is his religion and he could trust it. We told him we would pay for it and that Mom could go too. He finally said to me, 'You know, Rosemary, to be honest, I just could not eat that food.' They serve healthy vegetarian food and he likes meat and potatoes. Then I knew that he had made his choice. It was never the best choice as far as I was concerned, but my job is to support my father."

respective communities. Friends, family, and neighbors are the people in our care. Relationship naturally encourages service and mutual understanding. An impersonal system is replaced with the very personal support of one another. Healers by no means can be cast economically adrift—the need for a fair exchange will always be paramount—but neither should the cost of medical treatment ignore common reality.

## Paying for Health Care

Many today have come to view a health insurance system as rightfully footing the bill for medical care. Anyone without insurance coverage needs to somehow be able to get to the point where they can afford the monthly premiums, or else have coverage provided through government-funded universal care. Our preference is a personal program of *health assurance*.

Health care is delivered for profit in this country rather than for healing. Physicians' earnings top six figures, and the cost of technology does not recognize affordable limits. Administrative overhead is admitted to be 25 percent of the cost of our care.[4] Prescribed medications force a choice between drugs or food for some of the elderly. The drug companies, according to recent estimates, annually spend between $8,000 and $13,000 per physician to promote their products.[5] "Relationships between physicians and industry raise concerns about whether the patient's best interests will come into conflict with industry's focus on the bottom line," writes Robert M. Tenery, M.D., of the Council on Ethical and Judicial Affairs of the American Medical Association. "Even more troubling is the apparent lack of awareness of these adverse influences, even by the participants themselves."[6]

No one is to blame, and yet hardly anyone questions the fundamental inequity now so enmeshed with the very compassionate act of caring for people in need. Our societal focus instead gets directed toward third-party reimbursement for exorbitant medical costs that are viewed as inevitable as death and taxes.

Insurance companies dictate how medicine is practiced by their policies of reimbursement, both in the listing of accepted procedures and in the Health Management Organizations' (HMO) approval of specific procedures for each individual's situation. Coverage takes a bow to conventional allopathy in a big way. Science points to rational cures, which insurance actuaries find irresistible in defining what constitutes "extensive coverage." We all know what regard *small print* generally holds for choice and alternative thinking. We may not realize what it means to refuse standardized procedure in the midst of a medical emergency, however. Julie Manchester, who tells the story of her leg burns on page 269, relates how coverage for that emergency room visit was denied. "I accepted the tetanus shot but not the antiseptic, antibiotic cream, or the bandaging. Because I didn't follow accepted procedures, the insurance company doesn't want to pay the $156 for my ER trip. Who the hell are they to decide?" demands Julie. The devil, as one wise muse put it, always lies in the details.

Procedures are much more profitable for doctors. A physical examination and talking to the family are low-paying tasks by comparison. The money to be made in the operating room is three to seven times more than for consulting. Lab tests always include a standard markup toward the expense of running a fully staffed medical office. A series of tests ensures a series of markups. What seems a single medical treatment to the patient often amounts to a series of standardized procedures, each itemized separately. The incentives and nonpersonal nature of modern health care aren't going to make things more affordable any time soon. An overnight stay in a hospital can cost as much as a week in a plush Caribbean resort. Malpractice insurance exacts a hefty toll from every doctor, with obstetricians topping the scale at a whopping $100,000 a year in premiums. Who would want to deliver babies given that scenario?

Such an atmosphere of distrust has poisoned doctor/patient relationships, that every patient coming through the door is now seen as a potential plaintiff in a lawsuit. Doctors are more afraid than ever to deviate from conventional standards of practice. Excessive testing demonstrates lab-thoroughness, not time spent intimately understanding a person's life. We best understand how *third-party disconnect* affects medicine if as herbalists we think this is the direction to go.

"A great way to kill a healing profession is to get it insured. Look at our medical system. What makes doctors not be good doctors? The fear that your patient is going to sue you. This is what we want as herbalists?" asks Rosemary Gladstar. "Insurance is the number one thing that has taken healing out of the allopathic profession."

"I don't like mistrust," said Patch Adams in a recent interview. "As soon as you carry malpractice insurance you're in effect telling your patients, 'I'm afraid of you and I don't trust you because I'm afraid you might sue me.' So you live your entire professional career in fear and mistrust. Many doctors are afraid to do procedures, or stop doing parts of their practice, because they're afraid

they might get sued. And because malpractice insurance makes it easy to choose a scapegoat if something does go wrong, you can't build good teamwork among health care professionals."[7]

Those of us used to medical expenses apparently being paid by third parties need to apply our thinking caps. In truth, we all foot the bill, either through a workplace arrangement, directly out of pocket, or with tax dollars funneled into Medicare. The cost of catastrophic care understandably hooks us into taking the bait in the first place. Spot visits to the doctor's office for flu medication or a sprained ankle are not financially devastating. Fear makes a great salesman: We put up with the insurance game because of the more ponderous risk. An insurance plan offers little incentive to seek reduced costs by those with the coverage. Patients become claimants, not consumers—and certainly not human beings with highly relevant individual circumstances. The direct connection between health care providers and the people needing their services is severed. Quite obviously, this is a system that takes care of its own. Unfortunately, that excludes far too many.

Health insurance companies would squawk at people banding together collectively to insure each other against excessive medical costs. Never mind that this was the original concept of mutual insurance before the profit motive took control. Yet in Amish communities, families organize community funds in their respective church circles to keep such money matters centered at home. "Every baptized member of our church contributes $45 a month," says David Kline, an Amish farmer in central Ohio, "with each family paying no more than $180. Some months we don't need to collect, occasionally we need a double collection. The other churches help with really large bills." Such reciprocal caring gets returned many times over, of course, in much the same way we non-Amish picture these plain folk coming together to rebuild a neighbor's house or barn after a fire. Rising medical costs pose more perplexing questions, however, even for people with a sense of shared responsibility for the health of their community.

"Each family will pay the first $1,000 of their hospital bill in a given year, after which they pay a quarter of the costs. It's good if a person is involved and has to pay a little," says David, "as we tend to be more cautious that way." Not all families are in a financial position to handle the unexpected, and then the church steps in to offer help as well. Still, a hundred church circles consisting of twenty-five families apiece can struggle to cope in today's health care economy, just like the rest of us. David and his kin don't shy away from necessary medical treatment, but neither do they rush to the doctor at the first sign of illness. Amish medicine women are scattered throughout these farm communities, ready with time-tested remedies of herbs and nurturing care. "And besides," David observes with a wry smile, "it's normal to have some aches and pains. Our doctor told me he had never operated on a ruptured appendix before he came to our county. We bear our pains, thinking it will be better the next day. Sometimes that's just not the case, and then we go to the doctor."

Most significant of all in considering why a collective medical fund works for the Amish, perhaps, is the wholesome diet these families steward from the good Earth beneath their feet. "My wife and I are not pill poppers," says David, referring to the vitamins recommended to supplement foods lacking in vitality. "We feed the soil, which in turn nourishes our crops. These nourish our animals, which graze on open pasture. The foods we eat are filled with all this goodness."

Health assurance begins with common sense and personal responsibility. Eating wholesome foods, getting regular exercise and rest, sharing love and knowing joy all matter. Being well most of the time follows from there. Second, our bodies have this incredible, innate healing ability. Not slowing down to take care of ourselves is often the reason we get sick. Our bodies know their job well once we heed this feeling-ill cue. The occasional herbal nudge can go a long way toward getting the job done. Hardly any costs need be incurred for the majority of everyday ailments.

Connecting with a community herbalist or the neighborhood granny healer (in the case of the Amish) becomes a superlative deal when we view gentle treatment with proper accord. The cost of such day-to-day care should be negotiated directly with the folks who care for us and be paid out of pocket. The gladsome thing about a direct relationship—with the person you consult about your health or the plant from which you seek your medicine—is the one-to-one basis of understanding of circumstance. *Doctor, I realize your skill has great value but we're going to need a year to get some money to you each month. Y'all don't worry about that . . . I'd be more than honored to get a side of homegrown beef or have someone fix that sagging porch of mine.* Being considerate of each other's true needs is not as corny as that all may sound. We may not all wind up with yachts and plush vacation homes, but, hey, being fair is obviously going to tone down those materialistic urges, as we embrace a life on this good Earth from a loving perspective.

The catastrophic exception is when we need to rely on community health insurance. Creating a better solution in a secular society will mean trusting each other. Universal coverage could be fittingly limited to those horrific occasions when acute trauma dictates intensive care. The high cost of business as usual will be little affected by a universal payment plan, however, if we do not address the care-for-profit motive now dominating modern medicine. The benefits of technology quite frankly do not always justify the costs of technology. Nor do private insurance companies currently have cause to rediscover the service aspect of the services they're so willing to sell. Pooling community resources to mutually insure each other in dire circumstances does not need to be an opportunity to skim the cream off the top. Degenerative disease can consume one's life savings long before one's life ends. When bad times come, we need to be committed to providing the means for each other that allow holistic choices to be made. Cancer is among us for a reason that transcends personal causation and environmental abuse. No condition could inspire us more to seek collective answers. What we will achieve as human beings when we step beyond greed and selfishness will be miraculous.

## Real Community, Real Love

A welcoming sign at the Gesundheit Institute in West Virginia reads "Please Live a Healthy Life—Medicine Is an Imperfect Science." Doctor Patch Adams and a circle of caregivers continue to work toward creating a free community hospital there. The irresistible energy of this good man flourishes in his clowning—laughter heals when Patch goes into action—and finds expression in his compassionate vision of caring for one another. His insightful book on service and joy, *Gesundheit!*, definitely transcends the movie version of his life. "I'm for every person who wants to help people be healthy or ease their suffering in some way," says Patch. "I'm interested in that help being in a context of generosity and compassion, not in a paternalistic, arrogant context of, 'I know the answer, and if you have money you can get the answer.' So I'm for modalities that care about people."[8] He sees the caregiver as most important, not necessarily the medicines and techniques that we might or might not be able to use.

Making time for the healing relationship is integral. The inspiration behind any vision of care bespeaks intimacy as a healing force. As community herbalists, we do share love and human kindness as much as a vital knowledge for using the healing plants. The love and kindness we experience in turn from our neighbors blesses our lives equally. Learning to trust this caring interaction to meet our needs is one of life's big hurdles. The money aspects of health care start off as such a bone of contention, and understandably so. Forging a life path based on intimate connection and holistic care foremost involves trusting that gentle ways will work out right for everyone involved. We aren't provided with skills in this culture to consider one another's needs. Competition long ago replaced cooperation, much to our own chagrin. We struggle with local economy and finding a sound footing for a sensible agriculture precisely because we let the big picture of real community fall from sight. Counting pennies is fine until we realize our legal tender doesn't account for every worthy value.[9] Introducing a concept such as local medicine into our collective consciousness touches on these issues in a new way. The community experiences the plants not as native medicinal resources but as nearby friends. The community knows its healers not as a medical system but as loving individuals deserving of support.

Our society desperately seeks the healing only intimacy can offer. Wisdom on these matters does indeed recycle. What is forgotten by one generation is inevitably brought back by the next. Herbalists can serve their communities by rekindling the innate healing connections provided for all people. Benjamin Colby emphasized such a point in his 1848 *Guide to Health*:

> Those who make the practice of medicine a source of gain, will ridicule the idea of every man being his own physician. So have priests ridiculed the idea of letting every man read the Bible, and judge for himself of the important truths therein contained. As well might the village baker ridicule the idea of the good housewife making her own bread; alleging that it required a long course of study to make breads, and the people must not only buy all their bread of them at an exorbitant price, but pay them a fee for telling them what kind they must eat, and how much. The preparation and use of medicine to cure disease, requires no more science than the preparation and use of bread. Every head of a family ought to understand the medicinal properties of a sufficient number of roots and plants to cure any disease that might occur in his or her family, and teach their children the same.

The big cost structure of medicine falls apart when we empower ourselves to do the best we can. Giving body/mind/spirit all the natural advantages needed to promote good health and self-healing will reduce our reliance on a high-dollar system run aground. Something as accessible as organic food in a garden and plant medicines of a bioregion ask only our effort and appreciation. "Our health insurance is our garden," says herbalist Shatoiya de la Tour of Dry Creek Herb Farm in California. "Eating the wild plants as food kicks in the best preventive medicine going. Simply having the plants around us brings incredible joy."

"Herbal medicine is our birthright as human creatures of the planet," says Michael Tierra of the EastWest School of Herbology. "We need to cultivate and maintain everyone's appreciation and knowledge of herbs at all levels. The knowledge should never become the exclusive right of a professional elite class. People should be encouraged to grow medicinal herbs in their gardens and to learn at least a few basic healing plants that are practically ubiquitous around the planet. Thus, herbal medicine will have the ability to continually renew its practical knowledge base."

People need to take back this power. No one should run to any medical system too quickly for treatment of common ailments. Our children need care, yes, but they also need to experience the rudiments of personal responsibility as regards proper rest, good foods, and healing herbs. That gets learned from parents fully engaged in the same. A principal role for community herbalists is to teach the people just in time.

"If children were taught they needed clean air, clean water, and good food to grow big and strong, then our society would be headed in the right direction," suggests Kathleen O'Mara of the Herb Network. "If parents would teach their children as apprentices in life rather than send them to underpaid, overworked teachers, then society would be learning. If people said to their neighbors, 'This is my skill, let's work together so that we can all have a better life,' then the power

*Text continues on page 306.*

*What do we really need beyond this simple healer's hut?*

—Ryan Drum

# Rosemary Gladstar

You start people into the magic realm of plants in a very simple, pragmatic way: Here is how to make a tincture, use it when you get the flu. 'My God, this is working really well.' Then the Spirit connection happens," says Rosemary Gladstar. "The best way to make that happen is by dissolving the mystery on both ends. You say, 'Here is how you make a salve,' and, 'You can pick dandelion greens and dry them and make tea.' The key is getting people to shut their brains off and open up this inner pool of knowledge that they have." Rosemary's inspiration and charisma as an herbal teacher reach far. She truly seems to see only the good in people and knows how to draw that out and accentuate it. The magic and spirit and power of the plants she knows and loves so well flows from simple beginnings. "People don't feel that they can connect through Spirit anymore except through a preacher. That's been going on for several hundred years, so it is very hard to restore people's belief in themselves. Talking to plants is one way of talking directly to spirit.

"You have to work with the plants themselves to get the whole effect of herbalism. It is about more than herbs in bottles. You can make that part work, but you are losing the most important part. When I go down to the lady's slippers and sit with them, even if I never read that they are a superior herb for the nervous system, I would know it. They exude a calming effect. It's not because I'm an herbalist. I could take a stressed-out businessman down there and he would feel it too. It has to do with the totality: where they grow, how they grow, their responsibility to other plants around them. Herbalism is far more than chemical constituents."

"All of life is healing. I think animals have medicine power, and rocks have medicine power. Plants have medicine power, and humans have medicine power. Medicine power is a high for life. When you have a lot of life in you, then you have a lot to give out to others to help." Each of us knows when we experience such power, though right now, as a culture, we don't see it very clearly.

The pulsating heartbeat of existence is thwarted on this stressed Earth and in our stressed selves. Things are in survival mode. Immune systems are suppressed. Rosemary has observed this, not just in our country, but everywhere she travels. Much of life is struggling to find a way to live. Now, more than anything, we need hope and light and gracious magic. "Plants are one of the oldest forms of life on the planet," she explains. "They have extra *chi*, extra energy to give out because they have been evolving for so long. They are a very high form of life. We are a relatively new form of life. We don't have a lot of extra chi to give out. Plants have been developing that for literally billions of years. Our life—human life—is dependent on the life of the plant. You have a very high life-form that has developed enough energy within itself to survive and then can give it out to everything else, and you have a very young life-form that is very dependent on everything else to exist. We lean very heavily on the oldest and wisest life form. Depending on it for the air that we breathe, the food we eat, the clothes we wear, and the medicines that we use." The warp and woof of this incredibly interwoven tapestry of life is Spirit. Plants interact with us in the spiritual realm, offering a transformation beyond being stuck in a material world. "The plants have enough spirit to transform our limited vision," says our lady of the herbs. "Again, because of our inexperience of life, our inability to really know life. We seem to be going backward as a species in understanding this."

The vision of community herbalism is alive today, in part, because of the clarity Rosemary offers to her students and contemporaries of a better way. The models for such teaching come from the gentle elders who walked this green Earth long before many of us awoke to the call of the herbal path. "Adele Dawson—we called her Vermont's natural treasure—was an amazing example of a community herbalist or granny healer. Adele had an incredible influence over her community. People would come to her for herbs and teas, and she would go out into her garden and pick them. A granny healer helps others on every level, not just with herbal remedies. If someone needs soup, or is low on corn, or whatever—it is a wonderful concept that needs to continue.

"I have heard many stories in which Adele gave people remedies and helped them heal, but that really isn't her fame. Her place in her community came because she was such a gracious human being with a backyard full of herbs. She was like a fairy running around her plants. She was just like this magical being and *that* was her healing. That's why you went to see her. She had this wise spirit

and this very laughing, upbeat way of being. The herbs and the remedies were really secondary."

Rosemary beams in telling about another herbal mentor, her very dear friend, Juliette de Baïracli Levy. "Juliette is very well known around the world for her ability to heal animals and people. She served her village that way, and still does.

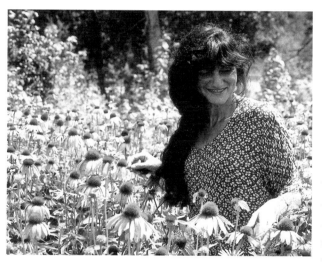

*The plants have enough spirit to transform our limited vision.*

—ROSEMARY GLADSTAR

People will come for advice— sometimes even several generations that have been raised on her book. They will bring these old books and say, 'I raised my kids on *Nature's Children*,' or 'My animal is alive because of *Herbal Handbook for Farm and Stable*.' Her healing is in her presence, her being. Juliette reminds people of something deeper inside themselves."

Most of us jot down all sorts of information about herbal remedies: *This herb is good for bedsores, and this herb is really good for a suppressed immune system.* We approach the plant not unlike a pharmacy. This way works, of course, and the herbs prove effective. Yet, as Rosemary likes to point out, there is an older way, a shamanic way. A traditional way. "The healer would go to the plant, and it didn't matter if that plant was for a specific remedy. There was an inner spirit in that plant that people could reach to make the deeper connection. Herbalists can use both techniques. This plant is good for this because it is rich in alkaloids or mucilaginous material—whatever it is—and then also reach into the spirit. That's why herbalism is really wonderful. Given one or the other, I would take plant spirit medicine because it jet-rockets you there."

Rosemary soars into many incredible moments, a young girl sharing her passage of womanhood as life gracefully presents sparkling wisdom. Have you ever known those people who can open their wallets to the moon to garner the real riches of this life? Have you ever whooped for beauty's sake? Have you ever held hands by a stream and prayed with deep love for someone else's pain which has only brushed you in passing? "The hardest thing for humans is to trust. Both the incredibleness of life and the dark shadow lands. To wake up every day like a child, and go, 'This is a new day. It's a gift. I'm alive!' You don't have to think this as much as it just comes. And then we need to realize the dark shadow lands bring just as many gifts as this bright and beautiful day." Rosemary shares this wonderful saying: *Love like you've never been hurt before, Dance like you do when nobody's watching, and Work like you don't need the money.* "I have this amazing world wrought with pain. That's the poet's life. The joy and sadness is intermingled. You have to grow and trust that. Tomorrow it can all be gone.

"The herbal world offers us a very real gift. Stephen Buhner and Elliot Cowan (authors of *Sacred Plant Medicine* and *Plant Spirit Medicine*, respectively) have brought this close to the surface so the rest of us can mine it easily: 'Remember that the plants are there to completely give to you.' Now expand that to all of life. Life is just rich with gifts. Air. Water. An incredible abundance of food. Each other. We have a choice every single time a pain comes to us. We can close down, become less thankful for the gift of life. We can become so fearful that, when we have a gift like the plants, we hold back from saying how great this really is because we know it may go. We fill our heart with so many holes," says Rosemary, "till eventually it becomes completely open once again."

The give-and-take of life fits into larger cycles that many of us overlook. Rosemary holds high hopes for our collective journey, while offering some helpful understanding. "We are all doing our very best, exploring different ways of thinking and being and how to integrate our beliefs about health and life. Out of this will come wholeness. There is a time when the apple tree is dying and a time when the apple tree is growing. History shows us to be in decay now, not in rise. Decay is what makes compost, what makes the soil, what creates the nutrients for new life to come. We can't see what we are holding up, we can only see what we are holding down. It is very important to remember that in this process there is holiness. Some people may say this is negative, but I don't see it as negative. It is like when the moon is waning. It is easy to celebrate when the moon in waxing, you feel it surging in your blood. Now the night of ceremony is upon us and the fairies are out, and we have to hold onto the energy before we rise to a new dawn." ℘

would return to the people. If saving local economy were more important than saving a penny, the world would have clean air, clean water, and good food for all."

"We need to come back to the model of the traditional healer," says Autumn Brennan from her Wisconsin seat on these herbal proceedings. Autumn's approach as the herbalist at the Wholistic Family Wellness Center in Viroqua broaches (as she puts it) *radical honesty with no fear attached.* People need to be empowered to take an active role in healing and face up to both personal and cultural reality. "The traditional healer can address imbalances of body, mind, and spirit," notes this spry woman. "The current medical system can't touch that! Using hands-on methods will bring more love to the planet."

"True health is based on medicine power. It belongs to God and Mother Nature and can be taken away at any moment," observes Matthew Wood. "There is no medical system or insurance that can guarantee it. It can be restored at any time, but it requires a tax be paid: spiritual change."

## ECO-HERBALISM

Herbal medicine requires plants. Sometimes the simplest statements accommodate the most reckoning: Respect for the well-being of the green world is the only way we humans will continue to share in its gifts of healing. Regardless of whether we're talking about local medicine or international herb traffic, corporate farming or wildcrafting euphoria, we need to be conscious how our health needs and personal livelihoods affect the plants on which we rely. Plant health depends on diversity—and, frankly, so does ours.

Increasingly, as our kind has greater and greater impact on this planet home, other species are losing out. Loss of habitat due to development, extensive timber harvesting, and animal grazing hits plant populations hard. Wildcrafters working hard to meet commercial demand for certain herbs and the people purchasing those herbs don't need to figure reverence into the transaction. Simply making people aware of this travesty in the making isn't enough.

When Rosemary Gladstar realized the impact that the herbal movement was having on the medicinal plant populations, she founded United Plant Savers, an organization working toward respect and conservation of medicinal plants. "My biggest concern is the health of the plants. The negative part of all this interest in herbalism is the declining plant populations and habitat destruction," explains Rosemary. "One of the reasons we see such an incredible number of people interested in herbs right now really isn't about our medicine. It's about Earth being our medicine and our need to take care of her."

All of us understand the healing power of Nature on one level or another. We seek out this experience even if only vicariously through a natural product. Now, with the natural environment shrinking so rapidly, people are facing the realization that we can't be healthy on an unhealthy planet. Unquestionably, the ultimate work of any herbalist centers on healing this precious Earth along with its human inhabitants.

United Plant Savers has birthed unprecedented interest in doing right by the plants. That herbalists can band together and build such positive momentum is a testament to healing connection. Focusing attention on those native North American herbs most at risk spearheads the plant-protection efforts. The UpS "At-Risk List" consists of those herbs that are broadly used in commerce and which, due to over-harvest or loss of habitat—or by nature of their innate rareness or sensitivity—are at risk of a significant decline in numbers within their current range. Other wild medicinal plants proposed for inclusion on this list but in need of further research make up the UpS "To-Watch List." Some of these plants may be abundant in one bioregion but quite rare in another. The lumping of all North American species in a genus (as indicated by the abbreviated term "spp." in the Latin name) highlights cases where there is reason to believe that various species within the genus besides the officially recognized medicinal species are being utilized. Such happens through misidentification on the part of the wildcrafter, and sometimes even deliberately if it's felt, for instance, that the buyer will recognize any echinacea as *Echinacea angustifolia*.

A concerted effort to step well beyond awareness and actually do something about plant conservation makes United Plant Savers so vital. The responsibility to be caring stewards lies with each of us: No one has any call to be exploiting endangered wild plants.

UpS emphasizes using cultivated plants instead, specifically asking manufacturers and consumers to insist on organically grown sources of at-risk herbs. The notion that the energetics of a wild herb somehow surpass those of a cultivated medicinal plant falls short when the prayerful intent of conscientious farming is taken into account. Wildcrafters are asked to consider the ecological impact of taking these herbs from the wild. Replanting is essential if the gathering trade is to continue. Wildcrafters are encouraged to provide seed and expertise to others on how to plant and grow these herbs (see page 47). Yet, some plants simply defy human efforts to intervene.

"We took an issue that was basically unheard of ten years ago and made it a major issue," says Rosemary. "Interestingly, I've found more resistance within the herb movement than in the herb industry. Industry recognizes the problem. We all grew up with the idea that there's endless supplies of everything. We have no idea of the concept of not enough. Or of long-term projection. We weren't here when the last buffalo thundered across the plains or the passenger pigeons filled the skies. We can walk out and find a whole swamp of sundew up in Alaska. It's incomprehensible to us that four big companies going up two years in a row can deplete that. Yet we're seeing this hap-

# UNITED PLANT SAVERS' AT-RISK PLANT LIST

| | |
|---|---|
| American Ginseng | *Panax quinquefolius* |
| Black Cohosh | *Cimicifuga racemosa* |
| Bloodroot | *Sanguinaria canadensis* |
| Blue Cohosh | *Caulophyllum thalictroides* |
| Echinacea | *Echinacea* spp. |
| Eyebright | *Euphrasia* spp. |
| Goldenseal | *Hydrastis canadensis* |
| Helonias Root | *Chamaelirium luteum* |
| Kava Kava | *Piper methysticum* (Hawaii only) |
| Lady's Slipper Orchid | *Cypripedium* spp. |
| Lomatium | *Lomatium dissectum* |
| Osha | *Ligusticum porteri* spp. |
| Peyote | *Lophophora williamsii* |
| Slippery Elm | *Ulmus rubra* |
| Sundew | *Drosera* spp. |
| Trillium, Beth Root | *Trillium* spp. |
| True Unicorn | *Aletris farinosa* |
| Venus Flytrap | *Dionaea muscipula* |
| Virginia Snakeroot | *Aristolochia serpentaria* |
| Wild Yam | *Dioscorea villosa* spp. |

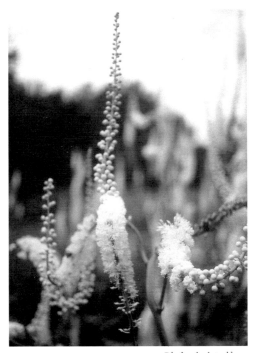

*Black cohosh in bloom*

pen. We have herbalists who live in plant-rich communities, totally resistant to the idea that osha or lomatium may be limited. If you look at market analysis and where projections go ten, fifteen years from now, you get a broader understanding. Many good, wise herbalists don't want to admit there are problems ahead for their favorite herbs.

"I'm treasuring my last bottles of immune formula that have osha. Once it's gone, I won't buy this herb anymore," pledges Rosemary. "I don't appreciate the argument that says, 'We have lots of this plant, I'm not going to stop using it,' when it's found growing nowhere else in the world except for the North American continent [at elevations of 9,000 feet or more] and you can't cultivate it. People are trying to learn how to cultivate osha, but aren't having any luck. Why do we keep using this in our medicine? We're very short-sighted."

The government is studying regulations on medicinal plants. One thought is to have the U.S. Forest Service certify herbalists in sustainable wildcrafting techniques as a prerequisite for being allowed to collect any plant species from public lands. As a part of this privilege, each person might also be required to help maintain the vigorous health of the plant stands from which they collect. New stands of herbs in appropriate areas of the forest could be encouraged. Stewardship in the long run, of course, needs to flow from individual hearts. Some herbalists understandably don't quite see government consciousness as the best answer going.

Certainly some wildcrafters acknowledge the finite tenderness of ecology. Common sense comes with the territory, so to speak, for people close to the land and the ways of Nature. Phyllis Light, in reflecting on her family's multigenerational tie to the land,

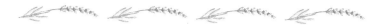

## UNITED PLANT SAVERS' TO-WATCH PLANT LIST

| | |
|---|---|
| Arnica | *Arnica* spp. |
| Butterfly Weed | *Asclepias tuberosa* |
| Cascara Sagrada | *Rhamus purshimia* |
| Chaparro | *Casatela emoryi* |
| Elephant Tree | *Bursera microphylla* |
| Gentian | *Gentiana* spp. |
| Goldthread | *Coptis* spp. |
| Lobelia | *Lobelia* spp. |
| Maidenhair Fern | *Adiantum pendatum* |
| Mayapple | *Podophyllum peltatum* |
| Oregon Grape | *Mahonia* spp. |
| Partridgeberry | *Mitchella repens* |
| Pink Root | *Spigelia marilandica* |
| Pipsissewa | *Chimaphila umbellata* |
| Spikenard | *Aralia racemosa, A. californica* |
| Stillingia | *Stillingia sylvatica* |
| Stoneroot | *Collinsonia canadensis* |
| Stream Orchid | *Epipactis gigantea* |
| Turkey Corn | *Dicentra canadensis* |
| White Sage | *Salvia apiana* |
| Wild Indigo | *Baptisia tinctoria* |
| Yerba Mansa | *Anemopsis californica* |
| Yerba Santa | *Eriodictyon californica* |

speaks of patches of plants in the Alabama woods that are kept secret and even guarded from intrusion. These wild patches were watched over and allowed to grow naturally without the influence of humans other than as wardens. "My cousin Calvin has watched over a ginseng patch for many, many years," says Phyllis. "It is his secret. He is connected to that patch of woods. Wildcrafters understand that indiscriminate harvesting results in loss for the years ahead. Unethical harvesting is a loss of plants, a loss of medicine, and a loss of income."

Nurturing the plants means we return more to the soil than we take. We acknowledge the inevitable ebb and flow of the seasons. Some years it may simply not be appropriate to harvest. And, we treat all species with a certain respect. "A true wildcrafter," adds Phyllis, "is a true guardian of our future."

The problem comes down to the fact that today there are so many more people. The escalating interest in herbs for alternative healing has fostered a big-business attitude toward this simple folk tradition. People caught up with the profit motive don't necessarily ever experience the plants growing in their natural habitat. Our responsibility toward these sentient beings begins with relationship. United Plant Savers makes its best case for conservation by simply inspiring people to get to know these precious herbs. In *Planting the Future*, America's most respected herbalists share in-depth information on using and growing thirty-three popular at-risk herbs. The real emphasis of this UpS book, however, lies in preserving wild stands of these plants. Recommendations are given for herb analogues for at-risk plants (other medicinal herbs that provide the same benefits and exist in plentiful amounts), as well as strict ecological guidelines for the at-risk plants. All author royalties go directly to fund the good work of United Plant Savers.

We strongly urge all herbalists to get involved by joining United Plant Savers. You'll find the address in appendix six. The eco-herbalism movement depends on its proponents to get the word out about plant conservation and land stewardship. A UpS education packet for presenters outlines a suggested talk about preserving our native medicinal plants. A slide show of at-risk plants (with eighty pictures of the roots,

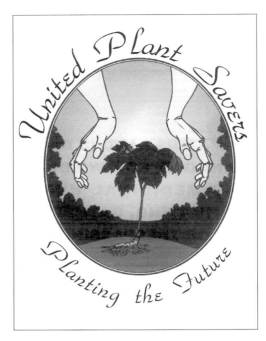

leaves, seeds, and flowers of these plants) with an informative script is also available. A directory of farms and nurseries that supply at-risk medicinal plants helps people find sources to follow through on the inspiration sure to be generated in a public presentation.

### Botanical Sanctuaries

United Plant Savers encourages people to designate their land as botanical sanctuaries. We can all create such places of protection and renewal, wherever we live. Sanctuary can be as small as a backyard or spread across acres and acres of wild land. "As we become ever more aware of the necessity to preserve our native wild plants," observes UpS board member Christopher Hobbs, "the realization that this task is impossible without first preserving habitat becomes equally clear. Each of us can contribute by viewing the land we live on as sanctuary—sacred, part of the great Earth Mother's heart—and caring for it in such a way."

The first botanical sanctuary came about when herbalist-farmer Paul Strauss donated

70 acres of his property in southeastern Ohio to United Plant Savers. Three decades of commitment to the land had instilled in Paul a profound desire to nurture Nature. Shortly thereafter, Michael and Judy Funk of Mountain People, a natural products distributor, made a considerable donation that enabled UpS to purchase 300 adjoining acres. This land portions equally between native hardwood forest and fields. More than 500 species of plants, more than 120 species of trees, and more than 200 species of fungi have been identified on the sanctuary. Half of the native medicinal plants on the At-Risk List thrive in abundance here. An annual series of workshops and work sessions brings herbalists to this land in Rutland (the sanctuary's hometown) to focus specifically on planting a sustainable future.

This is a story that gets far more exciting. Botanical sanctuary land does not need to be donated to United Plant Savers. People who choose to join the sanctuary network dedicate the privately held land in their stewardship to (I) active preservation of existing and introduced plant species; (2) an educational thrust that invites the public in for specific events; and (3) ongoing research on native medicinal plant conservation and cultivation. Land trusts can do the same. The goals go beyond serving as a rich depository for at-risk plants where seed stock can be generated and maintained. People willing to make a difference are needed. Restoring land to its richest diversity is foremost about love.

The guidelines for establishing a botanical sanctuary are available from United Plant Savers. Start by identifying the plants that are presently on your property. Consultants are available to help you learn more about your ecosystem and how to properly manage a native plant sanctuary. Offering educational opportunities can be as informal as teaching family and friends, holding classes for your community, or leading an herb walk. The two-year application requires a $100 fee ($50 per year) to cover the costs of listing each sanctuary, providing a sanctuary workbook and property signs, and promoting the concept in general.

Regenerating our lands is fulfilling work. Becoming a land steward lies at the heart of eco-herbalism. Only then does our work as herbalists become spiritually in tune with the plants and the community of all species.

## THE HERBALIST'S WAY

Herbalists can work with medical doctors and other health care providers to keep our respective communities in good health. Families can pursue responsibility for personal health. Local medicine can flow from a local agriculture centered firmly as the crown jewel of a bioregional economy. The plants can help restore sense to the human condition. This embrace of earthy reality will be good for what ails us.

One of Elliot Cowan's teachers had this to say about local medicine: "Anything that can be done with needles can also be done with herbs," said Professor Worsley. "But if you use herbs, for God's sake use local ones, because they are not only ten times stronger, they are not only a hundred times stronger, they are *one thousand times stronger* than plants that grow someplace else."[10]

It's striking, isn't it, how broad concepts such as community health and the energetics of plant medicine are rooted inextricably in local ground? We belong in our place, just like the plants, the rocks, the mountains and streams. Reestablishing roots grounds us in the earth consciousness we urge so strongly throughout this book. The local herbs referred to don't have stronger constituents per se, nor are they necessarily the most expedient medicine on the global shelf from a knowledge perspective. Being neighbors is what counts. The potency of herbs draws on the sun and rain and the stars shining down on our home turf, just as a healthy bacterial culture relies on interconnected balance in each gut, or the mycorrhizal fungi throughout the forest floor link tree to tree in the sharing of soil nutrients in each place. Our immune system does not resist the environment, but rather it leads a dance with the organisms encountered wherever we go. Our harmony with the land beneath our feet similarly weaves us into the web of life.

Cultural beliefs strongly influence what individuals believe. Land and community surround this issue of our health. Many of us have lost our biological roots in pursuit of the American Dream. We cast aside Nature to be rich and sated. That cultural choice in turn casts us out of the sacred hoop of Creation. We allow our physical selves to be isolated and alone when a caring natural world surrounds us. The diversity we find in Nature (when we're not disrupting the whole shebang) urges us to see how health flows in the interconnectedness of place. We need to recognize what we have in common, not only with the flora and the fauna, but with each other.

The good intention behind integrated medicine is one such step. The quest for the simple life is another. Extending the concepts of mind, body, and spirit to all aspects of the human condition opens the door for further understanding. We run into difficulty when we insist one reality dominates another. A Western doctor meeting up with native healers abroad can either acknowledge humbly virtues hitherto unforeseen or plow straight ahead with his "superior science." A constituency of pro-

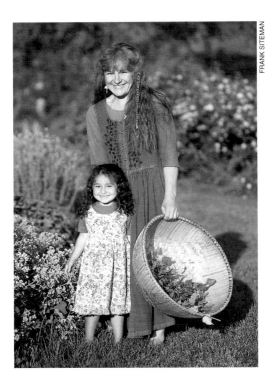

FRANK SITEMAN

fessional herbalists may eventually mandate that certain paths of education, an *accepted knowledge base,* so to speak, will determine who indeed may officially claim the title of herbalist. Sometimes only the names change in these long-standing debates of dominance, when what we really need is to be looking at the models and paradigms we wish to emulate. An indigenous system of health for our times will be embracing in the way only connection to place, and to each other, can be.

"The process is about changing our consciousness," says Pam Montgomery. "An herbal remedy is not going to save us. We need to change our consciousness. One person's healing experience at a time brings this about."

Therein lies the greatest hope. Awakening an awareness of that innate ability to heal in one person at a time is an easy thing to do. No complicated health campaigns need be undertaken, no missives need be

*Earth wisdom passes to each generation in turn. Gracie, having grown up knowing the healing plants, already has herbal skills to offer our community.*

issued on the government or industry levels. The ponderous questions of the twenty-first century are to be answered by the love and compassion that humans best can share with each other on a one-to-one basis. What flows so readily from the plants, and yet gets denied so vociferously in this culture, is the understanding that we are here for each other. That message, more than any other, lies in the heart and ways of every village herbalist since time immemorial.

"We can't force people to have the same ideals, even among the pure souls," Faye Burtch told Michael in his travels to meet with community herbalists. This comment certainly accounts for the many diverging opinions encountered on so many aspects of herbalism. We've alluded to the difficulties we face as a movement trying to incorporate the ideals of the herbal renaissance into the practical concerns of the day. Licensing requirements will not make the medicine of the people any more accessible. Strict standards set for corporate medicine making are not going to reacquaint people with their healing heritage. Fear to acknowledge our own human culpability is not going to make for a more loving society. These routes are simply not healing.

"Freedom to choose one's own health care was nearly added to the Bill of Rights, but wasn't, as no one thought it could ever be taken away," points out Joyce Wardwell. "Return us that right and watch the health care field truly blossom. To protect the plants from overharvesting and to ensure good-quality products, we must teach botany, gardening, ethnobotany, and cooking in our schools as well as at home. Anything that encourages hands-on experience and knowledge of plants." Like Joyce, we all intuitively know as Earth-loving herbalists what are the right courses of action. Herbal

medicine belongs to everyone. Despite our rancor and occasional confusion, we have to trust that something bigger is at work as we shape a holistic future. A medicine that strengthens the primary determinants of health—environment, nutrition, and behavior—clearly needs to be the goal.

## PLANTS GREENER THAN GREEN

MICHAEL TRAVELED Down Under for a year in the early 1980s. One day he took a municipal bus out of Christchurch, New Zealand, to the end of the line, and headed to Arthur's Pass toward the glorious Southern Alps. The Maori driver, a man nearing retirement age, turned to him—no one else was left on the bus at this point—and said, "I had this dream. A Greek-looking temple faced me. The broad steps led up to a pair of doors upon which were written the words *Love* and *Respect*. Like a complete code for living our lives, don't you think? I opened the door and saw not the inside of a building but a fabulous garden landscape. I saw people, all happy people, wearing white togas. One figure stood out from the rest. All the others basked in this presence of love. Then I noticed that everyone, when they ate, partook of a leafy plant, a plant greener than green. This seemed to nourish the people completely."

Then the bus driver focused his eyes deep into Michael's: "Perhaps that's why you are here, to find this plant that is greener than green."

Heady stuff for a youth headed for the hills, to be sure. Discovering a plant greener than green that offers such spiritual and physical nourishment seems more a community task. Twenty years later Michael is coming to an understanding of how this man's dream meshes with his own quixotic path. The underlying spirit of the plant world awaits us on a much deeper level than we've ever expected. We're intuiting a right direction as we open our hearts to the full circle of Creation. Our work with the healing plants themselves is what's *greener than green*.

"Local herb growers and tincture makers and those versed in the herbs of their region have the most to offer their communities," says Bob Liebert. "We need to decentralize and localize herb use as it's meant to be. Teach folks the value of herbs in their backyard over corporate herbs. No herb growing in the rain forest is necessarily better than what is growing at your feet. What is at your feet is fresher, more potent, and absolutely more in tune with you."

Such messages are carried to the people in our communities one at a time. The long and winding path that has brought us each so much personally, that paved the way for our becoming community herbalists, speaks clearly on this point: We must share what we know. Our influence extends around the globe, not in the fast sense introduced by technology, but in the hand-to-hand sense of people caring about people. Of people caring about plants. Of people caring about all species.

"We feel so held by the herbal community and such a part of it," says Kate Gilday. "There are little points of light all over the Northeast, all over North America, and all over the World, where people with like minds, with the compassion and desire to help the plants and all life-forms, can be found. It's a hundredth monkey sort of thing. People are deciding this is really going to be their life. This can really make an impact on the changes that are happening around us."

The work of the community herbalist is indeed timeless. The people that we become as herbalists, the work that we do in this bright new century, will be exactly the same as all other times when human hearts connect. Nurturing our loved ones and our communities, bestowing the gifts of the plants and of Spirit, is the way of the herbalist.

Let yours be a dance of blessing and merriment.

## NOTES

1. "An enlightened being who, out of compassion, forgoes nirvana in order to save others," *The American Heritage Dictionary* (New York: Houghton Mifflin, 1992 edition).

2. Ibid.

3. Patch Adams, *Gesundheit!* (Rochester, Vt.: Healing Arts Press, 1993, 1998), 49.

4. And to be fair to doctors who, after all, are on the front lines of healing, the directors of HMOs receive million-dollar salaries with stock options to boot. Such mega-greed is a hard act to follow.

5. Drug samples, continuing medical education, and conference travel exert a strong influence over physicians prescribing specific medications. See Ashley Wazana, M.D., "Physicians and the Pharmaceutical Industry, Is a Gift Ever Just a Gift?," *Journal of the American Medical Association*, Vol. 283: No. 3 (January 19, 2000), 373–80.

6. Robert M. Tenery, M.D., "Interactions Between Physicians and the Health Care Technology Industry," commentary in note 5.

7. "Patch Adams on Health and Healing," *Communities: Journal of Cooperative Living*, 102 (spring 1999), 38.

8. Ibid., 39.

9. Local currency can certainly be a more thoughtful medium of exchange. "Ithaca Hours" essentially equates an hour of anyone's labor as the basis of value in the Ithaca area of New York state. Paper "hour bills" can be exchanged with anyone networking in the system for his or her product or service. This type of wealth never leaves the community. For more on the concept and implementation of community currencies see Thomas H. Greco Jr., *Money: Understanding and Creating Alternatives to Legal Tender* (White River Junction, Vt.: Chelsea Green, 2001).

10. Elliot Cowan, *Plant Spirit Medicine* (Newberg, Ore.: Swan Raven & Company, 1995), 64.

# Terminology to Explain the Actions of Herbs

FOLLOWING ARE some of the most common terms used to describe the actions of herbs. These terms are an old and useful way to define herbs. The different actions indicate attributes of the herbs and help us choose remedies. Students relatively new to herbalism can create a practical learning tool by making a set of flash cards with the action on the front and the action word on the back.

**Adaptogen** A substance that helps us adapt to stresses, having a nourishing and tonifying effect. Examples include Siberian ginseng and nettles.

**Alterative** These herbs gradually restore proper functioning of the body, increasing health and vitality. Many aid the body in assimilating nutrients and supporting waste elimination. Some are antimicrobial. Examples include echinacea, red clover, cleavers, burdock, nettles, and dandelion.

**Analgesic/Anodyne** Herbs used to reduce pain. Examples include valerian, Jamaican dogwood, and passionflower.

**Antibiotic** Some have a direct germ-killing ability, others work by stimulation of the body's immune system. Examples include chaparral, echinacea, garlic, goldenseal, and thyme.

**Anticatarrhal** Herbs that help prevent and remove excess mucous buildup in the sinus area or elsewhere in the body. Examples include cayenne, ginger, goldenrod, sage, garlic, yarrow, and yerba santa.

**Anti-inflammatory** An herb that reduces and relieves inflammation. Examples include chamomile, calendula, witch hazel, and yarrow.

**Antispasmodic** Herbs that can prevent, reduce, and relieve muscle spasms or cramps. Examples include black cohosh, cramp bark, valerian, chamomile, wild yam, and skullcap.

**Astringent** These herbs contract tissues and thus reduce secretions and discharges. Examples include witch hazel, white oak bark, plantain, raspberry, yarrow, and uva ursi.

**Bitter** Herbs that taste bitter and stimulate the digestive system through a reflex via the taste buds. Examples include wormwood, gentian, goldenseal, hops, yarrow, and chamomile.

**Carminative** Herbs that are rich in volatile oils that stimulate the peristalsis of the digestive system and relax the stomach. They support digestion and help prevent and release gas. Examples include angelica, caraway, ginger, dill, cayenne, and peppermint.

**Demulcent** Herbs that are rich in mucilage. They soothe and heal irritated and inflamed tissue. Examples include comfrey, slippery elm, marsh mallow, chickweed, flax, and oats.

**Diaphoretic** Herbs that promote sweating and thus aid the body in the removal of wastes. Examples include catnip, elder, yarrow, boneset, peppermint, and ginger.

**Diuretic** Herbs that increase elimination of urine. Examples include cleavers, corn silk, dandelion, nettles, uva ursi, yarrow, and parsley.

**Emetic** Herbs that cause vomiting. Sometimes they must be taken at a relatively high dose. Examples include lobelia and ipecacuanha.

**Emmenagogue** Herbs that both stimulate and bring on menstrual flow. The term is also used in a generalized way for herbs that function as general tonics for the female system. Examples of herbs that help promote menstruation include pennyroyal, black cohosh, angelica, and blue cohosh.

**Emollient** Herbs that are applied to the skin to soften, soothe, and protect it. They act in a similar way externally as demulcents act internally. Examples include chickweed, comfrey, plantain, and marsh mallow.

**Expectorant** Herbs that help expel excess mucus from the respiratory system. Examples include elecampane, coltsfoot, garlic, goldenseal, and lobelia.

**Febrifuge** These herbs help the body to bring down a fever. Examples include boneset, elder flower, and yarrow.

**Galactogogue** Herbs that increase the secretion of mother's milk. Examples include fennel, blessed thistle, aniseed, and fenugreek.

**Hemostatic** Herbs that control or stop bleeding. Examples include yarrow, shepherd's purse, and white oak bark.

**Hepatic** Herbs that aid the liver. Their use helps tone, strengthen, and increase the flow of bile. Examples include dandelion, Oregon grape root, goldenseal, wild yam, and yellow dock.

**Hypnotic** Herbs that promote deep relaxing sleep (not a hypnotic trance). Examples include hops, skullcap, valerian, and passionflower.

**Laxative** Herbs that promote bowel movement. Laxatives are less drastic than purgatives. Examples include cascara sagrada, senna, flaxseed, yellow dock, and rhubarb root.

**Nervine** Herbs that have a beneficial effect on the nervous system. Examples include peppermint, skullcap, valerian, chamomile, catnip, and passionflower.

**Pectoral** These herbs have a general strengthening and healing effect on the respiratory system. Examples include coltsfoot, garlic, elecampane, mullein, and marsh mallow.

**Rubefacient** Herbs that increase the surface circulation, bringing blood flow to the skin and causing local irritation. They draw inflammation and congestion from deeper tissue. Examples include cayenne, horseradish, ginger, and mustard.

**Sedative** Herbs that calm the nervous system and reduce stress and nervousness throughout the body. Examples include valerian, skullcap, passionflower, hops, and wild lettuce.

**Stimulant** Herbs that increase the energy of the body by quickening and enlivening the physiological functions. Examples include cayenne, ginger, peppermint, ginseng, sage, prickly ash, and horseradish.

**Styptic** These herbs reduce or stop external bleeding by their astringent and coagulating effects. Examples include yarrow and shepherd's purse.

**Tonic** Herbs that strengthen, nourish, and enliven specific organs or the whole body. Examples include ginseng, dong quai, nettles, dandelion, raspberry, oats, and vitex.

**Vulnerarie** Herbs that help heal the body by promoting cell growth and repair. Applied externally to aid the body in healing wounds and cuts. Examples include aloe vera, comfrey, chickweed, plantain, calendula, and St. John's wort.

# APPENDIX TWO
# *Home Study Courses*

**Australasian College of Health Sciences**
5940 SW Hood Avenue
Portland, OR 97239
1-800-487-8839
www.achs.edu

**Clayton College of Natural Health**
2140 11th Avenue South, Suite 305
Birmingham, AL 35205
1-800-995-4590
www.ccnh.edu

**Dominion Herbal College**
7527 Kingsway
Burnaby, British Columbia, V3N 3C1, Canada
1-888-342-1220
www.dominionherbal.com

**EastWest School of Herbology**
Michael and Lesley Tierra
PO Box 275
Ben Lomond, CA 95005
1-800-717-5010
www.planetherbs.com

**Integrating Western Herbology and Ayurveda**
Candis Cantin
PO Box 1445
Placerville, CA 95667
530-626-9288
www.evergreenherbgarden.org

**Foundations in Herbal Medicine**
Dr. Tieraona Low Dog
4840 Pan American Freeway NE
Albuquerque, NM 87109
1-888-857-1976
www.fihm.com

**Foundations of Herbalism**
Christopher Hobbs
4731 East Fork Road
Williams, OR 97544
541-846-0702
www.foundationsofherbalsim.com

**The School of Natural Healing**
PO Box 412
Springville, UT 84663
1-800-372-8255
www.schoolofnaturalhealing.com

**Science and Art of Herbology**
Rosemary Gladstar
PO Box 420
East Barre, VT 05649
802-479-9825
www.sagemountain.com

**Spirit and Practice of the Wise Woman Tradition**
Susun Weed
PO Box 64
Woodstock, NY 12498
845-246-8081
www.susunweed.com

# Herb Schools and Apprenticeship Programs

*Programs that offer long-term, ongoing courses that meet several days per week:*

**California School of Herbal Studies**
James Green, director
PO Box 39
Forestville, CA 95436
707-887-7457
www.CSHS.com

**The College of Phytotherapy**
Rutherford Park, Marley Lane
Battle, East Sussex TN33 0TY
    United Kingdom
+44 (0)1424 776780
www.collegeofphytotherapy.com

**International College of Herbal Medicine**
Amanda McQuade Crawford,
    associate director
18-B Sirrah Street Wainui
Gisborne, New Zealand
805-646-6699 in the USA

**North American Institute of Medical Herbalism**
Paul Bergner, director
PO Box 20512
Boulder, CO 80308
303-541-9552
www.naimh.com/

**Northeast School of Botanical Medicine**
7Song, director
PO Box 6626
Ithaca, NY 14851
607-539-7172
www.7Song.com

**Southwest School of Botanical Medicine**
Michael Moore, director
PO Box 4565
Bisbee, Arizona 85603
520-432-5855
www.swsbm.com

**Tai Sophia Institute for the Healing Arts**
7750 Montpelier Road
Laurel, MD 20723
1-800-735-2986
www.tai.edu

**Wild Rose College of Natural Healing**
Terry Willard, director
#400, 1228 Kensington Rd.
    NW
Calgary, Alberta T2N 4P9
    Canada
1-888-953-7673
www.wrc.net

*Herb centers that offer long-term apprenticeships, herb intensives, weekend programs, and one-day classes. We have included just a sampling of the many quality programs available:*

**Avena Institute**
Deb Soule
219 Mill Street
Rockport, ME 04856
207-594-2403
www.avenaherbs.com

**Blazing Star Herbal School**
Tony(a) Lemos
PO Box 6
Shelburne Falls, MA 01370
413-625-6875
www.blazingstarherbalschool.org/

**Columbines School of Botanical Studies**
Howie Brounstein
PO Box 50532
Eugene, OR 97405
541-687-7114
www.botanicalstudies.net

**Dandelion Herbal Center**
Jane Bothwell
4803 Greenwood Heights Drive
Kneeland, CA 95549
707-442-8157
www.dandelionherb.com

**Earthsong Herbals**
Margi Flint
10 Central Street
Marblehead, MA 01945
781-631-4312
www.earthsongherbals.com/

**Heartsong Farm Healing Herbs
    and Educational Center**
Nancy and Michael Phillips
859 Lost Nation Road
Groveton, NH 03582
603-636-2286
www.herbsandapples.com

**Herbal Therapeutics**
David Winston
PO Box 553
Broadway, NJ 08808
908-835-0822
www.herbaltherapeutics.net

**Plant People**
Joyce Wardwell
3936 Mt. Bliss Road
East Jordan, MI 49727
616-536-2877

**Ravencroft Garden**
EagleSong and Sally King
PO Box 170
Startup, WA 98293
360-794-2938
www.ravencroftgarden.com

**Partner Earth Education Center**
Pam Montgomery
1525 Danby Mountain Road
Danby, VT 05739
802-293-5996
www.partnereartheducation
    center.com

**Prairie Wise Herbal School**
Kahla Wheeler
1156 West 103rd Street, #123
Kansas City, MO 64114
816-361-4081
www.prairiewise.com

**Sage Mountain Herbal Retreat
    Center and Botanical
    Sanctuary**
Rosemary Gladstar
PO Box 420
East Barre, VT 05649
802-479-9825
www.sagemountain.com

**Sacred Plant Traditions Center
    for Herbal Studies**
Kathleen Maier
313 2nd Street SE, Suite 211
Charlottesville, VA 22902
434-295-3820
www.sacredplanttraditions.com

**Sweetgrass School of Herbalism**
Robyn Klien
6101 Shadow Circle Drive
Bozeman, MT 59715
406-585-8006
www.rrreading.com

**Wise Woman Center**
Susun Weed
PO Box 64
Woodstock, NY 12498
845-246-8081
www.susunweed.com

**Woodland Essence**
Kate Gilday and Don Babineau
392 Tea Cup Street
Cold Brook, NY 13324
315-845-1515
www.woodlandessence.com

# Holistic Health on the World Wide Web

*Links can take one anywhere in cyber-space. We've included a few worthy places to go that guide our wide-ranging interests. Additional Web sites are listed elsewhere in these appendices.*

## INTERNET DIRECTORIES

**Health World Online**
www.healthy.net

**Health WWWeb**
www.healthwwweb.com/

**InfoMine: Biological, Agricultural & Medical Sciences**
http://infomine.ucr.edu/

**Internet Directory for Botany**
www.botany.net/IDB/botany.html

**Martindale's Health Science Center**
www.martindalecenter.com/

**National Center for Complementary and Alternative Medicine**
http://nccam.nih.gov/

**National Library of Medicine**
www.nlm.nih.gov/

**Rosenthal Center for Alternative/Complementary Medicine**
www.rosenthal.hs.columbia.edu/

**Virtual Library of Pharmacy**
www.pharmacy.org/

## PLANT MISCELLANY

**American Indian Ethnobotany Database**
http://herb.umd.umich.edu/

**James Duke's Phytochemical Database**
www.ars-grin.gov/duke/

**Medical Marijuana Research**
www.maps.org/mmj/?13,22

**Medicinal Herbs by Botanical Name**
www.nnlm.nlm.nih.gov/pnr/uwmhg/botnames.html

**Plants Database**
http://plants.usda.gov/plants/

**United Plant Savers**
www.plantsavers.org

## MORE HERB CONNECTIONS

**David Hoffman's Materia Medica on Health World**
www.healthy.net/clinic/therapy/herbal/herbic/herbs/index.asp

**European Scientific Cooperative on Phytotherapy**
www.escop.com/

**Everything Herbal**
www.herbnet.com/

**Henriette's Herbal Homepage**
www.ibiblio.org/herbmed/

**Herbal Hall**
www.herb.com/herbal.htm

**Herb Med**
www.herbmed.org/

**The Phytochemistry of Herbs**
www.herbalchem.net

## BOOK REFERENCES

**Classic Texts**
www.swsbm.com/homepage/

**Grieve's Modern Herbal**
www.botanical.com/botanical/mgmh/mgmh.html

**King's American Dispensatory**
www.ibiblio.org/herbmed/eclectic/kings/main.html

**The Merck Manual**
www.merck.com/pubs/mmanual/

**Robyn's Recommended Reading**
www.rrreading.com

# An Herbalist's Source List

## PLANTS AND SEEDS

**Fedco Seeds**
PO Box 520
Waterville, ME 04903
207-873-6411
www.fedcoseeds.com

**Garden Medicinals**
PO Box 320
Earlysville, VA 22936
434-964-9113
www.gardenmedicinals.com

**Horizon Herbs**
PO Box 69
Williams, OR 97544
541-846-6704
www.horizonherbs.com

**Land Reformer's Nursery**
35703 Loop Road
Rutland, OH 45775
740-742-3478

**NC Ginseng & Goldenseal**
   **Company**
300 Indigo Bunting Lane
Marshall, NC 28753
828-649-3536
www.ncgoldenseal.com

**Prairie Moon Nursery**
31837 Bur Oak Lane
Winona, MN 55987
1-866-417-8156
www.prairiemoon.com

**Richters Herbs**
Goodwood, Ontario, L0C 1A0
Canada
905-640-6677
www.richters.com

## ORGANIC GROWING SUPPLIES

**Earth Tools**
660 Mt. Vernon Ridge Road
Frankfort, KY 40601
502-226-5751
*United Plant Savers receives a donation
   for every purchase of a BCS tiller.*

**Peaceful Valley Farm Supply**
PO Box 2209
Grass Valley, CA 95945
1-888-784-1722
www.groworganic.com

## BULK HERBS

**Blessed Herbs**
109 Barre Plains Road
Oakham, MA 01068
508-882-3839
www.blessedherbs.com

**Frontier Herbs**
3021 78th Street
Norway, IA 52318
319-227-7966
www.frontiercoop.com/

**Healing Spirits**
9198 St. Rt. 415
Avoca, NY 14809
607-566-2701
www.infoblvd.net/healingspirits/

**Heartsong Farm Healing Herbs**
859 Lost Nation Road
Groveton, NH 03582
603-636-2286
www.herbsandapples.com

**Herb Pharm**
PO Box 116
Williams, OR 97544
1-800-348-4372
www.herb-pharm.com/

**Ryan Drum**
Island Herbs
PO Box 25
Waldron, WA 98297
206-499-0994
*Sea vegetables.*
www.partnereartheducationcenter.
   com/ryan/islandherbs.html

**Southern Virginia Herbals**
1107 Wooding Trail
Halifax, VA 24558
804-476-1339

**Zack Woods Herb Farm**
278 Mead Road
Hyde Park, VT 05655
802-888-7278
www.zackwoodsherbs.com

## MEDICINE MAKING WHEREWITHAL

**Aaper Alcohol**
PO Box 339
Shelbyville, KY 40066
1-800-456-1017
www.aaper.com

**Apothecary Products, Inc.**
11750 12th Avenue South
Burnsville, MN 55337
1-800-328-2742
www.apothecaryproducts.com/

**Desert Bloom Herbs**
1606 N. Florida
Silver City, NM 88061
1-800-583-2976
www.zianet.com/desertbloom
*Herbalist Richard McDonald handcrafts percolator bottles at low cost.*

**Jean's Greens Herbal Essentials**
1545 Columbia Turnpike
Schodack, NY 12033
518-479-0471
www.jeansgreens.com
*Herbs, essential oils, jars, tinctures, salves, books, beeswax, infused oils, and more.*

**Longevity Herb Company**
1549 West Jewett Boulevard
White Salmon, WA 98672
509-493-2626
www.tincturepress.com/
*The best tincture presses for a homegrown apothecary.*

**Morningstar Publications**
44 Rim Road
Boulder, CO 80302
1-800-435-1670
*Debra St. Claire's medicine making video.*

**Mountain Rose Herbs**
PO Box 50220
Eugene, OR 97405
1-800-879-3337
www.mountainroseherbs.com

**Sayfer Botanicals**
530 Oxford St. West
London, Ontario N6H 1T8,
   Canada
519-472-0011
www.herbmeds.com/

**Vita-Mix**
8615 Usher Road
Cleveland, Ohio 44138
1-800-848-2649

## FLOWER ESSENCES

**Flower Essence Society**
PO Box 459
Nevada City, CA 95959
1-800-736-9222
www.flowersociety.org

**Woodland Essence**
PO Box 206
Cold Brook, NY 13324
www.woodlandessence.com
*Specializing in at-risk North American forest and flower essences.*

## ESSENTIAL OILS

**Benzalco Essential Oil Equipment**
1291 Cumberland Avenue
West Lafayette, IN 47906
765-497-1313

**Essential Oil Company**
PO Box 206
Lake Oswego, OR 97034
1-800-729-5912
http://essentialoil.com/

Liberty Naturals
PO Box 66068
Portland, OR 97266
1-800-289-8427

## WORTHY CONNECTIONS

### Gesundheit! Institute
Patch Adams, M.D.
6855 Washington Blvd.
Arlington, VA 22213
703-525-8169
*Tax-deductible donations for a
free hospital are welcomed.
To volunteer directly at the
site, write Gesundheit!
Institute, HC 64, Box 167,
Hillsboro, WV 24946.*

### National Center for Preservation of Medicinal Herbs
33560 Beech Grove Rd.
Rutland, OH 45775
740-742-4401
http://home.frognet.net/~
rural8/

## BOOK CONNECTIONS

### American Botanical Council
PO Box 201660
Austin, TX 78720
www.herbalgram.org

### Eclectic Medical Publications
36560 SE Industrial Way
Sandy, OR 97055
1-800-332-4372
www.eclecticherb.com/emp

### Herbalist & Alchemist Books
PO Box 553
Broadway, NJ 08808
908-835-0822
www.herbaltherapeutics.net/

### Lloyd Library and Museum
917 Plum Street
Cincinnati, Ohio 45202
www.lloydlibrary.org/

### Miscellaneous Medica Herbarium Supply Company
PO Box 10966
Bozeman, MT 59715-
8420
1-800-348-2338
www.herbariumsupply.com

### SKS Bottling and Packaging Company
3 Knabner Road
Mechanicville, NY 12118
518-899-7488
www.sks-bottle.com

### Burch Bottle
430 Hudson River Road
Waterford, NY 12188
1-800-903-2830
www.burchbottle.com/

# Associations and Publications

## ASSOCIATIONS

### American Herbal Products Association
PO Box 30585
Bethesda, MD 20824
301-951-3207
www.ahpa.org
*National trade organization for herbal product manufacturers.*

### American Herbalists Guild
1931 Gaddis Road
Canton, GA 30115
770-751-6021
www.americanherbalistsguild.com/
*Peer reviewed professional organization. Publishes directory of herbal education and herbal practitioner directory.*

### Bio-Dynamic Farming and Gardening Association
25844 Butler Road
Junction City, OR 97448
1-888-516-7797
www.biodynamics.com

### Herb Growing & Marketing Network
PO Box 245
Silver Spring, PA 17575
717-393-3295
www.herbworld.com
*Publishes the* Herbal Green Pages *and helps with all sorts of business connections.*

### Herb Research Foundation
4140 15th Street
Boulder, CO 80304
303-449-2265
www.herbs.org/
*Provides online database searching and scientific articles.*

### Northeast Herb Association
PO Box 103
Manchaug, MA 01526
www.northeastherbal.org
*Publishes an excellent newsletter and promotes herbal camaraderie of the finest kind.*

### United Plant Savers
PO Box 400
East Barre, VT 05649
802-479-9825
www.plantsavers.org
*Organization working to save endangered medicinal plants. Publishes newsletters and sources for growing endangered and threatened medicinal plants.*

### Weston Price Foundation
PMB 106-380,
4200 Wisconsin Avenue NW
Washington, DC 20016
202-333-HEAL
www.westonaprice.org
*Publishes* Wise Traditions in Food, Farming and the Healing Arts *and connects one with Sally Fallon's good work.*

## PUBLICATIONS

**American Herb Association Quarterly Newsletter**
PO Box 1673
Nevada City, CA 9595
530-265-9552
www.ahaherb.com

**Herbs for Health**
Ogden Publications
1503 SW 42nd Street
Topeka, KS 66609
www.discoverherbs.com

**HerbalGram**
PO Box 201660
Austin, TX 78723
1-800-373-7105
www.herbalgram.org

**Medical Herbalism**
PO Box 20512
Boulder, CO 80308
303-541-9552
www.medherb.com

# *Herbal Recommendations*

Name: _____

Date: _____ Next Appointment Time:_____

Key physical areas of concern: _____

Key emotional areas of concern: _____

Key spiritual areas of concern: _____

## DIETARY RECOMMENDATIONS:

### 1. Reduce the following:

| | | | | | | |
|---|---|---|---|---|---|---|
| Wheat | Sugar | Dairy | White flour products | Fried foods | Meat | Processed foods |
| Alcohol | Coffee | Diet drinks | Caffeinated beverages | Foods with Aspartame | | Hydrogenated oils |

Other: _____

### 2. Increase these foods (organic when possible):

Whole grains: brown rice, millet, buckwheat,
    oats, barley, quinoa, spelt

Green vegetables: kale, collards, turnip, mustard
    or beet greens, broccoli, brussels sprouts,
    sea vegetables (kelp, dulse, nori)

Orange vegetables: carrots, squashes, yams,
    sweet potatoes

Fresh fruit in season:

Cold pressed oil: olive, sesame

Protein: fish, poultry, eggs, beans and rice, raw
    nuts, seeds

Spices: ginger, turmeric, cinnamon, basil, kelp,
    onion, garlic, miso

## POSSIBLE SUPPLEMENTS:

## HERBAL RECOMMENDATIONS:

| | FORMULA | HOW MUCH | HOW OFTEN |
|---|---|---|---|
| Teas: | | | |
| Tinctures: | | | |
| Capsules: | | | |
| Bath or footbath: | | | |
| External Applications: | | | |
| Essential Oils: | | | |

## EXERCISE:

Daily _____

Weekly _____

## OTHER POSSIBLE THERAPIES:

Chiropractic, Acupuncture, Massage, Reiki, etc.

Relaxation/Reflection: Prayer time, Yoga, Meditation, Gentle music, visualization, or other.

# Bibliography

Achterberg, Jeanne. *Woman as Healer.* Boston: Shambhala, 1990.

Adams, Patch, with Maureen Mylander. *Gesundheit!* Rochester, Vt.: Healing Arts Press, 1993.

Barasch, Marc Ian. *The Healing Path: A Soul Approach to Illness.* New York: Penguin, 1993.

Bergner, Paul. *The Healing Power of Garlic.* Rocklin, Calif.: Prima Publishing, 1996.

Buhner, Stephen. *Herbal Antibiotics: Natural Alternatives for Treating Drug-Resistant Bacteria.* Pownal, Vt.: Storey Books. 1999.

————. *Sacred Plant Medicine.* Boulder, Colo.: Roberts Rinehart, 1996.

Cech, Richo. *Making Plant Medicine.* Williams, Oreg.: Horizon Herbs, 2000.

————. *Medicinal Herbs Cultivation* Series (12 booklets). Williams, Ore.: Horizon Herbs, 1995.

Chevallier, Andrew. *Natural Health Encyclopedia of Herbal Medicine.* New York: DK Publishing, 1996.

Clayman, Charles, editor-in-chief. *The Human Body: An Illustrated Guide to its Structure, Function, and Disorders.* New York: DK Publishing, 1995.

Colbin, Annemarie. *Food and Healing.* New York: Ballantine, 1986.

Coleman, Elliot. *The New Organic Grower.* White River Junction, Vt.: Chelsea Green, 1989.

Cowan, Elliot. *Plant Spirit Medicine.* Newberg, Ore.: Swan Raven & Company, 1995.

Crellin, John K., and Jane Philpott. *Trying to Give Ease: Tommie Bass and the Story of Herbal Medicine.* Durham, N.C.: Duke University Press, 1989.

Ehrenreich, Barbara, and Deirdre English. *Witches, Midwives, and Nurses.* Old Westbury, N.Y.: Feminist Press, 1973.

Elliot, Doug. *Wild Roots: A Forager's Guide to the Edible and Medicinal Roots, Tubers, Corms, and Rhizomes of North America.* Rochester, Vt.: Healing Arts Press, 1995.

————. *Wildwoods Wisdom: Encounters with the Natural World.* New York: Paragon House,1992.

Engeland, Ron L. *Growing Great Garlic.* Okanogan, Wash.: Filaree Productions, 1991.

Falconi, Dina. *Earthly Bodies & Heavenly Hair.* Woodstock, N.Y.: Ceres Press, 1998.

Fallon, Sally, and Mary G. Enig. *Nourishing Traditions: The Cookbook that Challenges Politically Correct Nutrition and the Diet Dictocrats.* Washington, D.C.: New Trends Publishing, 1999.

Felter, Harvey Wickes. *The Eclectic Materia Medica, Pharmacology, and Therapeutics.* Cincinnati: John K. Scudder, 1922.

Findhorn Community. *The Findhorn Garden.* New York: Harper & Row, 1975.

Foster, Steven. *Herbal Renaissance: Growing, Using, and Understanding Herbs in the Modern World.* Salt Lake City: Gibbs Smith Publishing, 1993.

Foster, Steven, and James A. Duke. *Eastern/Central Medicinal Plants and Herbs.* Peterson Field Guides. New York: Houghton Mifflin, 2000.

Jacobs, Betty E. M. *Growing and Using Herbs Successfully.* Pownal, Vt.: Storey Books, 1976, 1981.

Gladstar, Rosemary, ed. *Planting the Future.* Rochester, Vt.: Healing Arts Press, 2000.

———. *Herbal Healing for Women.* New York: Fireside, 1993.

Green, James. *The Herbal Medicine-Maker's Handbook.* Forestville, Calif.: Simplers Botanical Company, 1990.

Grieve, Maude. *A Modern Herbal.* New York: Dover, 1971.

Griggs, Barbara. *Green Pharmacy: The History and Evolution of Western Herbal Medicine.* Rochester, Vt.: Healing Arts Press, 1981, 1997.

Hälvä, Seija, and Lyle E. Croker. *Manual for Northern Herb Growers.* Amherst, Mass.: HSMP Press, 1996.

Heinerman, John. *The Healing Benefits of Garlic.* New Canaan, Conn.: Keats Publishing, 1994.

Hobbs, Christopher. *Herbal Remedies for Dummies.* Foster City, Calif.: IDG Books, 1998.

Hobbs, Christopher, and Kathi Keville. *Women's Herbs, Women's Health.* Loveland, Colo.: Botanica Press, 1998.

Hoffmann, David. *The Complete Illustrated Holistic Herbal.* Boston: Element Books, 1996.

———. *An Elder's Herbal.* Rochester, Vt.: Healing Arts Press, 1993.

Hopman, Ellen Evert. *Tree Medicine, Tree Magic.* Custer, Wash.: Phoenix, 1991.

Keville, Kathi, and Mindy Green. *Aromatherapy: A Complete Guide to the Healing Art.* Freedom, Calif.: Crossing Press, 1995.

Kindscher, Kelly. *Medicinal Wild Plants of the Prairie: An Ethnobotanical Guide.* Lawrence, Kans.: University Press of Kansas, 1992.

Levy, Juliette de Baïracli. *Herbal Handbook for Farm and Stable.* Emmaus, Pa.: Rodale, 1952.

———. *Nature's Children.* Woodstock, N.Y.: Ash Tree, 1970.

Logsdon, Gene. *Good Spirits: A New Look at Ol' Demon Alcohol.* White River Junction, Vt.: Chelsea Green, 1999.

Lovel, Hugh. *A Biodynamic Farm.* Kansas City: Acres USA, 1994.

Mehl-Madrona, Lewis. *Coyote Medicine: Lessons from Native American Healing.* New York: Fireside, 1997.

Miller, Lucinda G., and Wallace J. Murray, eds. *Herbal Medicinals: A Clinician's Guide.* Binghamton, N.Y.: Pharmaceutical Products Press, 1998.

Mills, Simon. *Out of the Earth: The Essential Book of Herbal Medicine.* London: Viking, 1991.

Mills, Simon, and Kerry Bone, *Principles and Practice of Phytotherapy.* London: Churchill Livingstone, 2000.

Moore, Michael. *Herbal Materia Medica* (teaching manual). Bisbee, Ariz.: Southwest School of Botanical Medicine, 1995.

———. *Medicinal Plants of the Desert and Canyon West.* Sante Fe: Museum of New Mexico Press, 1989.

———. *Medicinal Plants of the Mountain West.* Sante Fe: Museum of New Mexico Press, 1979.

Northrup, Christiane. *Women's Bodies, Women's Wisdom.* New York: Bantam, 1994, 1998.

Onstad, Dianne. *Whole Foods Companion.* White River Junction, Vt.: Chelsea Green, 1996.

Painter, Gilian. *A Herbalist's Medicine-Making Workbook.* Auckland, New Zealand: 1998.

Parker, Trudy Ann. *Aunt Sarah: The 108 Winters of an Abenaki Healing Woman.* Lancaster, N.H.: Dawnland Publications, 1994.

Perone, Bobette, Henrietta Stockel, and Victoria Krueger. *Medicine Women, Curanderas, and Women*

*Doctors.* Norman, Okla: University of Oklahoma Press, 1989.

Potts, Billie. *Witches Heal.* 3d ed. Summit, N.Y.: Cohosh Corners Press, 1998

Preston, Thomas. *The Clay Pedestal: A Re-examination of the Doctor-Patient Relationship.* Seattle, Wash.: Madrona, 1981.

Romm, Aviva Jill. *Natural Healing for Babies and Children.* Freedom, Calif.: Crossing Press, 1996.

Root-Bernstein, Robert and Michèle. *Honey, Mud, Maggots, and Other Medical Marvels: The Science Behind Folk Remedies and Old Wives' Tales.* New York: Houghton Mifflin, 1997.

Sachs, Paul. *Edaphos: Dynamics of a Natural Soil System.* Newbury, Vt.: Edaphic Press, 1993.

St. Claire, Debra. *The Herbal Medicine Cabinet.* Berkeley, Calif.: Celestial Arts, 1997.

Soule, Deb. *The Roots of Healing: A Woman's Book of Herbs.* New York: Citadel, 1995.

Steiner, Rudolf. *Spiritual Foundations for the Renewal of Agriculture* (a course of lectures given in 1924). Kimberton, Pa.: Biodynamic Farming and Gardening Association, 1993.

Strol, Wolf D. *Culture and Horticulture.* Wyoming, R.I.: Biodynamic Literature, 1979

Sturdivant, Lee. *Herbs For Sale.* Friday Harbor, Wa.: San Juan Naturals, 1994.

Sturdivant, Lee, and Tim Blakley. *Medicinal Herbs in the Garden, Field and Marketplace.* Friday Harbor, Wash.: San Juan Naturals, 1999.

Tierra, Michael. *The Way of Herbs,* New York: Simon & Schuster, 1990.

Tierra, Michael, editor. *American Herbalism: Essays on Herbs and Herbalism by Members of the American Herbalists Guild.* Freedom, Calif.: Crossing Press, 1992.

Tilford, Gregory L. *From Earth to Herbalist: An Earth Conscious Guide to Medicinal Plants.* Missoula, Mont: Mountain Press Publishing Company, 1998.

Tilford, Gregory L. and Mary Wulff-Tilford. *All You Ever Wanted to Know About Herbs for Pets.* Irvine, Calif.: BowTie Press, 1999.

Tilgner, Sharol. *Herbal Medicine: From the Heart of the Earth.* Creswell, Ore.: Wise Acres, 1999.

Tompkins, Peter. *The Secret Life of Nature: Living in Harmony with the Hidden World of Nature Spirits from Fairies to Quarks.* San Francisco: Harper, 1997.

Walters, Charles, and C. J. Fenzau. *An Acres USA Primer.* Kansas City: Acres USA, 1979.

Wardwell, Joyce. *The Herbal Home Remedy Book.* Pownal, Vt.: Storey Books, 1998.

Weed, Susun. *Healing Wise.* Woodstock, N.Y.: Ash Tree Publishing, 1989.

Weiss, Rudolf Fritz. *Herbal Medicine.* Translation. Beaconsfield, England: Beaconsfield, 1988.

Weil, Andrew. *Eating Well for Optimum Health.* New York: Alfred A. Knopf, 2000.

———. *Eight Weeks to Optimum Health.* New York: Alfred A. Knopf, 1997.

White, Linda, and Sunny Mavor. *Kids, Herbs, Health.* Loveland, Colo.: Interweave, 1998.

Wood, Matthew. *The Practice of Herbal Wisdom: A Guide for Practitioners of Traditional Herbal Wisdom.* (A work-in-progress generously shared with us by the author.)

———. *The Book of Herbal Wisdom: Using Plants as Medicines.* Berkeley: North Atlantic Books, 1997.

Wrensch, Ruth D. *The Essence of Herbs: An Environmental Guide to Herb Gardening.* Jackson: University Press of Mississippi, 1992.

Yance, Donald. *Herbal Medicine, Healing and Cancer.* Chicago: Keats, 1999.

# Index

## A

Adams, Dr. Patch, 298, 300, 302
adaptogen herbs, 145
*Adverse Effects of Herbal Drugs,* 66
agrimony, 78, 171
alcohol, 231–33
alfalfa, 161, 204, 205, 228
alkahest, 231
alkanet, 171
allopathic medicine, 3–4, 295–99
*All You Ever Wanted to Know About Herbs for Pets,* 54
alternative medicine, 3, 8–11, 293
American Botanical Council (ABC), 10, 91, 266
*The American Eclectic Materia Medica and Therapeutics,* 225
American Herbalists Guild (AHG), 25, 26, 34, 94, 99, 101, 133, 134, 147, 295
American Herbal Products Association, 30, 265
*American Materia Medica Therapeutics and Pharmacognosy,* 85
anatomy, 143–46
*Anatomy and Physiology in Health and Illness,* 144
*The Anatomy Coloring Book,* 144
angelica, 164, 184, 202, 221
apothecary, 52–56, 212–13, 219–21
apprenticeships, 91–98, 287–91
aqueous ethanol alcohol, 231
Argus, Jean, 31, 32, 53, 252–53
arnica, 190, 246
aromatherapy, 244
Arvigo, Rosita, 79
ashwagandha, 17, 178, 179, 192, 202, 206, 273
assessment, 133–41
astragulus, 145, 228, 229, 251, 273
At-Risk List (UpS), 196, 307, 308
Aurora, 111
*Ayurvedic Healing,* 131

## B

Babineau, Don, 32, 169, 174, 285, 288–90
barberry, 146
bark, harvesting, 194–96
bartering, 110, 118, 122
Bass, Tommie, 32, 113
Bauer, Rudolf, 29
bearberry, 170, 255
Bear Creek Herbs, 52, 98, 264
belladonna, 17, 65
bergamot, 170
*Between Heaven and Earth,* 131
beverage tea, 225
bionomial nomenclature, 65
Birzneck, Ella, 291
black cherry, 195
black cohosh, 147, 174, 197, 273
black peppermint. *See* peppermint, black
Blakley, Tim, 170
blessed thistle, 184, 202
bloodroot, 174
blossoms, plucking, 190–92
blue cohosh, 174
blue vervain, 71, 205
boneset, 161
*The Book of Herbal Wisdom,* 13, 86
books, herbal, 84–91
borage, 145, 188, 205
botanical sanctuaries, 310–11
*Botany in a Day,* 67, 90
Bothwell, Jane, 75, 110, 278–79
*Breast Cancer? Breast Health!,* 87, 97
Brennan, Autumn, 306
Brooks, Svevo, 114
bugleweed, 197
Buhner, Stephen, 17, 24, 60, 77, 147, 306
burdock, 113, 191, 192, 229, 273
Burtch, Faye, 23, 30, 53, 57, 179, 198, 313
business, herbal, 208–215, 257–62
contracts, 210–12
expanding, 262

labeling, 224, 262–66
marketing, 210, 257–58, 275–77
pricing, 213–15, 258–59
product line, 259–61
supplies, 261

## C

Cabrera, Chanchal, 105, 125
calendula, 184, 190, 204, 222, 237, 245, 246, 248
capsules, 248–49
cascara sagrada, 221
Cate Farm, 180
catnip, 81–82, 155, 170, 178, 188, 196, 204, 209, 273
cayenne, 5, 178, 244, 273
Cech, Richo, 88, 162–63, 165, 174, 215
ceremonies, 60–61
certification, 23–27
certified herbalists, 37
chamomile, 82–83, 160, 169, 178, 191, 217, 255, 273
chaparral, 202
chaste tree, 53, 147
cherry, 195–96
black, 195
wild, 194, 234
chickweed, 221, 273
children, 89, 281–85
Christopher, John, 16
Clark's Rule, 256
*The Clay Pedestal,* 23–24
cleavers, 255
clinical herbalists, 37
Colbin, Annemarie, 21, 22
cold-pressed oils, 245
cold-water infusions, 226
Collins, Ken, 131
Colman, Sally, 186, 190
coltsfoot, 202, 273
combination menstruums, 234

Nature and Spirit Camp, 281–85
*Nature's Children*, 7, 87
nettles, stinging, 65, 68, 82, 145, 160, 161, 164, 175, 191–92, 207, 228, 229, 268, 273
*Newcomb's Wildflower Guide*, 68
New England Center for Integrative Health, 11, 296
*The New Organic Grower*, 169
Northrup, Dr. Christine, 87, 109
*Nourishing Traditions*, 20, 21

## O

oil-based medicines, 244–48
O'Mara, Kathleen, 303
organic agriculture, 18–22, 48–49
organoleptic method, 221–22
osha, 47, 48

## P

Packard, Candis Canton, 126, 131, 142
Palmer, Mary Pat, 103, 119, 148
Panti, Don Elijo, 79
Parvati, Jeannine, 114
pennyroyal, 255
peppermint, black, 82, 187, 221, 273, 292
percolation, 240–43
pessaries, 247
pharmacopoeia, 85
Pilarski, Michael, 171
pills, herbal, 249–50
pipsissewa, 197
plantain, 5, 187–88, 202, 268
plant allies, 75–79
*Planting the Future*, 91, 310
*A Plant Lover's Guide to Wildcrafting*, 198
plant sense, 175–79
*Plant Spirit Medicine*, 60
plant spirits, 59–62
pleurisy root, 255, 273
poke, 65
polypharmacy, 66, 148
poultices, 246, 250
*The Practice of Herbal Wisdom*, 137
*A Practicing Herbalist*, 137
preceptorship, 105
Price, Dr. Weston, 20
pricing, 213–15, 258–59
*Principles and Practice of Constitutional Physiology for Herbalists*, 137

*Principles and Practice of Phytotherapy*, 90
production gardens, 275
production records, 224
propagation, 164–75
pulse diagnosis, 133, 136, 137
Purple Shutter Herbs, 52–53

## R

red clover, 190, 204, 209–210, 273
Reisen, Andrea, 175, 189, 200, 204–206
Reisen, Matthias, 49, 175, 178, 183, 189, 200, 202, 204–206, 213, 214, 296
Reppert, Bertha, 279
Romm, Aviva, 25, 34–35, 36, 87, 127, 281
*The Root Children*, 156, 157
root division, 170–74
roots, 192–94, 200, 202
rose hips, 65, 149
Rude, Monica, 50, 59, 122, 178, 180, 192, 202, 210, 211
Rufsvold, Dr. Robert, 11, 296
Rundlett, Melanie, 219

## S

*Sacred Plant Medicine*, 60
sage, 170, 268, 273
Sage Mountain, 274, 286
salves, 246–47
sassafras, 31
saw palmetto, 27, 197
*Science and Art of Herbology*, 95, 280
Scudder, Dr. John, 138, 144
seeding, 165–70, 184–85
seeds, harvesting, 191–92
self–heal, 71
selling herbs. *See* business, herbal
senna, 254
7Song, 64–65, 101, 260, 290
shamanic journeying, 13, 131
Shaudys, Phyllis, 279
shepherd's purse, 52
Shiva, Vandana, 199
skullcap, 14, 71, 174, 237, 273
Slick, Karl, 274
slippery elm, 194, 251, 254
Soberg, Renne, 203, 210–11
soil, 156–64
solar drying, 200–202

solar infusions, 226
solid extracts, 228
Soule, Deb, 26, 33, 42, 44–45, 87, 214
soups, 229
*Specific Diagnosis and Specific Medicines*, 85, 144
*Specific Indications for Herbs in General Use*, 149
spilanthes, 179, 215, 273
spirit-based medicines, 229–30
St. Claire, Debra, 88, 243
St. John's wort, 9, 18, 27, 66, 125, 135, 147, 187, 189, 190, 191, 208, 237–38, 239, 245, 246, 248, 273
Stalbard, Granny, 7
standardization, 27–29
standardized extracts, 240
*Stella Natura*, 189
Stilwell, Linn, 270
stinging nettles. See nettles, stinging
stoneroot, 174
store. *See* apothecary
storing herbs, 206–208
Strauss, Paul, 214, 310
suppositories, 247
sweet flag, 171
synergy, 28, 146–49, 254
syrups, 227–28

## T

tea, 225–26
teaching, 36, 56–59, 267–91
    apprenticeships, 91–98, 287–91
    children, 281–85
    family members, 298
    marketing courses, 275–77
    workshops, 277–87
    teaching gardens, 271–75
Tenery, Dr. Robert M., 299
thistle
    blessed, 184, 202
    milk, 18, 27, 66, 191, 273
Thomson, Samuel, 5
Tierra, Lesley, 97, 100, 281
Tierra, Michael, 65, 86, 97, 100, 137, 148, 303
tinctures, 80, 208, 219, 229, 230, 235–40, 257
tongue diagnosis, 132, 136
*Tongue Diagnosis in Chinese Medicine*, 137
tools
    cleaning, 193–94
    harvesting, 182–83, 188, 190, 192, 207